CW01574705

Diagnostic Clusters in Shoulder Conditions

Puneet Monga • Lennard Funk
Editors

Diagnostic Clusters in Shoulder Conditions

Springer

Editors
Puneet Monga
Upper Limb Unit
Wrightington Hospital
WN6 9EP
Lancashire
United Kingdom

Lennard Funk
Upper Limb Unit
Wrightington Hospital
WN6 9EP
Lancashire
United Kingdom

ISBN 978-3-319-57332-8 ISBN 978-3-319-57334-2 (eBook)
DOI 10.1007/978-3-319-57334-2

Library of Congress Control Number: 2017953774

© Springer International Publishing AG 2017
This work is subject to copyright. All rights are reserved by the Publisher, whether the whole or part of the material is concerned, specifically the rights of translation, reprinting, reuse of illustrations, recitation, broadcasting, reproduction on microfilms or in any other physical way, and transmission or information storage and retrieval, electronic adaptation, computer software, or by similar or dissimilar methodology now known or hereafter developed.
The use of general descriptive names, registered names, trademarks, service marks, etc. in this publication does not imply, even in the absence of a specific statement, that such names are exempt from the relevant protective laws and regulations and therefore free for general use.
The publisher, the authors and the editors are safe to assume that the advice and information in this book are believed to be true and accurate at the date of publication. Neither the publisher nor the authors or the editors give a warranty, express or implied, with respect to the material contained herein or for any errors or omissions that may have been made. The publisher remains neutral with regard to jurisdictional claims in published maps and institutional affiliations.

Printed on acid-free paper

This Springer imprint is published by Springer Nature
The registered company is Springer International Publishing AG
The registered company address is: Gewerbestrasse 11, 6330 Cham, Switzerland

Dedicated to Archita, my better half, and to the two best daughters in the world, Arushi and Anika, for their innumerable sacrifices.

–Puneet

With thanks to my wife and children—my joy, my support and my sanity.

–Lennard

Rationale of Diagnostic Clusters

An accurate diagnosis is the foundation of Good Medical Practice.

The inspiration for this work has been to pull together the diagnostic knowledge, skills, and wisdom gathered over generations by the orthopaedic fraternity practising common sense orthopaedics. The relevance and need of such *common sense-based clinical practice* has been amplified by the pressures faced by the chaotic Internet information boom, easy access to radiology, corporatization of medical care, and the rapid pace of our life demanding binary answers to complex questions.

In routine clinical practice, the diagnosis of a particular shoulder condition is best made on history, clinical examination, and special tests, usually with the help of radiological investigations. It is often the case that all these subcomponents are to be used in conjunction with each other as "*clusters*" rather than in isolation. Current textbooks are focused on physical examination techniques or radiological examination and do not take into account this cluster approach one needs to use in everyday practice. The purpose of this book is to bridge this gap and serve as a practical guide to diagnosis in modern day clinical practice.

We are all familiar with the patients who have had a scan which shows a "tear," and having done their Internet research, they present with an expectation for such a "tear," often in the absence of relevant clinical symptoms, to be "fixed." This book is to serve as a reminder that a clinical diagnosis remains reliant on multiple sources. This reminder is particularly relevant in the current vastness of medical information available on the Internet for patients and clinicians alike. This work represents a body of collective experience and knowledge of carefully selected shoulder surgeons and specialist physiotherapists, who practice the cluster approach to making a diagnosis.

A focused history can tease out the diagnosis in a vast number of shoulder conditions. Also, the conventional examination of the shoulder joint follows a sequence of "look, feel, and move." This sequence is in line with the orthopaedic examination of other joints. The knowledge of shoulder conditions has vastly improved over the past two decades, with the "shoulder subspecialty" growing at a rapid pace regarding practitioner numbers, knowledge, evidence base, and procedures. One has seen the emergence of a vast variety of "special tests" to aid in the diagnosis of shoulder conditions. In conditions such as subacromial impingement, for example, over 12 special tests have been described. The multitude of special tests means that the clinician faces a vast choice of tests, with a broad range of sensitivities and specificities. At the same time, radiological techniques have advanced rapidly over the last decade with significant leaps in quality, speed, and indications. Such developments are so rapid that the clinical implications of radiological findings are frequently debated!

Hence, the four key pillars over which one constructs a diagnosis are a clinical history, the conventional examination sequence, special tests, and radiological investigations. Diagnosis of a particular condition relies on a varying degree of support from these individual pillars. The first section of the book defines these four key pillars. Each of these initial chapters describes the particular Pillar and provides a broad knowledge over which the subsequent chapters are then constructed. The reliability of a diagnosis is high when individual subcomponents are aligned. Equally, when different subcomponents are not overlapping and pointing in the same direction, the confidence in the diagnosis is lower. One needs to accept that the outcome of diagnostic assessment may well be a "probable diagnosis" which needs further clarification by invasive techniques such as arthroscopy (Fig. 1).

Pain, weakness, and instability are the three common reasons for which patients seek help for their shoulders. Further sections of the book have been structured around these three presentations rather than pathological processes. The book is a step in the direction of patient-centred medical literature and will serve to remind us to think about "what's the patient in clinic for?" Within these sections, specific conditions with their corresponding "clusters" comprise the bulk of the work. The authors have painstakingly extracted the relevant components from clinical experience, published work, clinical examination textbooks, radiology textbooks, and online resources.

This work is based out of the Wrightington Hospital, which provided a setting for the pioneering work of our forebear Late Sir John Charnley, the father of modern Hip Replacement. He continues to provide us with an unending source of inspiration. We are honoured to have the blessings of Dr. Ben Kibler for this work, who

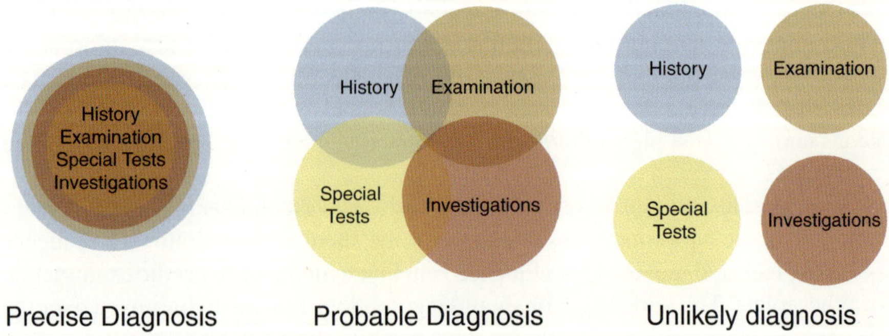

Fig. 1 Reliability of a diagnosis

challenged us to think about "what's relevant to the patient" throughout the preparation of this book. There is no doubt that you would notice a streak of common sense orthopaedics across each chapter, a tribute to the lessons learnt from Mr. Tim Meadows, retired Consultant Orthopaedic Surgeon, and also to our surgical trainers spread across the globe. We are grateful to the great support from the publishers, Springer, and in particular Liz Pope, Priya Vairamani and Andre Tournois in the editorial team.

The overall proposed style of writing for the book is a practical, well-referenced, easy-to-read resource for general practitioners, orthopaedic trainees, physiotherapists, orthopaedic surgeons, radiology trainees, radiographers, and musculoskeletal radiologists. As with all works addressing the complexity of diagnostic decisions, the knowledge is vast and fast evolving. We accept that any book of this nature cannot claim to be a comprehensive guide and we would welcome feedback from the readers. Each chapter starts with an illustrative case example signifying a "classic" patient presentation, the detailed description of individual diagnostic clusters, and finally a discussion of the case and a chapter summary with a tabulated summary of clusters. Subcomponents of clusters have been chosen based on evidence, experience, and applicability. Such a subdivision is designed for a quick read-through for a busy clinician, if they so wish.

We hope you enjoy reading this book as much as we have enjoyed compiling and editing "*The Shoulder Clusters*."

2017

Puneet Monga
Lennard Funk

Prologue: Making the Diagnosis

I am honoured to be asked to write a prologue for this book on diagnosis in shoulder disorders. Any book needs a strong rationale and definite application to be relevant. This book is relevant. It addresses an important topic at a timely point in the evolution of our knowledge of the treatment of shoulder injuries. It highlights the fundamental importance of the diagnosis in treatment, a point which is frequently undervalued or underappreciated.

The diagnosis is the key and critical aspect in health care. All treatment interventions are based on the information provided in the diagnosis. The diagnosis should be able to answer the question "why is the patient in your office," both from the patient's and the doctor's point of view. Most patients report they come to the office to be evaluated and treated for an alteration in their functional capability [1], while most doctors report they feel the patient has come to be assessed for a particular alteration of anatomy. The comprehensive diagnostic process can help the clinician assemble all relevant information necessary to address the functional problem. An effective diagnosis can be defined as "*that body of information, collected through the process of evaluating the patient's health problem, that determines the content and timing of the treatment of the health problem*"[2]. The diagnostic process may be short or long, may involve several steps, or may require outside consultation, but the goal is to produce a more precise and complete understanding of the patient's health problem.

In the USA, the Institute of Medicine (IOM), now named the National Academy of Medicine (NAM), has recognised the central importance of the diagnosis in health care and the problems associated with inefficient diagnoses. In September 2015, the IOM produced the latest report in its highly regarded Quality Chasm Series, titled "Improving diagnosis in health care" [2]. The report documented troubling deficiencies in the effectiveness of developing the diagnosis in all health care disciplines. They called these deficiencies "diagnostic errors." Diagnostic errors may be defined as "*the failure to develop the information required to establish an accurate and timely explanation of the patient's health problem, and the failure to meaningfully communicate the information to the patient*" [2]. The information must be accurate (not differing from the actual patient problem, or imprecise or

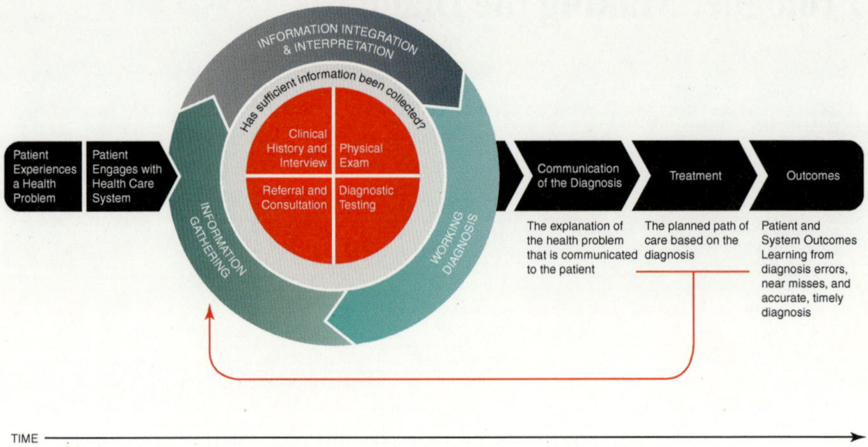

Fig. 2 The Diagnostic process as presented by Balough et al. (2015)

incomplete) and timely (not delaying the correct treatment). It also must be communicated to the patient in understandable terms so the patient can participate in the determination of the treatment plan. Diagnostic errors can be harmful in several ways. They can prevent or delay appropriate treatment, they can lead to inappropriate or unnecessary treatment, and/or they increase medical expenditures and waste financial and medical resources.

In addition to documenting the presence and incidence of diagnostic errors, the report described a general model of the diagnostic process that was designed to systematically address the components of the diagnostic process, in order to bring a more unified approach to the process (Fig. 2) [2].

The general suggestions made in the IOM report have specific application for orthopaedics and shoulder surgery. There are multiple studies in the orthopaedic literature that support the report's conclusions regarding the imprecision and lack of effectiveness of the diagnosis for shoulder injuries [3–11]. Also, the general model described in the IOM report for the diagnostic process can be used as a framework for re-envisioning the process in orthopaedics. The model is very similar to the rationale for diagnostic clusters that forms the basis for this book. Several points can be made regarding the applicability of the model to orthopaedics and shoulder surgery, and for use in applying the principles advocated in this book. First, it is sequential, starting with the patient experiencing some alteration of their normal functional status. In this book, the main alterations are pain, weakness, and instability, but there may be others that need to be elucidated by interaction with the patient. Second, it emphasises the key role for comprehensive information gathering from multiple sources, a point emphasised strongly in this book in the four key pillars. I would add two other supporting resources: (1) including patient-determined factors and expectations, such as the apprehension of the injury and treatment and problems with job status, and (2) information from arthroscopic or other surgical observations that can be helpful in confirming the comprehensive diagnosis. Each of these dimensions must be evaluated in every patient. Third, it emphasises the involvement of patient preferences and concerns in determining treatment after a diagnosis has been made. Fourth, the treatment that results from the diagnosis includes content and timing of the interventions based on the deficits found. Fifth, the treatment results in outcomes, which the IOM report describes as patient outcomes (observed/measured by clinicians, reported by patients) and system outcomes (quality, cost, safety, efficiency, public confidence in the system). Finally, in this model, there is a linear, almost cause and effect relationship between the diagnosis and the treatment outcome. Effective treatment is therefore shown to be dependent on a comprehensive diagnosis.

Unfortunately, there are well-demonstrated deficiencies in the diagnostic process and the resulting diagnoses in many shoulder injuries. In general, the diagnostic errors often result in imprecise and incomplete information which may frequently lead to unreliable treatments and outcomes. The final diagnoses recorded often fail to identify the actual anatomical lesion and the associated physiological and biomechanical alterations, fail to include patient-reported factors and expectations, do not adequately define what functional loss exists, are inconsistent in guiding treatment, and only infrequently are associated with predictability of outcomes. Examples can be given for labral injury [3, 4], impingement [5, 6], rotator cuff disease [7, 8], AC joint injury [9], clavicle fractures [10], and instability [11]. There is also anecdotal but widely believed evidence of overutilization of imaging in the diagnostic process and overdiagnosis of many shoulder problems [12]. We as clinicians must accept responsibility for improving our diagnostic capabilities. We must ask more pertinent questions in the history, develop expertise in the clinical exam as we do in surgical techniques, and must use imaging wisely. This will require a certain amount of time and effort but must be seen as wise expenditures. Without that effort, the patient may not receive the optimal care.

Many methods have been advocated over the years to establish a firm, reliable, and accurate diagnosis in health care, and most doctors and medical clinicians use specific questions, and tests they feel will develop the best information. Careful study, however, demonstrates that in a disturbingly high percentage of cases, the diagnostic process results in suboptimal outcomes. This book attempts to better systematise the diagnostic process for identification of the comprehensive set of alterations that represent the patient's unique health problem. It makes excellent points regarding how to effectively make the diagnosis and can give clinicians guidance in improving their capabilities. Whatever method each clinician chooses to use, I would recommend that the method adheres to a comprehensive set of principles I call the "5 A's." At the end of the individual patient diagnostic process the information gathered should reflect:

- *Accuracy*—all anatomical, physiological, and biomechanical alterations that accompany the health problem should be evaluated and categorised
- *Assessment*—patient-derived factors and expectations, and meaningful communication to ascertain patient acceptance and involvement

- *Agreement*—the process should result in high inter-rater reliability for the process and the content of the evaluation
- *Applicability*—the process should lead to reliable guidance for the content and timing of all the aspects of the comprehensive treatment plan
- *Accountability*—the information should be able to relate to predictions of outcome reasonably

In summary, the diagnosis is the key element in developing effective medical care. Much effort is currently being made to identify, quantitate, and improve the value associated with the outcomes of treatment of medical conditions. Outcomes are typically defined as how did the patient do after an intervention and may be termed "value on the back end" of the treatment process. There has not been the same amount of effort related to improving the process for making the diagnosis, the "value on the front end" upon which the treatment is based. As doctors and clinicians continue to search for methods to improve the quality, safety, efficacy, and value of treatment, devising better surgical techniques or more precise measurements of outcomes will not necessarily be of maximal benefit unless equal attention is placed on improving the diagnosis upon which the techniques and subsequent measurements depend.

W. Ben Kibler, M.D.

References

1. Smith-Forbes EV, Moore-Reed SD, Westgate PM, Kibler WB, Uhl TL. Descriptive analysis of common functional limitations identified by patients with shoulder pain. J Sport Rehabil. 2015;24:179–88.
2. Balogh EP, Miller BT, Ball JR. Improving diagnosis in healthcare. Washington: National Academies Press; 2015.
3. Kibler WB, Sciascia A. Current practice for the diagnosis of a superior labral anterior to posterior (SLAP) lesion: systematic review and physician survey. Arthroscopy. 2015;31(12):2456–69.
4. Hegedus EJ, Goode AP, Cook CE, Michener L, Myer CA, Myer DM, et al. Which physical examination tests provide clinicians with the most value when examining the shoulder? Update of a systematic review with meta-analysis of individual tests. Br J Sports Med. 2012;46:964–78.
5. Ketola S, Lehtinen J, Rousi T, Nissinen M, Huhtala H, Konttinen YT, et al. No evidence of long-term benefits of arthroscopic acromioplasty in the treatment of shoulder impingement syndrome: five-year results of a randomised controlled trial. Bone Joint Res. 2013;2(7):132–9.
6. Alqunaee M, Galvin R, Fahey T. Diagnostic accuracy of clinical tests for subacromial impingement syndrome: a systematic review and meta-analysis. Arch Phys Med Rehabil. 2012;93:229–36.
7. Unruh KP, Kuhn JE, Sanders R, An Q, Baumgarten KM, Bishop JY, et al. The duration of symptoms does not correlate with rotator cuff tear severity or other patient-related features: a cross-sectional study of patients with atraumatic, full-thickness rotator cuff tears. J Shoulder Elbow Surg. 2014;23(7):1052–8.
8. Wylie JD, Suter T, Potter MQ, Granger EK, Tashjian RZ. Mental health has a stronger association with patient-reported shoulder pain and function than tear size in patients with full-thickness rotator cuff tears. J Bone Joint Surg (Am). 2016;98:251–6.

9. Cho CH, Hwang I, Seo JS, Choi CH, Ko SH, Park HB, et al. Reliability of the classification and treatment of dislocations of the acromioclavicular joint. J Shoulder Elbow Surg. 2014;23:665–70.
10. Jones GL, Bishop JY, Lewis B, Pedroza AD, Shoulder Group M. Intraobserver and interobserver agreement in the classification and treatment of midshaft clavicle fractures. Am J Sports Med. 2014;42(5):1176–81.
11. Kuhn JE, Helmer TT, Dunn WR, Throckmorton TW. Development and reliability testing of the frequency, etiology, direction, and severity (FEDS) system for classifying glenohumeral instability. J Shoulder Elbow Surg. 2011;20(4):548–56.
12. Weber SC, Martin DF, Seiler III JG, Harrast JJ. Superior labrum anterior and posterior lesions of the shoulder: Incidence rates, complications, and outcomes as reported by American Board of Orthopedic Surgery part II candidates. Am J Sports Med. 2012;40(7):1538–43.

Acknowledgment

Make things as simple as possible, but not simpler

–Albert Einstein.

Thanks to the contributing authors for sharing our passion in the quest for making things as simple as possible.

Contents

Contributors

Sohail Akhtar Wrightington Hospital, Wigan, UK

Subh Basu Wrightington Hospital, Wigan, UK

Andreas Baumann Royal Preston Hospital, Preston, UK

Jonathan A. Baxter St George's Hospital, London, UK

Simon Boyle York Teaching Hospital, York, UK

Usman Butt Salford Royal Hospital, Salford, UK

Nicholas J. Dedy Krankenhaus Barmherzige Brüder Regensburg, Regensburg, Germany

Lennard Funk Wrightington Hospital, Wigan, UK

Jeremy Granville-Chapman Heatherwood and Wexham Park Hospital, Slough, UK

Emmet Griffiths Norfolk and Norwich University Hospital, Norwich, UK

Richard Heasley Pennine Acute Hospitals, Bury, UK

Daniel Henderson Alps Surgery Institute, Annecy, France

Gareth Howell Royal Preston Hospital, Preston, UK

Arpit Jariwala Ninewells Hospital and Medical School, Dundee, UK

Amit Kapoor Royal Oldham Hospital, Manchester, UK

W. Ben Kibler Lexington Clinic Orthopedics-Sports Medicine Center, Lexington, KYUSA

Amar Malhas Royal Berkshire Hospital, Reading, UK

Avanthi Mandaleson Department of Orthopaedic SurgeryAustin Hospital, Heidelberg, VICAustralia

Puneet Monga Wrightington Hospital, Wigan, UK

Barnes Morgan Stepping Hill Hospital, Stockport, UK

Sedeek M. Mosaid Harrogate District NHS Foundation Trust, Harrogate, UK

Chye Yew Ng Wrightington Hospital, Wigan, UK

Dariush Nikkhah Barts and The Royal London Hospital, London, UK

Chris Peach University Hospital of South Manchester, Manchester, UK

Abbas Rashid University College London Hospitals NHS Foundation Trust, London, UK

Pradyumna Raval Ninewells Hospital and Medical School, Dundee, UK

Sarah Russell Wrightington Hospital, Wigan, UK

Marlis Sabo Section of Orthopaedic Surgery, Cumming School of Medicine, Calgary, AB, Canada

Apurv Sinha Chesterfield Royal Hospital NHS Foundation Trust, Chesterfield, UK

Suresh Srinivasan Leicester General Hospital, Leicester, UK

R. Steve Bale Wrightington Hospital, Wigan, UK

Charlie Talbot Harrogate District NHS Foundation Trust, Harrogate, UK

Fraser J. Taylor Gold Coast University Hospital, Brisbane, Australia

David Temperley Wrightington Hospital, Wigan, UK

Jill Thomas Wrightington Hospital, Wigan, UK

Ian A. Trail Wrightington Hospital, Wigan, UK

Santosh Venkatachalam Northumbria Healthcare, North Shields, UK

Rajat Verma Salford Royal Hospital, Salford, UK

Julia Walton Wrightington Hospital, Wigan, UK

Michael Walton Wrightington Hospital, Wigan, UK

Phil Wright Bradford Royal Infirmary, Bradford, UK

Part I
Basic Ingredients

Chapter 1
Clinical History

J.A. Baxter and M. Walton

The key to successful management of a patient with shoulder symptoms is establishing an accurate diagnosis. On occasion this is straightforward but in diagnostic challenges, time spent teasing out a good history is always rewarded. Taking a history, on many occasions, is a matter of pattern recognition. Most diagnoses are made by the history with examination and investigations serving to confirm one's suspicions. Table 1.1 is Pain Severity from Shoulder Conditions.

A. **Demographic**

   Age of the patient
   Hand dominance
   Occupation
   Leisure activities

B. **Presenting Complaints**

   General

   Duration of symptoms
   Traumatic/Atraumatic
   Onset—Acute/Gradual
   Progression—Slow/Rapid
   Loss of Function; Daily activities, Work & Sport

J.A. Baxter (✉)
St George's University Hospitals NHS Foundation Trust, First Floor Flat, Chiswick, London W4 1PQ, UK
e-mail: jonabaxter@doctors.org.uk

M. Walton
Consultant Shoulder Surgeon, Wrightington Hospital, Wigan, UK

© Springer International Publishing AG 2017

P. Monga, L. Funk (eds.), *Diagnostic Clusters in Shoulder Conditions*,
DOI 10.1007/978-3-319-57334-2_1

Table 1.1 Pain severity

Pathology	Mean VAS
GHJ arthritis	7.83
Subacromial impingement	7.80
Calcific tendinitis	7.50
Rotator cuff tears	7.05
Instability	6.72
ACJ pathology	6.43

VAS Visual Analogue Scale, *GHJ* Glenohumeral joint, *ACJ* Acromioclavicular joint [5]

Pain

Location
Radiation
Severity
Night pain, rest pain, constant/intermittent
Aggravating/Relieving factors/positions
Is the shoulder pain related to neck movements?
Red Flag Signs

Instability

History of giving way/clicks/jerks
Frequency of symptoms
Ligamentous laxity in other joints
Was there a frank dislocation?

Age of the first dislocation
Ease of reduction
Position of instability
Cumulative time in the dislocated position

Weakness

Muscular
Neurological symptoms, paraesthesias

Stiffness

Duration of onset
Preceding pain
Past injuries

C. **Previous Treatment**

Non-operative; medications, injections, physiotherapy
Operative; location, timing, procedure

D. **Past Medical History**

Associated medical conditions
Systemic disease including diabetes and connective tissue disorders
Previous trauma
Previous surgery (problems with anaesthetic)
Smoking status

E. **Patient Factors**

Timelines of return to sports for athletes
Expectations from treatment
Apprehensions related to medical care
Influence of potential treatment on work and hobbies

The key questions one needs to consider when taking a clinical history are as follows

How Old Is the Patient?

Most shoulder conditions are related to specific age groups. Pathology in children and adolescents is almost always traumatic in origin leading to fractures around the shoulder girdle (usually clavicle) or less commonly dislocations. Atraumatic pain in this age group is a concerning feature and should raise concerns for primary bone tumours. Young adult pathology is also usually traumatic in onset and related to glenohumeral joint and acromioclavicular joint (ACJ) instability. From middle age, one begins to develop degenerative tendinopathy, and the more elderly suffer from degenerative joint disease (osteoarthritis) and rotator cuff arthropathy. Rotator cuff tendinopathy is the most common shoulder condition presenting to the general practitioner [1, 2].

How Did the Symptoms Start?

A key discriminator in shoulder pathology is be the presence of an initial traumatic event or if the symptoms were of gradual or insidious onset. In combination with the age of the patient, this will often separate acute from degenerative conditions.

If the patient confirms that an injury heralded the onset of symptoms, further information should be sought. These include the date of the injury, the mechanism including arm position, direction and magnitude of the load, whether there was a fracture, dislocation or soft tissue injury. It is useful to ask about how it was managed, by whom and was any imaging obtained at the time. The degree to which the symptoms resolved after the initial injury is also necessary.

Is the Shoulder the Source of the Discomfort?

It is pertinent to ascertain if the pain is arising from the shoulder girdle or referred from adjacent or sometimes distant structures. Neck pain and radiculopathy are often referred to the shoulder region [3]. Such referral applies in particular to the C5/6 dermatome, and it is essential that this should be actively ruled out as a cause of symptoms.

Neck pain is often referred to the scalp region and medial scapula. It can be associated with trapezius muscle pain and secondary shoulder discomfort. Nerve root impingement leads to radiculopathy, which can be felt over the shoulder itself but is often described as radiating more distally down the arm to the elbow and into the hand. It can be associated with altered sensation and paraesthesia and is often described as "burning" in nature. Such pain may be exacerbated by neck movement. Less commonly one might come across right shoulder pain due to gallbladder inflammation and left shoulder tip pain due to cardiac pathology.

What Exacerbates the Pain?

Shoulder pain usually occurs during functional activities. Pain at rest is a significant symptom and should trigger further enquiry about the "Red Flag" symptoms. Pain when reaching above the head, tucking in a shirt or scratching the back is common. The position of the arm at which any pain begins can give clues as to the underlying cause. Such position dependent pain is often referred to as the "painful arc" and, the range, in the mid or high zones, can be as a result of different pathology.

Pain on elevation in the "mid-arc" of the scapular plane is commonly seen in patients with subacromial or rotator cuff pain [4]. Pain is classically described as beginning at 70° often easing above 130°, as the scapula is responsible for the majority of the further movement. Often patients will complain of increased pain on bringing their arm down from an elevated position within this arc. It will often be made worse by internal rotational movements.

Pain at the top of elevation or "high-arc," is often seen in those with ACJ pathology. Patients may complain of discomfort when locking out an overhead press during exercise or when across chest activities are being performed such as washing under the opposite arm. This pain is usually well localised by the patient.

A painful restriction in movement is often seen in patients with adhesive capsulitis. The severity of pain and loss of range is variable, but typically a limitation in external rotation is often present early in the disease process. Patients often complain of difficulty during activities such as brushing their hair. The patients complaining of pain and restriction on all movements, especially with associated crepitus, may be suffering from glenohumeral joint arthritis.

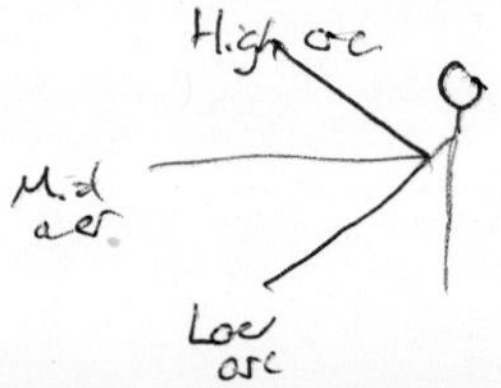

What Is the Location and Nature of Pain?

Individual conditions classically present with pain at a particular location over the shoulder with varying degrees of referred pain to the neck or down the arm. Shoulder pain mapping techniques have been very useful in demonstrating shoulder pathologies present with differing and reproducible patterns of pain distribution [5] (Table 1.1 and Figs. 1.1–1.3).

Pain from ACJ pathology is predominantly sharp and stabbing over the ACJ itself. It tends to be well localised to the joint and not to be referred to the arm. The presence of popping, clicking, or catching in the history should raise suspicion of instability or the presence of a SLAP lesion [6]. The pain felt with instability is often a mixture of sharp and dull in nature without radiation past the elbow [5].

In patients with subacromial impingement and rotator cuff tears, pain is less well localised. It is often described as sharp in nature at the anterior aspect of the shoulder with a dull, aching pain radiating to the upper arm and forearm. Patients with subacromial impingement may describe pins and needles affecting the hand [5]. A proportion of patients may also present with varying degrees of chronic neck pain [7]. Pain in the

Fig. 1.1 The visual analogue scale

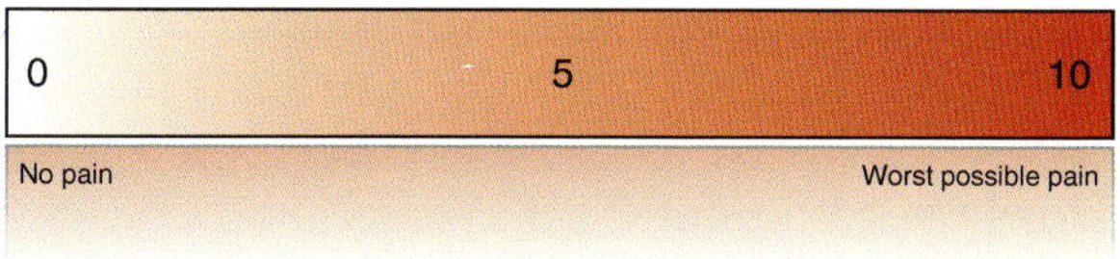

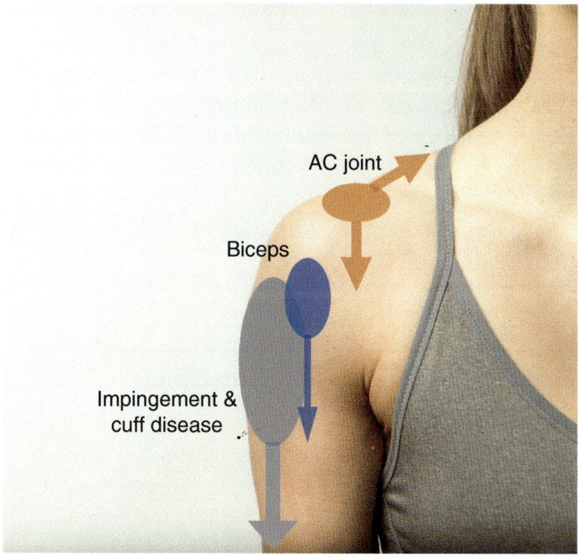

Fig. 1.2 Location of anterior pain. Image Published under License from www.shoulderdoc.co.uk and www.shoulderpedia.org

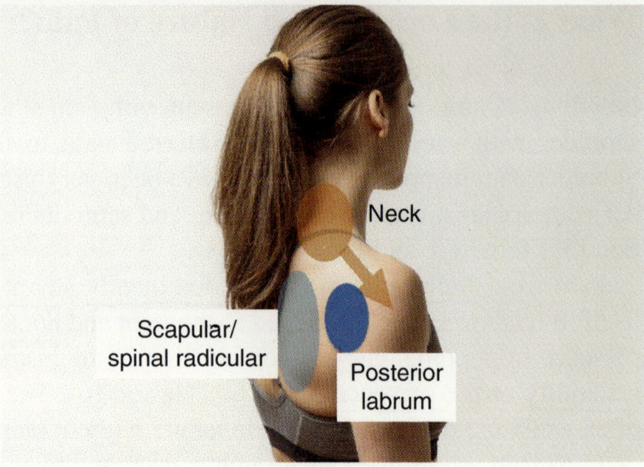

Fig. 1.3 Location of posterior pain. Image Published under License from www.shoulderdoc.co.uk and www.shoulderpedia.org

presence of calcific rotator cuff tendonitis can be severe and is often shooting in nature over the lateral aspect of the shoulder without radiation past the elbow.

Sternoclavicular joint pathology is often described as a well localised dull ache over the joint itself. It can, however, be referred to the ipsilateral anterior neck and along the length of the clavicle to the shoulder [8].

Does the Shoulder Feel Weak?

In older patients, true weakness is a feature of rotator cuff dysfunction either by pain inhibition or a structural tendon tear. In younger, active patients such as manual workers and gym goers, subjective weakness can also be a feature of underlying apprehension or instability. The position of weakness in this group can be associated with the direction of instability i.e. weakness in abduction, and external rotation would suggest anterior instability whereas weakness in cross body adduction or weight bearing (press-up position) is more suggestive of posterior apprehension [9].

Rarely weakness will be due to an underlying neurological or muscular disease (myopathy). A family history is significant for this group to exclude potential inherited disorders.

Does the Shoulder Feel Unstable?

The majority of shoulder dislocations are initially traumatic in origin. A clear description of the original event, the direction of dislocation and subsequent management are essential to understanding the pathology. Following this, it is important to ascertain what the patient means when they state that their shoulder is unstable. They will often describe the shoulder feeling 'loose' as if it wants to 'slip' or 'come out' of joint. Progressive reduction in energy required for recurrent dislocation to occur implies a worsening of the pathological lesion. The number of dislocations and the cumulative time in the dislocated position may influence the amount of bone loss, and these details should be identified in the history.

Does the Shoulder Feel Stiff?

It is important to ascertain what the patient means by the term stiffness. True stiffness, as associated with frozen shoulder, degenerative joint disease and occasionally a missed dislocation is due to a mechanical block. This leads to a reduction in the active and passive range of motion, which cannot be overcome. Patients, however, may use the term to describe a reduced range of active motion due to pain inhibition in the absence of a physical block to movement. It is often challenging for the patient to differentiate between true and apparent stiffness and the distinction requires clinical examination. The pseudoparalysis of a cuff deficient shoulder may also be described as stiffness by the patient.

Red Flag Signs

The "Red Flags" are signs and symptoms that raise concern that the shoulder pain is due to a serious underlying pathology. These necessitate more expedient investigation and management to exclude potential tumours or intra-articular infection. The signs include severe, unremitting pain present at rest and night. Other symptoms include a history of cancer, signs of systemic disease such as weight loss, generalised joint pains, fever, lymphadenopathy and concerning local features such as a mass lesion [2].

Further Medical History

While the shoulder is the focus of the patient's complaint, a complete medical history should be taken in all patients. All comorbidities should be recorded as well as medications, allergies and problems with previous anaesthetics. Many associated medical conditions can have a bearing on the threshold for surgical intervention and also influence access and practicality of various treatment options. Some specific medical conditions also increase the risk of developing certain shoulder pathology. Adhesive capsulitis is more likely if the patient has a history of diabetes [10], thyroid disorder [11] or Parkinson's disease [12]. Rotator cuff tears are more common in the presence of obesity in both men and women. A body mass index (BMI) >30 increases the odds of having a rotator cuff tear requiring surgery. The odds are even greater with a BMI >35 [13]. Glenohumeral joint arthritis is more likely if the patient has a previously dislocated the shoulder [14], is aged >70 years or has a diagnosis of knee osteoarthritis [15].

Individual Lifestyle Factors

Once a diagnosis has been made, in order to achieve a good outcome, it is important to have a clear understanding of the patients' individual lifestyle requirements. These include occupation, hand dominance, leisure activities and importantly, expectations of treatment. These can give both clues to the diagnosis but importantly the effects of any intervention.

Certain occupations and lifestyles are associated with pathology. For example, a diagnosis of rotator cuff tear is more likely with a history of heavy lifting, above shoulder work and work involving handheld vibration tools [16]. Acromioclavicular joint arthritis is more often seen in weightlifters [17], and posterior labral tears are more common in contact athletes such as American football or rugby players [18].

The management of the pathology is then dictated by the required patient-specific functional requirements. Tendon ruptures to the biceps or pectoralis major may well be treated conservatively in the low demand patient, but there is a lower threshold for operative intervention in the younger, active patient to facilitate work or recreational activities. Younger patients and those involved in contact sports may have a lower threshold to opt for stabilisation procedures to continue with their chosen sports. It would indeed be paramount in the scenario of the professional athlete where injuries can be career limiting.

Similar pathologies can have different symptoms and the same interventions different implications. It is imperative for the clinician to spend the time to understand how the shoulder symptoms are impacting their individual patients' life and plan treatment accordingly. Often neglected, but critical, are the implications of the post-intervention rehabilitation process. The duration and limitations of which will have a profound impact on a patient's lifestyle and their ability to work and earn.

The process of understanding the individual's requirements enables the clinician and patient to share decision making in their specific management plan. Such a process should result in realistic goals, the achievement of which, will lead to higher patient satisfaction.

Specific Conditions Are Dealt with in the Individual Chapters in This Book, and the Following Examples Provide Some "Classic Stories".

Traumatic Instability/Capsulolabral Pathology

A 20-year-old male presents with shoulder discomfort. He states that he remembers the shoulder 'popping out' the year before while playing rugby but he did not attend the emergency department. He continued to improve and has returned to sports but has lost confidence in his shoulder in certain positions. He describes the feeling that the shoulder 'slips out' in the absence of a frank dislocation.

Traumatic instability/labral pathology is often seen in patients aged 15–35. A clear history of dislocation should be sought. Symptoms often include anxiety that the shoulder may dislocate with certain positions known as apprehension. The classic symptoms of anterior instability may follow an anterior inferior dislocation resulting in a Bankart lesion. However, SLAP tears are often seen in those participating in contact and overhead sports. Posterior labral pathology is commonly seen in rugby players landing on their elbow with a resultant high-energy, posteriorly directed force, which disrupts the posterior labral complex.

Atraumatic Instability

17-year-old female presents with recurrent dislocation of both shoulders. She denies a previous history of trauma stating that she has always been able to dislocate her shoulders. She states that she is very flexible. She has had many days off school over the last six months and is anxious about her upcoming examinations.

Atraumatic instability is seen in younger patients. Most commonly adolescent females but can occur in males and older patients. Symptoms of instability are present in the absence of a traumatic injury. This condition is often bilateral and accompanied by general ligamentous laxity of other joints. Symptoms of pain, weakness, numbness, crepitus on certain movements and instability that can occur at night may be present. It may also be seen as subclinical instability in the overhead athlete. In this particular group, an appreciation of the psychosocial elements to the symptoms is important.

Subacromial Impingement

A 40-year-old female presents with severe pain over the lateral aspect of her shoulder radiating down the arm. She denies previous trauma but thinks she may have overdone her shoulder exercises in the gym. This pain has been worsening over the past six months and now disturbs her sleep.

Impingement is commonly in patients aged 35–75. Pain is often described as lateral to the acromion and is exacerbated by elevation. When severe the pain can become burning in nature and affect the area distal to the lateral acromion down the lateral aspect of the upper limb. There is often troublesome night pain. Patients may describe abnormal sensation overlying this area, and careful differentiation between these symptoms and those of a cervical spine radiculopathy is needed.

Rotator Cuff Tear

A 56-year-old builder presents complaining of pain and weakness in the dominant shoulder. He states that three weeks previously he slipped on some steps and grabbed a railing to prevent his fall. He felt a tearing sensation in the shoulder immediately that has been replaced by a dull ache.

Acute rotator cuff tears usually occur in patients over 40 with a history of an recent injury preceding the symptoms. They can happen, however, in younger patients with high-energy injuries especially contact athletes. Pain is usually described lateral to acromion and weakness in arm elevation may be present. The size and location of the tear will determine the symptoms present. These can range from small tears causing impingement symptoms to large tears causing reduced shoulder function and pseudoparalysis. Tears involving the subscapularis tendon may present with symptoms of the long head of biceps pathology due to the effect that these tears have on the role of this tendon in the bicipital groove.

Acromioclavicular Joint Disease

A 39-year-old gentleman presents with a gradual onset, well-localised pain over the top of their shoulder. It has been present for approximately 12 months. He first noticed the pain after heavy lifting in the gym but he is now restricted in most overhead activities and when reaching across his chest.

The Acromioclavicular joint disease leads to pain that is well localised over the AC joint itself. If it is present in isolation, the patient may point directly to this area with one finger, but it is often associated with rotator cuff pain. ACJ discomfort is classically exacerbated by movements such as cross body adduction and is often worse in the high arc due to compression of the joint in these positions.

Frozen Shoulder

A 55-year-old female diabetic patient presents with a four-month history of pain and stiffness affecting her shoulder. She is now unable to comb her hair or fasten her bra. She struggles to sleep on the affected side at night.

Patients presenting with a frozen shoulder are usually aged between 40 and 60 years old. They describe a reduction in the active and passive range of movement especially external rotation. An initial pain predominant phase with diffuse discomfort lasting between 6 weeks and 9 months often precedes the stiff phase. The stiff phase can last over 12 months followed by the thawing phase with a gradual return of motion over a period of 6–24 months. Associations include diabetes, thyroid disorders, previous surgery (shoulder, breast, lung), prolonged immobilisation and extended hospitalisation.

Glenohumeral Joint Arthritis

75-year-old female presents with severe pain on movements affecting her right shoulder. It has worsened over the past year, and she now suffers from constant background pain including night pain. She complains of grinding within the joint on movement.

Patients with arthritis are often aged over 60 with reduced active and passive range of movement especially external rotation. Unlike frozen shoulder, there is often no acute painful phase with a gradual onset of symptoms culminating in rest and night pain. A history of previous trauma, surgery, rheumatoid arthritis, connective tissue disease and spondyloarthropathies should be sought.

Internal Impingement

A 28-year-old female, national standard heptathlete presents with discomfort over the posterior aspect of her shoulder when training and competing. Her pain is worsened during and after throwing events.

Internal impingement is a less common cause of shoulder pain but can be seen in the overhead or throwing athlete. The pathology affects the articular surface of the rotator cuff but can include superior labral lesions, posterior capsular and posterior glenoid cartilage damage. Diffuse pain develops along the posterior border of the deltoid and may radiate to the upper arm similar to rotator cuff pain. The pain is often exacerbated by the throwing action; with the extreme external rotation of late cocking and early acceleration are often the positions of maximal discomfort.

Suprascapular Nerve Entrapment

A 32-year-old Olympic standard volleyball player presents with weakness affecting the dominant shoulder. They report a general ache and think they have lost muscle mass at the back of the shoulder.

Suprascapular nerve pathology is a rare cause of shoulder discomfort but can be seen in the overhead athlete, in particular, volleyball players. Often the patient reports vague posterior shoulder pain. As the nerve has both sensory and motor function, symptoms of pain and weakness may be present depending on the level of the nerve affected. More proximal lesions are more likely to cause pain and limited function with atrophy of supraspinatus and infraspinatus muscles. If the nerve is compressed at the level of the spinoglenoid notch isolated atrophy of the infraspinatus tendon may be evident in the presence of little pain.

Conclusion

A focused history is frequently the most important pillar leading to a diagnosis. Pathology causing symptoms around the shoulder girdle can be split into discrete groups based on age, the presence of trauma and the acute or gradual nature of the onset. The chief complaints are of pain, stiffness, weakness and instability. All have an associated loss of function the character of which is fundamental to formulating a patient-specific management plan.

References

1. van der Windt DA, Koes BW, de Jong BA, Bouter LM. Shoulder disorders in general practice: incidence, patient characteristics, and management. Ann Rheum Dis. 1995;54:959–64.
2. Mitchell C, Adebajo A, Hay E, Carr A. Shoulder pain: diagnosis and management in primary care. BMJ. 2005;331:1124–8.
3. Bokshan SL, DePasse JM, Eltorai AE, Paxton ES, Green A, Daniels AH. An evidence-based approach to differentiating the cause of shoulder and cervical spine pain. Am J Med. 2016;129:913–8.
4. Neer CS. Anterior acromioplasty for the chronic impingement syndrome in the shoulder: a preliminary report. J Bone Joint Surg Am. 1972;54:41–50.
5. Bayam L, Ahmad MA, Naqui SZ, Chouhan A, Funk L. Pain mapping for common shoulder disorders. Am J Orthop (Belle Mead NJ). 2011;40:353–8.
6. Michener LA, Doukas WC, Murphy KP, Walsworth MK. Diagnostic accuracy of history and physical examination of superior labrum anterior- posterior lesions. J Athl Train. 2011;46:343–8.
7. Gorski JM, Schwartz LH. Shoulder impingement presenting as neck pain. J Bone Joint Surg Am. 2003;85-A:635–8.
8. Hassett G, Barnsley L. Pain referral from the sternoclavicular joint: a study in normal volunteers. Rheumatology (Oxford). 2001;40:859–62.
9. Owen JM, Boulter T, Walton M, Funk L, Mackenzie TA. Reinterpretation of O'Brien test in posterior labral tears of the shoulder. Int J Shoulder Surg. 2015;9:6–8.
10. Thomas SJ, McDougall C, Brown ID, et al. Prevalence of symptoms and signs of shoulder problems in people with diabetes mellitus. J Shoulder Elb Surg. 2007;16:748–51.
11. Milgrom C, Novack V, Weil Y, Jaber S, Radeva-Petrova DR, Finestone A. Risk factors for idiopathic frozen shoulder. Isr Med Assoc J. 2008;10:361–4.
12. Riley D, Lang AE, Blair RD, Birnbaum A, Reid B. Frozen shoulder and other shoulder disturbances in Parkinson's disease. J Neurol Neurosurg Psychiatry. 1989;52:63–6.
13. Wendelboe AM, Hegmann KT, Gren LH, Alder SC, White GL, Lyon JL. Associations between body mass index and surgery for rotator cuff tendinitis. J Bone Joint Surg Am. 2004;86-A:743–7.
14. Marx RG, McCarty EC, Montemurno TD, Altchek DW, Craig EV, Warren RF. Development of arthrosis following dislocation of the shoulder: a case-control study. J Shoulder Elb Surg. 2002;11:1–5.
15. JH O, Chung SW, CH O, et al. The prevalence of shoulder osteoarthritis in the elderly Korean population: association with risk factors and function. J Shoulder Elb Surg. 2011;20:756–63.
16. Seidler A, Bolm-Audorff U, Petereit-Haack G, et al. Work-related lesions of the supraspinatus tendon: a case-control study. Int Arch Occup Environ Health. 2011;84:425–33.
17. Scavenius M, Iversen BF. Nontraumatic clavicular osteolysis in weight lifters. Am J Sports Med. 1992;20:463–7.
18. Escobedo EM, Richardson ML, Schulz YB, Hunter JC, Green JR, Messick KJ. Increased risk of posterior glenoid labrum tears in football players. AJR Am J Roentgenol. 2007;188:193–7.

Chapter 2
The Conventional Examination

I.A. Trail

Introduction

To make the correct diagnosis for a condition of the shoulder as in other areas of medicine is mostly based on the taking of an accurate and relevant history. Indeed the old maxim that once the history is complete, a treating clinician should have at the very least a differential diagnosis which is then clarified by examination or investigation is very true.

Of all the symptoms pain is predominant. Indeed it is almost always the reason a patient attends for treatment. As such, it is important for the clinician to spend time getting patients to describe their discomfort. Of particular relevance being the onset, site, radiation, precipitating or aggravating factors of the pain experience. Pain can either be acute or chronic depending on the history of a precipitating event. Plainly an acute onset would indicate some structural deficit and chronic would tend towards a degenerative aetiology. The site of the pain is also important. Is the pain localised to the acromioclavicular joint, glenohumeral joint, subacromial space or biceps tendon? It is also important to remember that pain from the glenohumeral joint can radiate down the upper arm, although rarely past the elbow. Added to that, pain from the pathology of the cervical spine can also radiate to the shoulder and then down the arm to the fingers with associated neurological symptoms. As a consequence, assessment of the cervical spine would be seen as mandatory when considering pathology of the shoulder. About aggravation, it is important to note whether the pain is present all the time or made worse by certain activities and exposure to cold. The latter would tend to indicate a degenerative process specifically osteoarthritis,

I.A. Trail, M.D., F.R.C.S.
Hand and Upper Limb Surgery, Wrightington Hospital,
Hall Lane, Appley Bridge, Wigan, Lancashire WN6 9EP, UK
e-mail: upperlimb@wrightinhton.org.uk

© Springer International Publishing AG 2017

P. Monga, L. Funk (eds.), *Diagnostic Clusters in Shoulder Conditions*,
DOI 10.1007/978-3-319-57334-2_2

whereas constant pain is more likely to be due to inflammatory conditions such as rheumatoid arthritis or frozen shoulder. Pain aggravation on elevation is more related to a problem with the rotator cuff. Finally, it is also useful to try and grade the level of pain. This can be done simply using a visual analogue score; 0 being no pain and 10 the worst pain ever experienced. While this can take various formats, such as pain after activity, pain at night, etc., it is only necessary to ask one question provided consistency is maintained. It may also be appropriate to ascertain whether the patient is having problems sleeping and some idea of how much analgesia is being taken. Again its changes rather than absolute measurements that are relevant.

As well as pain, it is important to ascertain stiffness or loss of movement. Global loss of movement, particularly internal and external rotation would indicate pathology involving the glenohumeral joint, e.g., osteoarthritis or frozen shoulder. Pain on elevation and abduction would tend to indicate a problem with a rotator cuff. However, this is not absolute, and cross-over is relatively common. For example, patients with rotator cuff pathology can often have secondary capsulitis.

The experience of weakness in the shoulder, again either global or with specific activities can be useful. For example, weakness of abduction and external rotation may indicate upper nerve root pathology, whereas weakness on elevation and abduction would indicate a tear or non-function of the rotator cuff. Weakness on internal rotation would mean pathology affecting subscapularis. Global weakness, however, would tend to indicate a pathology affecting the glenohumeral joint. Finally, any history of swelling or neurological symptoms should be taken. A record of instability with either true dislocation or a feeling of giving away should also be noted. Indeed patients can often describe these feelings of instability in detail, often indicating the direction of instability.

Examination initially would take the form of an inspection (look), thereafter palpation (feel) and finally an assessment of both active and passive movements. The final section of an examination would be "special tests". That is specific tests that are positive in certain clinical scenarios.

What should not be forgotten, however, is an evaluation of the effect of the shoulder symptomatology on function. After pain, loss of function is of great importance to the patient. Any assessment would involve effects on work but also household tasks as well sporting activities etc.

Inspection (Look)

Much can be gained by the simple observation of the head, neck, scapula and shoulder as well as the upper arm generally. Traditionally the patients should stand with the best views obtained from the rear. Some clinicians have the patient standing in front of a long mirror, so they are also able to see the front and face simultaneously. It is also useful to correct any obvious asymmetry and to note any effect this has on patient symptomatology. Any increase in pain suggests that asymmetry has been adopted for pain relief. Conversely, any improvement may help with future

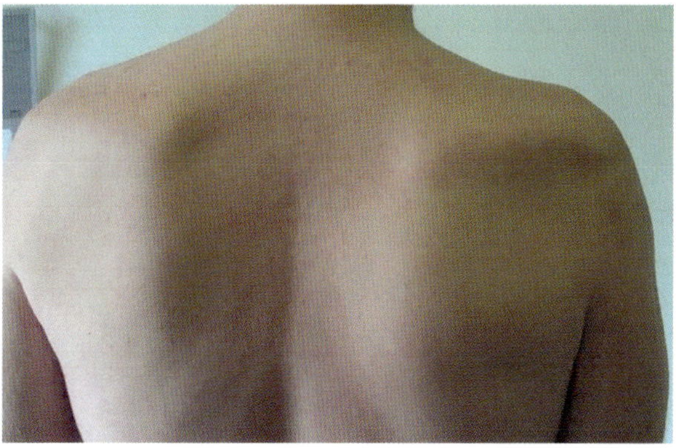

Fig. 2.1 Wasting of Supraspinatus and Infraspinatus. Image Published under License from www.shoulderdoc.co.uk

treatment. In this regard assessment of the cervical, upper thoracic but also scapular positioning is crucial. Exaggeration of the upper thoracic kyphosis and as a consequence over correction by way of extension of the cervical spine would indicate a degenerative condition affecting the cervical spine.

After that, any muscle wasting should be noted. Specifically wasting of the rotator cuff muscles (supra and infraspinatus) would indicate long-standing rotator cuff pathology (Fig. 2.1). Wasting of the deltoid can usually be clearly seen and would again indicate long-term disuse of the glenohumeral joint. Such disuse would typically be seen in frozen shoulder or glenohumeral arthritis but also after surgery. Generalised muscle wasting affecting both the peri-scapular and glenohumeral musculature would represent a more proximal pathology involving the cervical spine or brachial plexus. As would be appreciated, however, muscle wasting can also be seen in cases of prolonged disuse. Finally, any signs of rupture of the long head of biceps should noted. This is classically described as a 'Popeye' sign.

Thirdly scarring either post-traumatic or surgical should be noted. These would be indicators of either previous pathology or ongoing treatment. Finally, any swelling or redness should be noted. Swellings can include cysts arising for example from the acromioclavicular joint but also marked effusions can sometimes be seen with severe glenohumeral arthritis. Redness could indicate the presence of infection and may be particularly important after previous surgical procedures.

Palpation

Palpation which elucidates localised tenderness can be extremely useful for narrowing down the site of pathology (Figs. 2.2 and 2.3). This should include palpation of the cervical and thoracic spine although it is important to remember that older patients particularly can suffer from dual pathology. That is both problems in the neck and shoulder. Around the scapula, localised tenderness, particularly over the supra-medial border, may be associated with scapular dyskinesis which can include

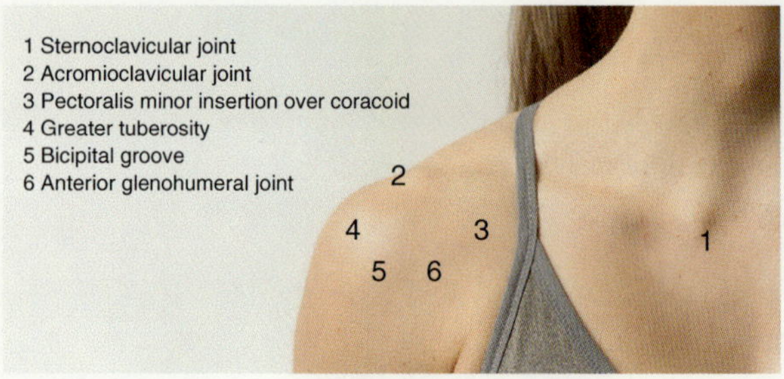

Fig. 2.2 Anterior localised tenderness points. Image Published under License from www.shoulderdoc.co.uk and www.shoulderpedia.org

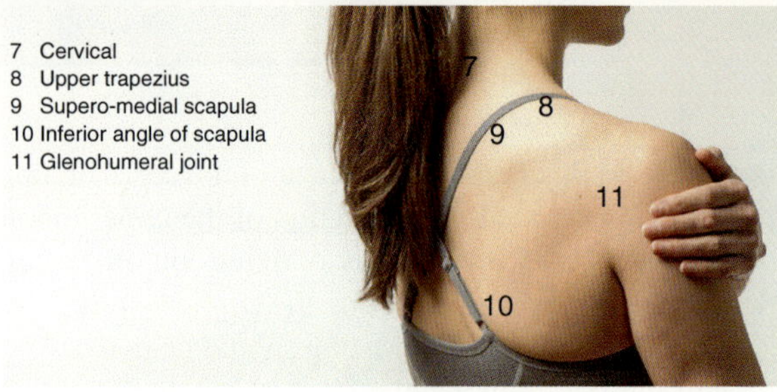

Fig. 2.3 Posterior localised tenderness points. Image Published under License from www.shoulderdoc.co.uk and www.shoulderpedia.org

a cracking sensation on movement. The acromioclavicular joint, however, is the easiest to assess by palpation. Specifically the joint is easy to identify, and localised palpation will elicit pain and discomfort. At the glenohumeral joint palpation of the rotator cuff and biceps tendon together with subscapularis if uncomfortable can indicate localised pathology. Indeed the author has found localised palpation particularly useful in diagnosing bicipital tendonitis.

Range of Motion (Movement)

Any assessment of movement of the shoulder that is of both the glenohumeral and scapular thoracic articulations should be undertaken actively and passively [1, 2]. Actively again the best position for observation is from the rear. It is, however, important to remember when standing behind a patient that it is not possible to monitor their face and as such acknowledge when movement is becoming painful. It is also useful to include an examination of movements of the cervical spine. At the shoulder, there are five modalities of movement; flexion, extension, abduction, internal and external rotation.

Active movement is assessed by asking the patient to firstly flex or elevate the shoulders until it becomes painful (Fig. 2.4). The degree of movement or deficit can then be assessed by simple observation or more accurately by a goniometer. Once extremes of active movement have been achieved then an assessment of passive movement can be undertaken. Again it is important to remember that if an examiner

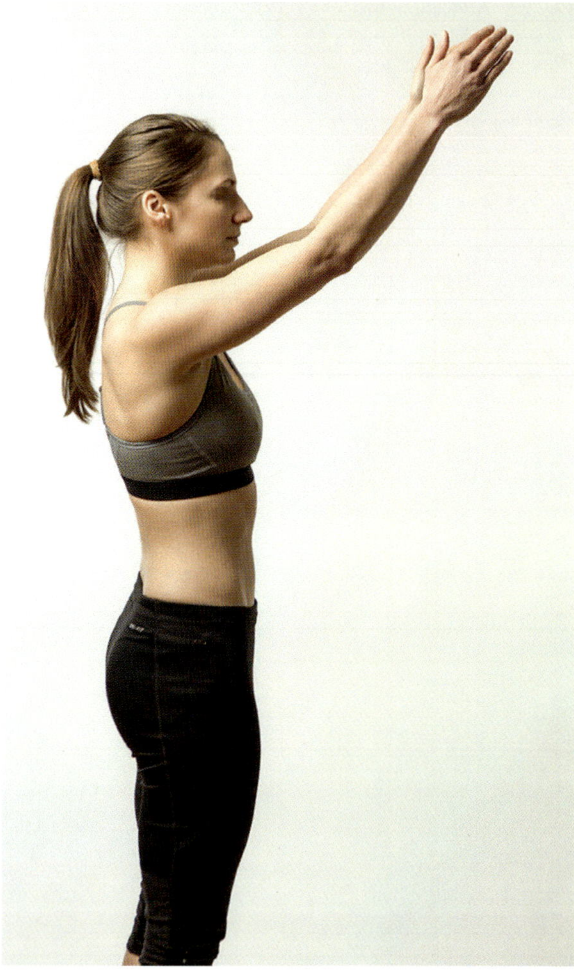

Fig. 2.4 Forward flexion. Image Published under License from www.shoulderdoc.co.uk and www.shoulderpedia.org

is standing behind the patient, it can be difficult to assess pain. Any improvement with passive motion is noted. If there is a significant increase with a passive examination, this will tend to indicate pathologies affecting the structures around the glenohumeral joint rather than the joint itself. For the latter in conditions such as glenohumeral arthritis, passive and active movements tend to be similar.

There are similar examination techniques for abduction (Fig. 2.5), specifically when standing behind the patient and asking them to elevate their arms in line with the chest. A comparison can be made with the contralateral side. Again a passive assessment should follow. It is important, however, to remember that patients can compensate for stiffness in the glenohumeral joint by compensatory scapulothoracic motion. Roughly two-thirds of shoulder abductions occur at the glenohumeral joint and one-third at the scapular thoracic articulation. Obviously, however, this movement is synchronous and can only be assessed by inspection from behind.

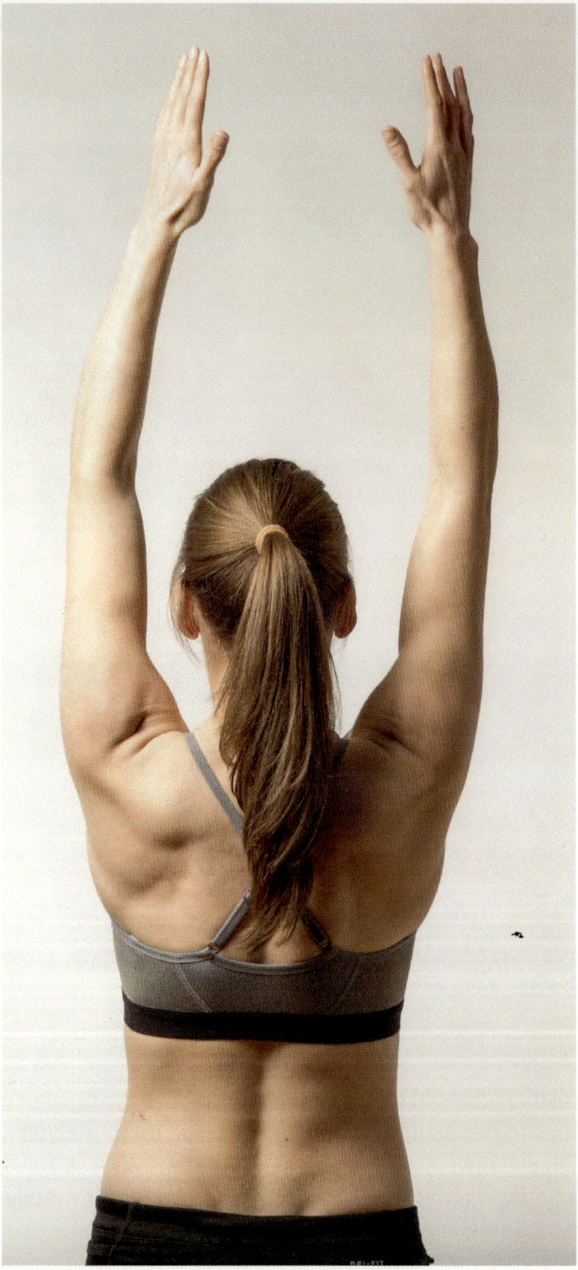

Fig. 2.5 Abduction. Image Published under License from www.shoulderdoc.co.uk and www.shoulderpedia.org

No Scap Movement

The next modality of movement to be evaluated is external rotation. For this, the patient is instructed to bend the elbows to 90° and tuck them into the side. Passive stabilising of the arm against the trunk reveals the true glenohumeral external rotation and eliminates scapulo-thoracic compensation (Fig. 2.6). Again it is useful to compare both sides passively and actively. Passive limitation in external rotation occurs

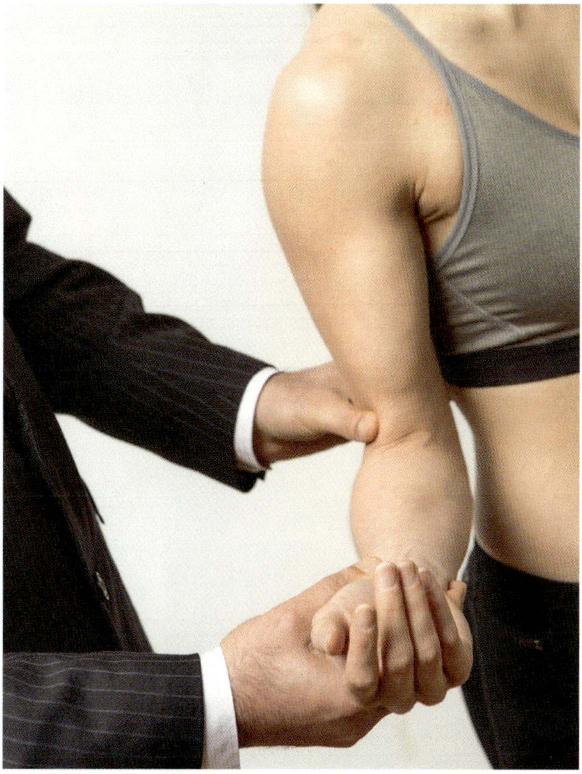

Fig. 2.6 Glenohumeral External rotation. Image Published under License from www.shoulderdoc.co.uk and www.shoulderpedia.org

most commonly in patients with frozen shoulder or osteoarthritis. Any difference between active and passive would indicate that the external rotators (teres minor and teres major) of the shoulder are deficient. Next, we test for internal rotation (Fig. 2.7). The easiest way is to ask the patient to put their hands up their back and touch their spine. Ideally, this should be one arm at a time. A good measure is to test how high up the spine the patients can place their hand. As you will appreciate, this not only checks internal rotation but also elbow flexion. Again limitation in the passive movement would indicate a structural abnormality of the shoulder, while the difference between passive and active would show weakness of the internal rotators.

Specific Tests

Subacromial Impingement

Impingement syndrome is characterised by pain experienced through an arc of elevation as the shoulder abducts. It should be appreciated that this is a condition that is associated predominantly with active movement of the shoulder. The two most commonly used tests for impingement are Neer's Sign and the Hawkins-Kennedy test [2, 3].

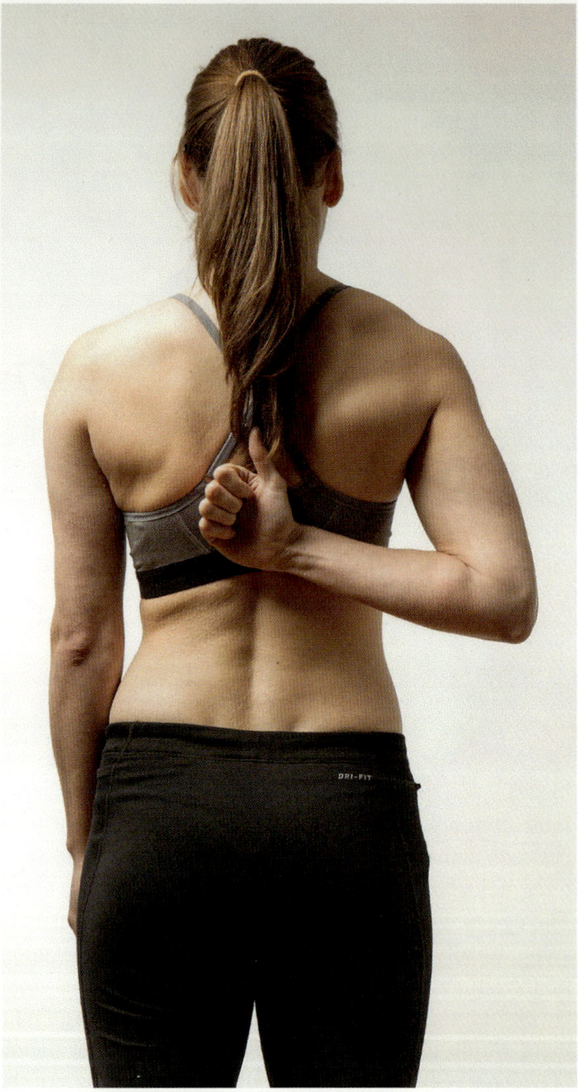

Fig. 2.7 . Image Published under License from www.shoulderdoc.co.uk and www.shoulderpedia.org

Neer's Sign

This sign allows demonstration of pain during passive elevation of the arm with the scapula stabilised, the examiner lifting the arm in the scapular plane with the arm internally rotated. As a supplementary part to this manoeuvre, the effect on the pain following an injection of local anaesthetic placed into the subacromial space is called Neer's test. A significant reduction or abolition of the pain is seen as a positive test [2].

Hawkins-Kennedy test

This is a passive test, with the examiner positioning the patient's arm at 90° elevation, the elbow bent to 90°, and the arm taken passively into internal rotation. Creation of pain during this manoeuvre is indicative of a positive test [2].

Rotator Cuff Disease

A large number of tests have been described to assess the rotator cuff. However, to evaluate individual muscles is almost impossible as there is significant overlap in function and compensation can occur [4]. The exception appears to be with subscapularis.

Pain elicited from these tests may be as a result of either tendinopathy/tear or subacromial impingement. Differentiation between tendinopathy and a small tear (partial thickness or full thickness) is often difficult if not impossible. Tears that involve a significant proportion of a tendon will tend to show signs of weakness. The clinician must be aware, however, that, even in the presence of a large or massive rotator cuff defect, the patient may still only demonstrate mild or subtle signs. This is a result of the ability of the shoulder to compensate for the absence of part of the rotator cuff with residual intact cuff and surrounding intact muscles [2].

Supraspinatus (Jobe's 'Empty Can' Test)

This test sets out to preferentially test supraspinatus, the most commonly affected tendon when considering degenerative cuff disease. It positions of the arm such that the supraspinatus tendon is placed under maximal stress as the arm is pushed down, attempting to invoke pain, weakness, or both.

The arm is flexed to 90° in the scapular plane and the forearm maximally pronated, so internally rotating the shoulder joint (the classical 'thumbs down' position). This position of internal rotation disadvantages the action of the deltoid, so improving the accuracy of testing supraspinatus. Pressure is applied to the arm and any pain or weakness recorded [2].

Infraspinatus (External Rotation Lag Sign)

This test sets out to examine the posterosuperior and posterior cuff elements. The arm is held in slight flexion with the elbow bent to 90°. The forearm is passively externally rotated to its maximal range and released. If the arm drops back towards its starting position, even by a few degrees, it is said to have a lag ('the lag sign') [2]. Conversely, the ability of the patient to maintain the arm fully externally rotated implies that infraspinatus is intact.

Teres Minor

Examination of the posterior cuff is to identify the "Hornblower sign". The arm is placed passively by the examiner in 90° of elevation and maximal external rotation. The patient is instructed to attempt to maintain the hand in space when the examiner releases the hold on the wrist. If the patient's arm falls forwards, this is a positive test, and indicates significant weakness of infraspinatus and usually teres minor. If the patient can maintain the position of the arm, this would suggest that teres minor is intact [2].

Subscapularis

Testing subscapularis involves the evaluation of the patient's ability to forcibly internally rotate the humerus. This can be achieved either in front (the belly-press test and bear-hug test) or behind (Gerber's lift-off test) the body. It must be appreciated that to make a satisfactory examination, the patient must be able to comfortably position their arm in the required position [2].

Belly Press Test (Napoleon Sign)

This involves the hand being placed flat on the abdomen, and the patient is requested to press the hand onto the stomach. If the patient is unable to maintain the elbow forward, so extending the shoulder and flexing the wrist to achieve the desired pressure, this indicates a positive test [2].

Bear-Hug Test

This involves the arm reaching across the body and, with the elbow held forward of the body, the strength of the resistance to the hand being pulled away from the body is evaluated [2].

Gerber's Lift-Off Test

The dorsum of the hand is placed on the sacrum, and the patient is asked to take the hand off the back, while the examiner maintains a fixed angle of elbow flexion. In addition to this test, one needs to look for a lag sign. With the arm held away from the sacrum by the examiner, so maximising the internal rotation of the humerus, the patient is then asked to maintain that position as the hand is released. If the hand falls back onto the sacrum, it indicates a weakness of subscapularis [2].

Biceps Evaluation

A biceps tendon is not always clearly palpable. The pathology involved with it should be considered if the patient complains of tenderness in and around the anterior lateral aspect of the shoulder just under the acromion. A number of provocative tests have been described including Yergason and Speed tests.

Yergason's Test

With this, the elbow is flexed to 90°. Holding the patient's wrist, the patient is then instructed to actively supinate against resistance. Localised pain over the bicipital groove suggests pathology affecting the long head of biceps.

Speed Test

With the elbow extended and the forearm supinated, forward elevation of the humerus is resisted. A positive result would be when this elicits pain again over the bicipital groove.

Superior Labral Anterior and Posterior Labral Detachment

Several tests have been described to elicit symptoms related to the pathology of the superior glenoid labral/biceps anchor. Unfortunately, while these tests often have sensitivity, they may not always have significant specificity.

Active Compression Tests (O'Brien Test)

The examiner stands behind the patient and stabilises the shoulder. Resistance is tested with the arm forward, flexed to 90° and adducted to 10° with the thumb pointing downwards. The patient is asked to determine the site of the pain. If the patient has a superior labral detachment, the pain will be superior to the glenohumeral joint.

Glenohumeral Instability

Assessment of glenohumeral stability requires the reproduction of symptoms of subluxation and/or apprehension by placing and stressing the shoulder in positions of compromise [5].

Glenohumeral Translation (Load and Shift Test)

This is assessed with the arm in 20° of abduction and slight forward flexion. The humeral head is loaded anteriorly and posteriorly translating the head on the glenoid fossa. An assessment of the degree of translation is then made by comparing it to the contralateral side. Passive translation or reproduction of symptoms would be a positive sign.

Apprehension Test

The most common direction of instability is anterior. With the patient sitting, the examiner stands behind the shoulder and externally rotates the arm with the shoulder at 90° abduction. Additional pressure can be applied with the thumb placed posteriorly pushing in the humeral head anteriorly. Any feeling of apprehension (apprehension sign) or instability would be regarded as a positive test and would indicate a tear of the anterior labrum.

Relocation Test

The relocation test will be described as positive if the symptoms of instability and apprehension are relieved during tests for apprehension when pressure is applied to the front of the shoulder pressing posteriorly. In other words, the load is taken off the anterior labrum. Again this would indicate the pathology of the anterior labrum.

Posterior Instability

Frequently this can be demonstrated by the patient. However, posterior translation can be easily assessed by passively translating the humeral head posteriorly on the glenoid and comparing the contralateral side.

Inferior Instability

This is manifest when traction on the arm reproduces symptoms and demonstrates a sulcus sign that is a gap between the acromion and humeral head.

Scapulothoracic Muscles

Impairment of the scapula muscles can occur in isolation or association with pathology of the glenohumeral joint, particularly the rotator cuff. Simple testing can be undertaken. For example serratus anterior by pushing against a wall, and trapezius by raising and rotating the scapula against gravity and load.

References

1. Armstrong A. Diagnosis and clinical assessment of a stiff shoulder. Shoulder Elbow. 2015;7(2):128–34.
2. Phillips N. Tests for diagnosing subacromial impingement syndrome and rotator cuff disease. Shoulder Elbow. 2014;6(3):215–21.
3. Walton J, Russell S. Physiotherapy assessment of shoulder stiffness and how it influences management. Shoulder Elbow. 2015;7(3):205–13.
4. Moser J. Physiotherapy assessment of patients with rotator cuff pathology. Shoulder Elbow. 2014;6(3):222–32.
5. Barrett C. The clinical physiotherapy assessment of non-traumatic shoulder instability. Shoulder Elbow. 2015;7(1):60–71.

Chapter 3
Special Tests

R. Steve Bale

This chapter will deal with the place of Special Tests as a pillar of diagnosis. The subsequent chapters will go into greater detail of the use of special tests for specific diagnoses. The value for the individual tests and clusters of tests will be discussed on a statistical basis.

What are Special Tests?

The four main pillars of diagnosis are History, Clinical Examination, Special Tests and Diagnostic Imaging. These pillars are essential in helping to make a correct diagnosis and arrive at a definitive plan for treatment.

Orthopaedic Special Tests can be used to provide additional useful information to the preceding pillars and when used appropriately can reduce the requirements for elements of the next pillar, diagnostic imaging, which may be uncomfortable and invasive to the patient, costly and logistically inconvenient.

How Many Special Tests Have Been Described?

There has been an enormous multiplication in the number of special tests described. There are well over one hundred described in the literature relating to shoulder surgery, but while the use of the tests is championed by the proponents, there has been

R. Steve Bale
Wrightington Hospital, Hall Lane, Appley Bridge, Wigan WN6 9EP, UK
e-mail: r.steve.bale@gmail.com

© Springer International Publishing AG 2017
P. Monga, L. Funk (eds.), *Diagnostic Clusters in Shoulder Conditions*,
DOI 10.1007/978-3-319-57334-2_3

far less critical analysis of the real value of these tests. Details on how to perform individual tests appear in subsequent chapters respectively.

Why Are the Tests Used?

Special tests may be used singularly or in groups or clusters to confirm a diagnosis, help with the differential diagnoses and help the clinician to distinguish between different pathologies which may be present in different anatomic structures coincidentally and also make sense of atypical presentations.

Many clinicians know a large number of tests and apply them as they feel appropriate without understanding how they can be used more effectively, often in specific combinations, to reach a diagnosis which has a statistically higher chance of truly being present.

The most important consideration is the clinical utility of the special tests, and the value of the test or combination of the tests is best considered in an evidence-based approach.

What Is the Statistical Basis for the Special Tests?

To consider the value of special tests, it is important to understand some of the statistical methods used to evaluate the tests.

The chance of a patient having a particular condition is based on prevalence and can be deemed the pre-test probability. Special tests are then chosen that determine the post-test probability of the patient having the condition. Whilst diagnostic certainty is nirvana, the clinician understands that this is not attainable. However, the clinician strives to reach a level of certainty where it is considered reasonable to offer treatment (Fig. 3.1). This is known as the treatment threshold.

Tests can be described as reliable when they produce information which is reproducible, and tests which provide an accurate diagnosis can be used to discriminate between patients who have the pathology from those who do not.

When considering reliability in special tests, there needs to be an agreement between observations. This can be measured between different examiners (inter-observer) and between the same examiner at different time points (intra-examiner). Kappa analysis allows us to gauge the agreement between observations when chance has been excluded such that values less than 0.1 have no reliability, ranging from slight, fair and moderate to substantial reliability with values over 0.81.

Tests are unlikely to be 100% accurate. The accuracy is determined by the level of agreement between the test being used and the reference standard which maybe findings on MRI or the objective observations at surgery itself. The accuracy of a test is described in terms of sensitivity, specificity, positive and negative predictive values and likelihood ratios. A typical contingency table can be used to determine the clinical utility of a test (Table 3.1).

Accuracy is given by

$$100\% \times (a + d) / (a + b + c + d)$$

But overall accuracy does not determine the clinical utility of the test. PPV is the likelihood of a person with a positive test result having the disease and NPV is the likelihood that an individual with a negative test does not have the disease.

Sensitive tests can detect patients who actually have a problem and are good at ruling out a problem. When a test has a high sensitivity, a negative result rules out the problem (SNout). Likewise, tests with a high specificity are good at ruling in a disorder when the result is positive (SPin).

Unfortunately, few tests have the combination of high sensitivity and high specificity. Therefore the use of likelihood ratios has been promoted. Likelihood ratios can be either positive or negative with a +LR shifting the probability in favour of having the problem while a −LR moves the probability in favour of not having the problem. Likelihood ratios are easily calculated if the test sensitivity and specificity are given within the description of the study results.

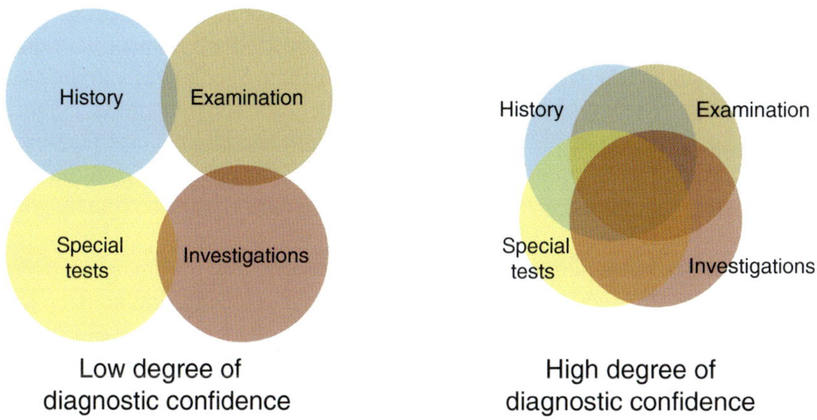

Fig. 3.1 Degree of diagnostic confidence. Image Published under License from www.shoulderpedia.org

Table 3.1 Contingency table.

	+ve ref. standard	−ve ref. standard	
+ve clinical test	True positive	False positive	$PPV = a/(a + b)$
−ve clinical test	False negative	True negative	$NPV = d/(c + d)$
	$Sens = a/(a + c)$	$Spec = d/(b + d)$	

$$+LR = sens / (1 - spec)$$
$$-LR = (1 - sens) / spec$$

Likelihood ratios less than one decrease the odds, given a negative test and values greater than one increase the odds, given a positive test. The important factors to consider are the magnitude of the shifts. Positive LRs greater than ten and negative LRs close to zero are believed to represent significant shifts.

Consideration also needs to be given to pre-test and post-test probability. Pre-test probability is the probability that a patient will have a disorder before the examination takes place. The value is often based on prevalence rates from the literature and represents the clinicians' starting point. Tests should ideally be chosen which have the potential to modify the pre-test probability. The post-test probability is the likelihood of having the problem after the examination. Decisions then rest around when the post-test probability is low enough to rule a problem out or high enough to rule the problem to be present.

What Is the Quality of the Literature on Special Tests?

While many papers are reporting to show the diagnostic accuracy of tests, usually by the authors proposing the use of the individual test, there is much less quality literature to support the appropriateness of Orthopaedic Special Tests in the overall clinical setting. Poor quality literature reporting tests showing good diagnostic accuracy can lead to premature incorporation of tests into clinical examination performance. Where functionality is not confirmed in quality follow-up studies, there is a risk that inaccurate diagnosis can ensue resulting in poorer management decisions.

Evidence-based medicine is the watchword for directing how we practice and systemic reviews of literature play a vital role in that evidence gathering. Various assessment tools have been developed to help better understand the quality of studies relating to diagnostic accuracy and reliability. QUADAS is a widely used assessment tool in diagnostic accuracy studies. It was initially described in 2003 [1] and then modified in 2011 [2]. It is a 14 point score, and 'quality' studies have been considered of higher merit where scores have been between 7 and 14 though some authors have used a higher range of scores to indicate a studies' worth. Other useful tools include QUAREL which is an appraisal tool for diagnostic reliability.

There is a paucity of systemic review data and meta-analysis relating to Orthopaedic Special Tests pertaining to the shoulder. The most relevant reviews will be summarised.

Hegedus et al. [3] published a systemic review and meta-analysis which assessed English language papers relating to diagnostic accuracy studies specific to the shoulder. Abstracts were reviewed and included if the reference standard was surgery or MRI, at least one special test was studied, and sensitivity or specificity was reported or could be deduced from the data. QUADAS was used to define study quality with scores of 10 used as the lower cut-off. Data was only pooled when both sensitivity and specificity data was given and were available for Neer's test for impingement, Hawkins test and Speed's test for labral pathology. In this study, 45 articles were assessed.

The paper reported that the Empty Can Test and the Infraspinatus Test was confirmatory for impingement. In the meta-analysis, only Neer's Test and Hawkins Test had enough data for consideration of pooling. The results showed Neer's test to have a sensitivity = 0.79 and specificity = 0.53, and Hawkins had sensitivity = 0.79 and specificity = 0.59. Neither test had diagnostic utility for impingement. The Internal Rotation Resistance Strength Test was found to improve the post-test probability of detecting impingement by more than a moderate amount, but this was derived from one article with a QUADAS score of less than ten.

When testing for rotator cuff integrity the External Rotation Lag Sign and Drop Arm Test were deemed of value for cuff tears, and Supine Impingement Test was reported to possibly rule out cuff tear when negative. Belly Press Test and Bear Hug appear valuable when positive for ruling in a subscapularis defect. External Rotation Lag Sign was diagnostic of Infraspinatus tear and Hornblowers Sign diagnostic of severe degeneration or tear of teres minor.

Detecting pathology of the labrum showed diagnostic value for the use of the Kim and Jerk Tests for posterior labral pathology and there appeared to be a value of Biceps Load II test for SLAP tears, but caution was recommended due to poorer performance in studies away from the originator. Meta-analysis was only possible on pooled Speed's Test data which showed no diagnostic utility. Apprehension, Relocation and Anterior Release Tests appeared diagnostic in anterior instability particularly if the feeling of apprehension was used as positive though the Anterior Release Test was valuable when either apprehension or pain was used.

The Active Compression test was thought likely to be diagnostic of ACJ pathology.

The first study described above looked at papers from 1966 to 2006. Hegedus et al. [4] published a second report in 2012 to include papers from 2006 to 2012, an additional 32 papers. Data was again pooled where appropriate, and Neer's Test showed sensitivity = 0.72 and specificity = 0.60 and Hawkins sensitivity = 0.79 and specificity = 0.60.

When used appropriately the relocation test had the best sensitivity for SLAP tear (0.52) and Yergasons had best specificity (0.95) with Compression Rotation Test showing the best +LR (2.81). The Passive Distraction Test for SLAP with a specificity of 0.85 and +LR more than five may rule in SLAP when positive. Interestingly the Biceps Load II Test introduced with high diagnostic statistics described in the first paper had no further replication of good results.

Other useful tests were emerging including the Belly-Off and Modified Belly Press for subscapularis pathology and Bony Apprehension for bony instability. The paper recommended the greater use of test combinations.

More recently Beiderwolf et al. [5] reviewed the literature to appreciate the utility of special tests. The pre-test probability was assumed to be 50%, and ruling in a problem was set at a post-test probability of 80% and ruling out at 20%. Papers were assessed from 1974 to 2013, and a score of seven on QUADAS was deemed sufficient to represent adequate quality. Where papers reported different results for tests, the inferior result was used. The pathology was divided into the cuff, Intra-articular and extra-articular problems.

A single test was used to rule in or out for intra and extra—articular pathology. The Internal Rotation Resisted Strength Test was used. One might notice from Hegedus et al. (2012) above that this was reported in a paper scored at less than the ten points used as the cut off in his series. This test had specificity of 0.96 and sensitivity of 0.86 with +LR 22 and −LR 0.13 which suggested the chance of having problems when the test was negative was 6%.

For impingement, the cluster of Hawkins, Infraspinatus Muscle Test and Painful Arc Sign had the best utility with 95.5% if all positive and 91% if two positive.

For rotator cuff tears Drop Arm Test, Internal Rotation Lag, External Rotation Lag and Hornblowers Signs had the best utility with post-test probabilities when positive of 100, 92.4, 88.8 and 87.7% respectively. Many of the commonly used tests did not meet diagnostic threshold used individually.

In anterior instability, the tests with the best utility were the Apprehension Test and the Anterior Release Tests with post-test probabilities of 91 and 80.7%. Diagnosing a Bankart tear was best with the cluster of Crank, Apprehension, Jobe, Load and Shift Test with Sulcus Test with a post-test probability of 75%. The Jerk and Kim test were deemed best at diagnosing posterior labral disruption with post-test probabilities of 94.8 and 86.9%. SLAP tears were best diagnosed with Biceps Load I and II tests with post-test probability of 93.8%.

Internal impingement is best diagnosed by Posterior Impingement Sign. For ACJ pathology the cluster of ACJ Resisted Extension, Cross-body adduction and O'Brien's tests were best with 80.5% post-test probability when all three were positive.

The concept of using combinations or clusters of special tests is gathering momentum [6]. It is clear that clustering has to be used correctly to improve on post-test probability and this recent work describes the best clusters from the literature. For rotator cuff pathology using age more than 60, painful arc, drop test and infraspinatus tests the +LR was 28 and −LR 0.09. In traumatic anterior instability, apprehension test and relocation test gave +LR 39.68 and −LR 0.19. Combining tests and also using demographic and subjective data can be shown to further enhance the diagnostic accuracy.

Summary

It is evident from the literature that excessive reliance on a single "special test" is not recommended. Indeed, to improve diagnostic accuracy, a cluster of tests should be used. Further research is needed to look at the utility of the special tests and is to consider how the tests can be used in combinations to aid diagnosis. Research into all aspects of the main pillars of diagnosis will eventually provide the physician with diagnostic algorithms supporting decision making, achieving thresholds for treatment and delivery of appropriate treatment.

References

1. Whiting PF, et al. The development of QUADAS: a tool for the quality assessment of studies of diagnostic accuracy included in systemic reviews. BMC Med Res Methodol. 2003;3:25.
2. Whiting PF, et al. QUADAS – 2: a revised tool for the quality assessment of diagnostic accuracy studies. Ann Intern Med. 2011;155(8):529–36.
3. Hegedus EJ, Goode A, Campbell S, Morin A, Tamaddoni M, Moorman CT 3rd, Cook C. Physical examination tests of the shoulder: a systematic review with meta-analysis of individual tests. Br J Sports Med. 2008;42(2):80–92.
4. EJ H, Goode AP, Cook CE, Michener L, Myer CA, Myer DM, Wright AA. Which physical examination tests provide clinicians with the most value when examining the shoulder? Update of a systematic review with meta-analysis of individual tests. Br J Sports Med. 2012;46(14):964–78.
5. Biederwolf NEA. proposed evidence-based shoulder special testing examination algorithm: clinical utility based on a systematic review of the literature. Int J Sports Phys Ther. 2013;8(4):427–40.
6. Hegedus EJ, Cook C, Lewis J, Wright A, Park JY. Combining orthopedic special tests to improve diagnosis of shoulder pathology. Phys Ther Sport. 2015;16(2):87–92.

Chapter 4
Radiological Investigations

S. Basu and D. Temperley

Radiological studies of the shoulder can assist in the diagnostic pathway in a wide variety of conditions. The appropriate imaging studies will depend on the nature of the suspected pathology, and the correct radiological investigation should be guided by accurate clinical history and examination. Plain X-ray is frequently the initial imaging investigation of choice, with more advanced imaging techniques e.g. ultrasound, MRI and CT selected, dependent upon the clinical and plain X-ray findings. This chapter aims to highlight and review the imaging modalities available to assess the various shoulder pathologies, describing their common indications as well as their clinical applications.

Plain X-ray

Plain film X-ray of the shoulder is the most commonly performed initial imaging investigation in patients presenting with shoulder trauma or chronic symptoms including pain, weakness and instability. It is useful to diagnose or exclude common shoulder pathologies, including fractures and dislocations in the context of acute trauma, or arthritic and degenerative changes in the context of patients presenting with chronic shoulder pain.

There are three commonly acquired X-ray views: anteroposterior (AP), lateral view of the scapula and an axial view (taken from inferior to superior or superior

S. Basu
Wrightington Hospital, Wigan, UK

D. Temperley (✉)
Department of Radiology, Wrightington Hospital,
Hall Lane Appley Bridge, Wigan WN6 9EP, UK
e-mail: david.temperley@wwl.nhs.uk

© Springer International Publishing AG 2017

P. Monga, L. Funk (eds.), *Diagnostic Clusters in Shoulder Conditions*,
DOI 10.1007/978-3-319-57334-2_4

and inferior with the arm in an abducted position). Modified views may need to be performed when the patient cannot move the arm particularly in the context of trauma and severe a result of trauma or pain.

Impingement and Rotator Cuff Tears

While plain X-ray cannot diagnose impingement or rotator cuff tears directly, there are useful secondary signs which should be reviewed as an adjunct to the clinical diagnosis.

Morphological changes in the shape of the acromion may have an association with impingement or rotator cuff tears, although such associations are not universally accepted. The most commonly described variations in acromion shape are lateral downsloping of the acromion (seen on the AP view) and variations of the curvature in the undersurface of the acromion as seen on the lateral scapular view or sagittal MRI sequence. Three morphological appearances to the acromion process were described by Bigliani [1]; Type I (flat undersurface), Type II (curved/concave undersurface), and Type III (anterior hook-shaped). Type III is said to have an increased association with impingement and rotator cuff tears, although other authors have not found a clear association. The presence of an unfused os acromiale is also important in the context of impingement and should be identified on imaging which aids the surgeon in operative planning.

Acquired degenerative changes are also important. Acromioclavicular joint (ACJ) osteoarthritis is common and can be a significant additional pain generator as well as associated inferior osteophytes which may be implicated in impingement to the rotator cuff. Degenerative cystic changes in the humeral head give an assessment of overall severity of the disease process.

In cases with advanced rotator cuff tear, the supraspinatus tendon tears and retracts, allowing the humeral head to migrate superiorly, thus narrowing the normal acromio-humeral distance. When this subacromial space is severely narrowed or obliterated, osteoarthritis type change can develop between the superior margins of the humeral head and the undersurface of the acromion. This is often associated with glenohumeral joint (GHJ) osteoarthritis (Fig. 4.1). This condition is known as 'rotator cuff arthropathy' and signifies an irreparable rotator cuff [2].

Arthritis

Osteoarthritis

Primary osteoarthritis of the GHJ is less common than secondary degenerative changes associated with rotator cuff disease, or ACJ osteoarthritis. As in other joints, the typical findings of osteoarthritis are osteophyte formation, subarticular

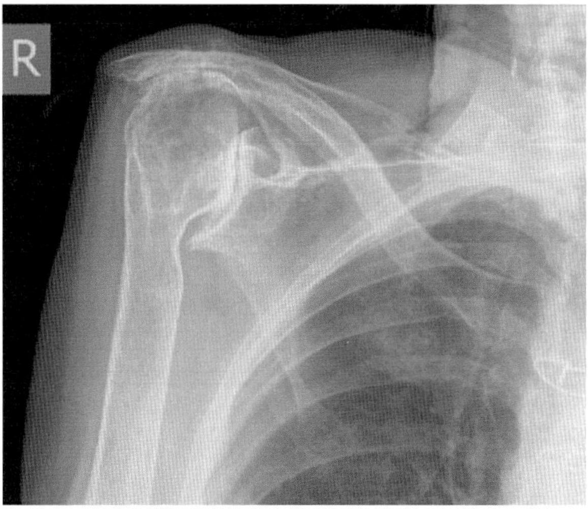

Fig. 4.1 X-ray rotator cuff arthropathy

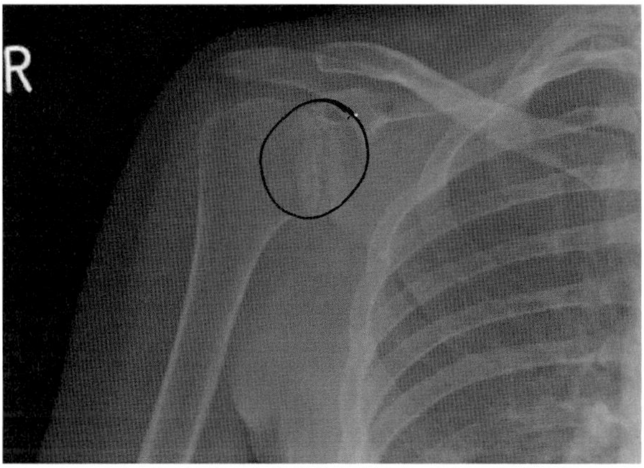

Fig. 4.2 X-ray glenohumeral osteoarthritis

sclerosis and joint space narrowing (Fig. 4.2). Subarticular cysts, or geodes, are often found. These defects, or erosions found in erosive arthritis, may be important quantitatively, as they can reduce the bone stock of the glenoid and it is, therefore, important to recognise in the context of surgical planning for shoulder arthroplasty.

Inflammatory Arthritis

The shoulder joint may be involved in inflammatory arthritides, particularly rheumatoid arthritis. This is a chronic multisystem disease which most commonly involves inflammation of the synovium with consequent bone erosion and cartilage loss. In the shoulder, the most common manifestations are marginal erosions within the humeral head and GHJ space loss. Erosion of the ACJ is common, particularly to the lateral clavicle. Also, there may also be associated rotator cuff tears.

Crystal Arthritis

Deposition of monosodium urate, calcium pyrophosphate or hydroxyapatite crystals may occur in or around the shoulder, although gout of the shoulder is uncommon. Of particular note is the condition Milwaukee shoulder syndrome. This is a condition of rapidly progressive and destructive arthritis, usually found in elderly women. It is uncommon but shows recognisable X-ray features with often gross bony destruction particularly in the humeral head and an effusion containing amorphous calcification. It is associated with hydroxyapatite crystals, although these are not necessarily causative [3].

Septic Arthritis

As with other joints, the X-ray is typically normal in the early stages of septic arthritis apart from possibly showing soft tissue swelling due to effusion. With the progression of any infection, bone demineralization and erosion with a destruction of the joint space can be seen.

Calcific Tendinitis

Calcific tendinitis results from the deposition of calcium hydroxyapatite crystals within the substance of the rotator cuff tendons, most commonly supraspinatus. The condition is typically encountered in the fourth and fifth decades and is usually self-limiting, as the calcification is resorbed spontaneously. However, the condition is often painful and may last for months or even years. X-ray shows a focus of calcification within the rotator cuff tendons, usually supraspinatus (Fig. 4.3). This may be well-defined, but can be ill-defined if there is extravasation into the overlying subacromial bursa.

Other Conditions

Instability

Assessment of instability often requires advanced imaging and in particular MRI or MRI arthrogram investigations. The X-ray should be reviewed for signs of glenoid fracture e.g. bony Bankart lesions, and humeral head fractures, particularly Hill-Sach's defects, which represent the consequence of previous dislocations. An axial

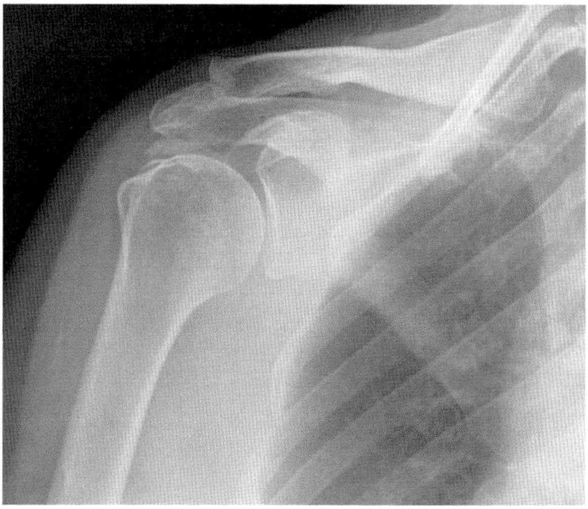

Fig. 4.3 X-ray calcific tendonitis

plain X-ray view of the shoulder can identify subtle displacements in position of the humeral head in relation to the glenoid.

Adhesive Capsulitis (Frozen Shoulder)

Often, a plain X-ray of the shoulder is normal in cases of adhesive capsulitis; the usefulness is to exclude any alternative causes e.g. Osteoarthritis, calcific tendinitis or even tumours.

Ultrasound and MRI may show non-specific features such as thickening of the coracohumeral ligament, and MRI may show besides, thickening to the inferior joint capsule at the inferior axillary recess, pericapsular oedema, and soft tissue thickening/scarring within the rotator interval, but ultimately the diagnosis is often made clinically.

Ultrasound

Musculoskeletal ultrasound is most commonly used to assess tendon pathology and to look for and describe excess fluid or abnormal fluid collections. Its use in the shoulder is no exception; ultrasound is commonly used to evaluate rotator cuff abnormalities and biceps tendon pathology, and fluid collections such as effusions, bursal fluid collections and cysts [4]. It is sensitive in the diagnosis of rotator cuff calcification. Ultrasound can be used to guide injections and other treatments. In the context of the acute presentation, ultrasound can distinguish and guide the aspiration of fluid collections for potential infection.

Ultrasound is less useful in the context of pathology associated with dislocation or instability; labral or SLAP tears will not usually be seen. While abnormalities have been described related to adhesive capsulitis, ultrasound will not typically add to the clinical assessment of this condition [5].

Ultrasound is a rapid examination which is performed with clinical correlation and can be used as an adjunct to clinical examination. Unlike other imaging modalities, a dynamic examination can be performed. While MRI provides a more global assessment of the shoulder and surrounding soft tissues, ultrasound is less time consuming and can give an answer to a focused clinical question which can be as accurate as with MRI.

Indications for Ultrasound

1. Assessment of rotator cuff pathology

   Advantages

   – Accurate assessment of rotator cuff tears
   – Quick examination; can be performed at the time of initial clinical assessment.
   – Dynamic assessment possible (e.g. assessment of impingement)

   Disadvantages

   – 'Operator dependent'- ultrasound images cannot be optimally reviewed independently afterwards, so the examination is dependent on the operator's interpretation.
   – Less accurate than MRI in diagnosing and grading muscle atrophy.
   – Cannot assess intra-articular or intrinsic bony pathology.
   – The examination may be limited if patient shoulder range of movement is reduced.

2. Assessment of long head of biceps tendon pathology

   – Can readily diagnose biceps tendon tears and dislocations.
   – The whole biceps tendon and muscle can be assessed if necessary.

3. Assessment of calcific tendinitis.

   – Ultrasound is the most sensitive imaging modality for calcific tendinitis.
   – Can be used to guide therapeutic injections e.g. Barbotage procedures

4. Assessment of instability and labral pathology.

   – Not useful in the intra-articular assessment of ligaments, labrum and articular chondral surfaces.

5. Assessment of fluid collections around the shoulder.
   - Accurate in the diagnosis of effusions, fluid in the subacromial/subdeltoid bursa and other fluid collections around the shoulder.
   - Can be used to guide aspirations.
6. Ultrasound-guided interventional procedures. Common procedures include
   - Injection of subacromial/subdeltoid bursa with steroid and local anaesthetic.
   - ACJ and/or GHJ injections.
   - Suprascapular nerve block or ablation.
   - Injection of calcific tendinitis.
   - Aspiration of collections where infection is suspected

Clinical Uses of Ultrasound

Impingement and Rotator Cuff Tears

Ultrasound of the shoulder in patients presenting with impingement or rotator cuff tears is often undertaken when the patient has failed to respond to initial conservative management including physiotherapy and possibly injections. A high-frequency linear array transducer is used. A full description of the technique of ultrasound is beyond the scope of this book; briefly, the long head of biceps tendon is usually examined first with the arm in a neutral position. The subscapularis tendon is assessed with the arm in external rotation, while the supraspinatus is examined with the humerus in extension and internal rotation. These changes of movement bring the relevant tendon anterior to the humeral head, where they can be examined clear of the acromion and clavicle. The ACJ is examined, and the muscle bellies, particularly supraspinatus, are reviewed to assess for atrophy [6]. Dynamic examination for impingement involves scanning while abducting the arm to assess for thickening or bunching of the subdeltoid bursa as it passes under the coracoacromial ligament.

A full-thickness cuff tear is a defect in the tendon which extends, at least for a small area, across the height of the tendon from the articular side to the bursal aspect of the tendon. Small full-thickness rotator cuff tears are seen as small defects in the rotator cuff tendon or subtle loss of the normal convexity of the bursal surface of the tendon. In large rotator cuff tears with tendon retraction, the supraspinatus tendon may appear absent with the deltoid muscle almost apposing or sagging upon the humeral head. Rotator cuff tears most commonly start in the supraspinatus tendon and may extend into the other rotator cuff muscles particularly infraspinatus and subscapularis. Assessment for subscapularis tears is of particular importance, as this may alter the surgical approach as well as becoming an increasing recognition for morbidity and failed shoulder surgery.

Partial-thickness tears are identified as a defect in the tendon that does not extend across its complete width. In rotator cuff tendinopathy, the tendon will be thickened and amorphous, with loss of the normal low signal and striated tendon pattern. Increased Doppler flow may be seen.

Ultrasound is accurate in the assessment of full-thickness tears, with a sensitivity of 92% and specificity of 93% in a recent meta-analysis [7]. This is compatible to MRI. Ultrasound is less sensitive than MRI in the detection of partial-thickness rotator cuff tears, but with similar specificity. (Ultrasound: Sensitivity 52%, specificity 93%. MRI: Sensitivity 74%, specificity 93%).

Biceps Tendon Pathology

The long head of biceps tendon is easily visualised within the bicipital groove. In a complete tear of the long head of biceps tendon, the tendon will not be seen in the bicipital groove; the retracted end can be identified by scanning inferiorly. High-grade partial-thickness tears may be difficult to distinguish from a complete tear. The long head of biceps may sublux or dislocate from the bicipital groove; in this case, the tendon will be identified medial to its normal site and is classically seen in the context of full-thickness subscapularis tendon tears with disruption to the overlying transverse humeral ligament. Partial-thickness tears will be seen asa focal hypoechoic areas within the tendon. Fluid in the biceps tendon sheath may indicate tenosynovitis of the tendon or may be part of generalised GHJ effusion.

Calcific Tendinitis

In calcific tendinitis of the rotator cuff, calcification most commonly occurs within the supraspinatus tendon but may happen in other rotator cuff tendons. The presence of calcification is readily identified on ultrasound scanning, which is more sensitive than X-ray. Calcific tendinitis presents on ultrasound as calcification at any site in the body; usually an echogenic 'line' with a posterior acoustic shadowing (ultrasound artefact).

Ultrasound-Guided Injections

Injections can be performed under ultrasound guidance; the transducer is held in one hand while injecting with the other. By scanning in the correct plane, the needle tip can be seen to advance in 'real-time' while scanning. Thus the tip of the needle can be placed in a fluid collection or effusion for aspiration for biochemical or microbiological analysis, or an injection of local anaesthetic for diagnosis or of steroid for treatment can be made into the intended site under direct visualisation.

Ultrasound-guided injections are commonly given into the subacromial space, bicipital tendon sheath, GHJ or ACJ. The suprascapular notch can be identified on ultrasound, and the suprascapular nerve can be injected with local anaesthetic and steroid for diagnosis and temporary pain relief (suprascapular nerve block) [8] or permanently ablated using pulsed radiofrequency ablation, particularly in the context of rotator cuff arthropathy.

Ultrasound can be used to guide treatment of calcific tendinitis. An attempt can be made to aspirate the calcified deposits, or the calcification can be 'dry needled' by passing a needle through the calcification with several passes. This is to attempt to break up the calcification which may encourage healing by promoting a localised inflammatory/vascular response leading to an earlier reabsorption of the calcification than would spontaneously occur. Ultrasound-guided needling and lavage have been shown to give significantly better results than a subacromial corticosteroid injection only [9].

Magnetic Resonance Imaging (MRI)

Magnetic resonance (MR) imaging provides a comprehensive and accurate assessment of the osseous and soft tissue structures involving the shoulder [10]. Standard radiography is often used as a primary imaging modality to assess the osseous anatomy of the shoulder however its limited capability to evaluate the soft tissues often leads to MR imaging being utilised.

Conventional MR imaging is used to characterise a range of conditions from rotator cuff disease and acromioclavicular (AC) joint pathology in impingement disorders to glenoid labrum pathology and the capsular structures in instability utilising contrast-enhanced MR arthrography.

Protocols for Imaging of the Shoulder

- Patient's arm should be positioned with patient supine and the arm by the side parallel to the body with the shoulder in neutral to mild external rotation.
- Coronal oblique images are performed parallel to the course of the supraspinatus tendon.
- Coronal oblique Proton Density Fat-Suppressed sequences are sensitive to rotator cuff degeneration although it can be difficult to differentiate between severe cuff tendinosis and partial-thickness tears
- Coronal oblique or sagittal oblique T2 sequences are required to distinguish between severe tendinosis and partial tears with the presence of fluid high signal.
- Axial sequences are used to assess the AC joint, as well as capsular and labral anatomy.

- Sagittal oblique sequences are used to evaluate the acromial anatomy, rotator interval, the cuff muscles and the capsulolabral complex.

MRI Arthrography

The procedure involves the instillation of dilute gadolinium-based para-magnetic contrast agent to distend the glenohumeral joint via needle placement under fluoroscopic or ultrasound guidance.

- Typically T1, proton density or T2 fat-suppressed sequences may then be performed using axial, coronal oblique and sagittal oblique sequences.
- An additional abduction external rotation (ABER) view can be utilised in MR arthrography to evaluate for labral tears or in the integrity of the post-operative labrum.

Indications for MRI

1. Assessment of rotator cuff and long head of biceps pathology and tears.

   Advantages:

   – Accurate assessment of rotator cuff tendinopathy, partial-thickness and full-thickness tears.
   – Accurate assessment of biceps tears and dislocations.
   – Atrophy and fatty infiltration of rotator cuff muscles can be readily viewed and graded.
   – Underlying bone and intra-articular pathology can be assessed.

   Disadvantages:

   – Relatively expensive and time-consuming procedure.
   – Some patients cannot be scanned as a result of claustrophobia.

2. Assessment of instability and labral or articular cartilage defects.

   – Accurate assessment of labral and cartilage defects, including SLAP tears
   – Assessment of underlying bony pathology.

   Currently, in most centres, assessment of labral pathology and SLAP tears requires intra-articular contrast injection, turning a non-invasive examination into a minimally invasive study. More powerful magnets (3 T and above) may obviate the need for intra-articular injection in the future.

3. Assessment of bone tumours and infections.

   – The most accurate imaging modality for assessing the extent of the pathology.

Clinical Uses of MRI

Rotator Cuff Tears

MRI offers a detailed, global and accurate assessment of the shoulder in cases of impingement and suspected rotator cuff tears. Full-thickness rotator cuff tears can be accurately diagnosed and characterised, and distinguished from partial-thickness rotator cuff tears and tendinopathy (Fig. 4.4). Rotator cuff muscle atrophy is seen, and its severity can be graded (Fig. 4.5). Causes of impingement can be assessed; the presence of acromion and AC joint osteophytes and the assessment of acromion morphology are useful in the planning of surgery. Tears, tendinopathy and tenosynovitis of the biceps tendon are also well seen. Underlying bone pathology and arthritis will also be visualised to advantage on MRI scanning.

MRI and ultrasound can both be used to assess for rotator cuff tears. Compared with ultrasound, MRI offers an overall view of the shoulder and surrounding soft tissues. MR is also better at evaluating the rotator cuff muscles for atrophy than ultrasound, while ultrasound can be performed alongside clinical assessment, and offers an excellent opportunity for dynamic evaluation of the shoulder.

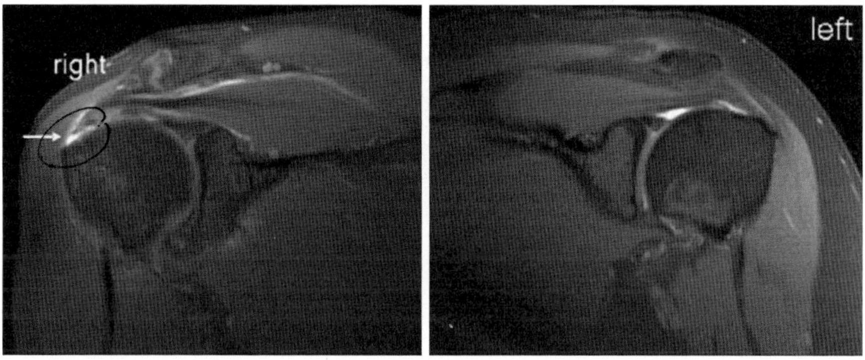

Fig. 4.4 MRI rotator cuff tear

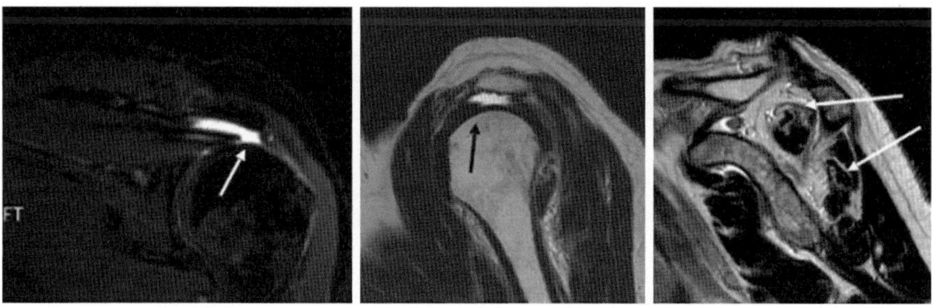

Fig. 4.5 MRI large rotator cuff tear with wasting and atrophy

Cochrane review [7] shows sensitivity and specificity of 94 and 93% respectively for full-thickness tears on MRI. For partial-thickness tears, the sensitivity and specificity values were 74 and 93% respectively. MR arthrography can also be used to assess for rotator cuff tears. While the images may give improved detail compared with plain MRI, the Cochrane review shows no significant advantage in the sensitivity and specificity, and for this reason, plain MRI is usually preferred to assess for rotator cuff pathology.

Instability

Injection of dilute paramagnetic contrast into the shoulder joint before MRI (MR arthrography) distends the shoulder joint and allows clear visualisation of the internal soft tissue structures of the shoulder joint which are sometimes not clearly distinguished on plain MRI [11]. Thus the articular cartilage, glenoid labrum, capsular ligaments and rotator interval are better assessed with MR arthrography.

In patients with instability, tears of the glenoid labrum, articular cartilage and capsular ligaments can be diagnosed and described before consideration of surgery (Fig. 4.6). Studies have shown that MR arthrogram is significantly more accurate in assessment of labral tears than plain MRI. Underlying bony glenoid and humeral head defects can readily be seen. MR arthrogram studies can be used to assess for associated rotator cuff tears, and it has been suggested that partial-thickness rotator cuff tears may be more easily identified in the younger age group with MR arthrograms. Contrast outlines the biceps and bicipital-labral complex to also aid in the detection of superior labral anterior to posterior (SLAP) lesions (Fig. 4.7). MRI arthrography can also be used to assess symptomatic recurrence in the shoulder previously operated for instability.

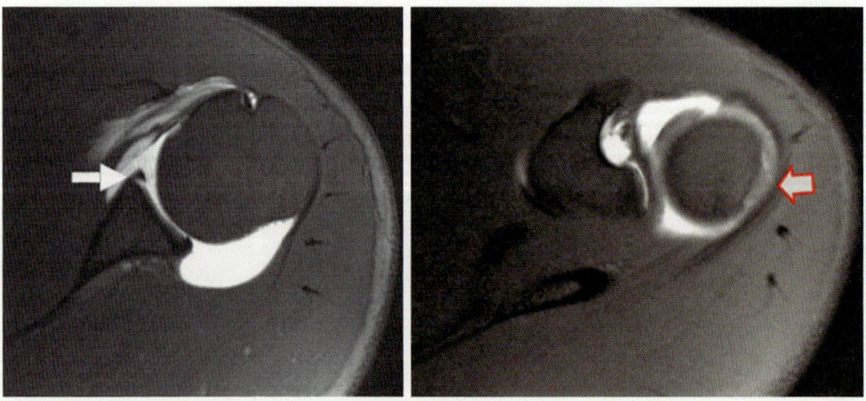

Fig. 4.6 MRA glenoid labral tear and Hill Sachs defect

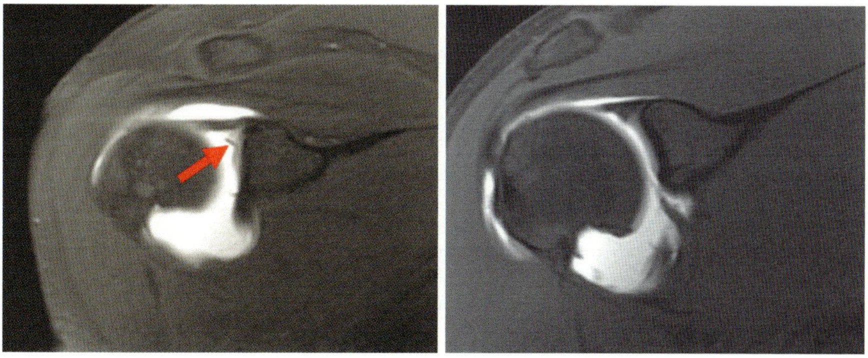

Fig. 4.7 MRA superior labral tear (**a**) compared with normal (**b**)

Other Clinical Indications

- MRI can be used to diagnose, describe and characterise bone and soft tissue tumours around the shoulder.
- The assessment of infections around the shoulder joint; to distinguish fluid collections from inflammation, and to assess for the presence of osteomyelitis
- In cases of complex osteoarthritis or inflammatory arthritis where X-ray does not give sufficient information. MRI is particularly useful in the assessment of effusions, fluid collections and bony involvement.

CT

CT (Computed Tomography, Computerised Tomography) involves passing X-ray beams at different angles through the patient in an axial 'slice'. The X-ray source continually rotates around the patient as the patient is moved through the scanner. X-raying the patient at multiple different angles allows the data to be reconstructed to give a density at each point (pixel) so that a 3-D picture can be obtained.

Images are usually displayed as successive 2-D 'slices' to build up a 3-D image. Modern multislice CT scanners produce images with a very thin (0.5 or 1 mm) slice thickness, enabling coronal, sagittal or oblique reconstructions to be made from the axial data with minimal loss of resolution. 3-D reconstructions can also be obtained, using all the data from the scan to produce a 3-D image which can be rotated to view from any angle.

As CT is an X-ray based imaging modality, the greatest advantage and most common use in orthopaedic imaging is to assess bony pathology. Bone outline, bony trabeculae and joint surfaces are easily visualised with high spatial resolution because of the inherent density difference between bone and other tissues. In general, there is a low difference in density between different soft tissues, and soft tissue pathology is less well visualised than on ultrasound or MRI. However intravenous iodine-based contrast administration can help particularly when MRI is contraindicated, and intra-articular contrast can be used as an alternative to MRI arthrogram to study cartilage defects and labral tears.

Indications for CT

1. Fractures. 3-D assessment of complex fractures and dislocations.
2. Arthritis. Assessment of glenohumeral arthritis and rotator cuff arthropathy preoperatively.
3. Instability. CT arthrogram can be used instead of MRI arthrogram to assess labral and bony defects.
4. Rotator cuff disease. Useful to evaluate the bony anatomy and fatty infiltration/atrophy of the rotator cuff musculature, but not helpful in the diagnosis of rotator cuff tears.

Clinical Uses of CT

Fractures

CT is ideally suited to give precise 3-D representation in cases of complex fractures and dislocations (Fig. 4.8). Healing of fractures can be studied with CT scanning; the degree of callus formation and bone union can be assessed in detail.

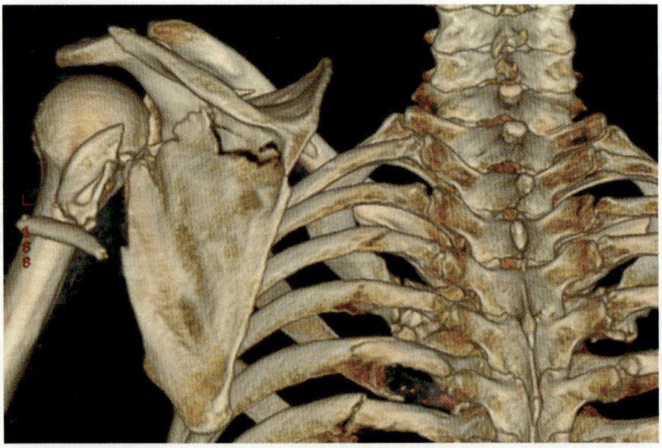

Fig. 4.8 CT 3D reconstruction of a scapula fracture

Arthritis

CT gives a detailed image of articular surfaces, showing joint space narrowing and subarticular erosion associated with arthritis. Glenohumeral, A/C joint arthritis and rotator cuff arthropathy can be assessed. CT scanning is most commonly used before shoulder surgery and in particular joint replacement. Review of glenoid bone stock is necessary preoperatively to evaluate the feasibility of glenoid prosthesis implantation and technical planning. This cannot be achieved on plain X-ray but is easily visualised on CT.

Symptomatic shoulder joint replacements can also be assessed with CT. Beam hardening artefact degrades the image a standard CT, but utilisation of extended Hounsfield unit scale and metal artefact reduction post-processing software should be used to give images where, for example, subtle loosening can be seen right up to the edge of the metallic prosthesis [12].

Instability—CT Arthrogram

Contrast medium is injected into the shoulder before a standard CT scan examination. The contrast distends the joint and outlines the articular cartilage, fibrocartilaginous labrum and glenohumeral ligaments. This allows defects in the structures, including labral and SLAP tears to be diagnosed and characterised. CT arthrography can be used as an alternative to MRI arthrography, with CT having the advantage of greater spatial resolution as opposed to the higher contrast resolution of MRI. CT is particularly useful in assessing the postoperative labrum, where MRI might be degraded by metal artefact. CT is also the preferred choice to evaluate the integrity of bone stabilisation procedures.

Rotator Cuff Disease

CT is not accurate in the assessment of rotator cuff tendon tears, and MRI or ultrasound should be used for this purpose. However, CT may be useful, especially when MRI is contraindicated, to assess the rotator cuff muscles for atrophy in cases of rotator cuff tears. The Goutallier classification, commonly used to determine the degree of degeneration and fatty infiltration of rotator cuff muscles in the context of rotator cuff tears, was initially described in shoulder CT but is also applicable to MRI [13].

Other Bony and Soft Tissue Pathology

CT gives explicit detail of bony erosion or destruction in cases of infection or tumour. The glenohumeral joint and scapula can be assessed in cases of dysplasia, particularly to look for the glenoid area, depth and version.

As discussed above, CT of the soft tissues is limited by the inherent lack of contrast, but masses and fluid collections can be assessed with the aid of intravenous iodinated contrast enhancement. However, MRI or ultrasound is preferred.

Nuclear Medicine

Nuclear medicine techniques involve injecting small amounts of radioactive substances, often bound to biologically active molecules. The gamma photons produced by the radioactive isotope are detected in the gamma camera with a crystal constructed of sodium iodide.

Technetium (Tc) 99 m MDP bone scintigraphy is the traditional isotope scanning technique to assess for increased osteoblastic activity and has been in use since the 1960s. Increased activity will be detected in bone tumours, infections, fractures, arthritis and other forms of increased metabolic activity such as Paget's disease. The investigation is, therefore, sensitive, but not specific.

Nuclear medicine imaging with^{111}Indium-Oxide or more recently anti-granulocyte scintigraphy using (99 m)Tc-labeled monoclonal antibodies (MoAb) provide a high degree of specificity in imaging osteomyelitis. In a patient presenting with chronic shoulder symptoms (pain, weakness or instability) nuclear medicine imaging does not have a place on the diagnostic workup unless an infection is suspected.

Conclusion

There is a broad range of imaging techniques available to investigate patients with shoulder pain, weakness and instability. The initial radiological investigation will usually be with a plain X-ray. Further studies—ultrasound, MRI, MRI arthrogram and CT scanning—will be dependent on the clinical presentation and the information required from the scan. This chapter has given an introduction to the different imaging modalities, their indications and the abnormal findings that can be seen with each technique. Specific imaging pathways will be further discussed in the relevant chapters to follow.

References

1. Bigliani LU, Morrison DS, April EW. The morphology of the acromion and its relationship to rotator cuff tears. Orthopaedic. Transactions. 1986;10:228.
2. Nam D, Maak TG, Raphael BS, Kepler CK, Cross MB, Warren RF. Rotator cuff tear arthropathy: evaluation, diagnosis and treatment. J Bone Joint Surg Am. 2012;94(6):e34.
3. Nguyen VD. Rapid destructive arthritis of the shoulder. Skelet Radiol. 1996;25(2):107–12.
4. Petranova T, et al. Ultrasound of the shoulder. Med Ultrason. 2012;14(2):133–40.
5. Moosikasuwan JB, Miller TT, Burke BJ. Rotator cuff tears: clinical radiographic and US findings. Radiographics. 2005;25:1591–607.
6. Teefey SA. Shoulder sonography, why we do it. J Ultrasound Med. 2012;31(9):1325–31.
7. Lenza M, Buchbinder R, Tagwoingi Y, Johnston RV, Hanchard NCA, Faloppa F. Magnetic resonance imaging, magnetic resonance arthrography and ultrasonography for assessing rotator cuff tears in people with shoulder pain for whom surgery is being considered (review). Cochrane Database Syst Rev. 2013; (9). Art. No.: CD009020. doi: 10.1002/14651858.CD009020.pub2
8. Harmon D, Hearty C. Ultrasound-guided suprascapular nerve block technique. Pain Physician. 2007;10:743–6.
9. deWitte PB, Selten JW, Navas A, Nagels J, Visser CP, Nelissed RG, Reijnierse M. Calcific tendinitis of the rotator cuff: Randomised controlled trial of ultrasound guided needling and lavage versus subacromial corticosteroids. Am J Sports Med. 2013;41(7):1665–73.
10. McNally EG, Rees JL. Imaging in shoulder disorders. Skelet Radiol. 2007;36:1013–6.
11. Magee T, Williams D, Mani N. Shoulder MR arthrography: which patient group benefits most? AJR. 2004;183:969–74.
12. Buchsbaum. orthopaedic hip implants, extended hounsfield units, and artefact reduction: Evaluation of a commercial CT System. Researchgate.net/publication/274946722.
13. Goutallier D, Postel JM, Bernageau J, et al. Fatty muscle degeneration in cuff ruptures. Pre- and post operative evaluation by CT. Clin Orthop Relat Res. 1994;304:78–83.

References

Part II
Shoulder Pain Clusters

Chapter 5
Subacromial Impingement Syndrome

Andreas Baumann and Barnes Morgan

Case Example

A 56-year-old female office worker is referred to the orthopaedic clinic by his GP with a four-month history of right-sided shoulder pain. There was no history of preceding trauma, but her symptoms started shortly after the patient had been re-decorating her house. She gets pain with any activities above chest level and struggles to tuck shirts in and do her bra behind her back. Pain often wakes her when she rolls onto the affected shoulder in bed. Despite Paracetamol, her symptoms have gradually deteriorated. She is in good health and has never had any problems with her shoulder in the past.

Introduction

Subacromial impingement syndrome is the most commonly diagnosed painful shoulder disorder [1]. It can be defined as ***symptomatic irritation of the rotator cuff and subacromial bursa within the subacromial space***. Subacromial impingement comprises a spectrum of pathologies, ranging from subacromial bursitis to rotator cuff tendinopathy and full-thickness rotator cuff tears. Despite its high incidence, the aetiology of subacromial impingement syndrome remains controversial. Both extrinsic compression and intrinsic degeneration may play a role.

A. Baumann
Royal Preston Hospital, Preston, UK

B. Morgan (✉)
Stepping Hill Hospital, Poplar Grove, Stockport, Cheshire SK3 7JE, UK
e-mail: barnesmorgan@doctors.org.uk

© Springer International Publishing AG 2017

P. Monga, L. Funk (eds.), *Diagnostic Clusters in Shoulder Conditions*,
DOI 10.1007/978-3-319-57334-2_5

The four muscles of the rotator cuff—the subscapularis, infraspinatus, teres minor and supraspinatus provide dynamic stability to maintain the humeral head within the glenoid fossa and form a force couple with the deltoid. Dysfunction of the rotator cuff can lead to *pathologic contact and compression of the supraspinatus tendon near its insertion on the greater tuberosity with the under-surface of the anterior edge of the acromion and coracoacromial (CA) ligament*—this is termed Impingement.

In 1972 Neer proposed that mechanical compression of the rotator cuff tendons occurred due to a narrowing of the subacromial space and he described the following three stages of impingement (Table 5.1) [2]:

From cadaveric studies, Neer concluded that impingement of the rotator cuff against the acromion occurs anterior rather than lateral. Acromial morphology was analysed, and certain acromial types have been correlated with the incidence of subacromial impingement—according to Bigliani and Morrison, a curved (type II) and a hooked (type III) acromion predisposes to impingement (Fig. 5.1) [3].

Intrinsic factors that may lead to rotator cuff failure include poor vascularity of the supraspinatus tendon, ageing and excessive tensile forces [4]. Lohr and Uhthoff

Table 5.1 Neer's 3 stages of subacromial impingement

• Stage 1: Oedema and haemorrhage, age <25, reversible
• Stage 2: Fibrosis and tendinitis, age 25–40, recurrent pain with activity
• Stage 3: Bone spurs and tendon rupture, age >40, progressive disability

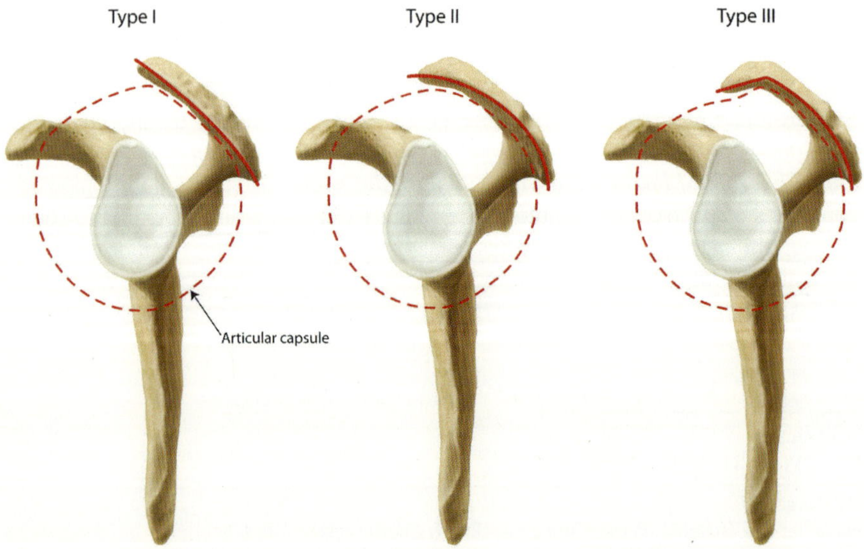

Fig. 5.1 Acromial shapes. Image Published under License from www.shoulderdoc.co.uk

found a hypovascular or critical zone close to the insertion of the supraspinatus tendon into the footprint [5]. They concluded that the poor vascularity of the tendon in this area could be a significant factor in the pathogenesis of rotator cuff degeneration and that subacromial impingement develops secondary to cuff weakness where the humeral head ascent against overlying structures.

Pillar 1: History

Patients presenting with subacromial impingement are almost always over the age of 40 and commonly complain of night pain, which is exacerbated when lying on the affected shoulder. There is usually an insidious onset of shoulder pain over a period of weeks to months, and the pain is typically localised in the bursal distribution. Lateral and/or superolateral pain radiates down towards the elbow is common. The range of motion is generally well preserved. Pain is often aggravated with an abduction of the arm and when reaching behind the back. In some cases, minor trauma to the shoulder or strenuous exercises precedes the onset of symptoms.

Pillar 2: The Conventional Examination

The examination should always include evaluation of the active and passive range of motion (ROM), rotator cuff strength and provocative tests. With subacromial impingement syndrome, inspection and palpation of the shoulder can sometimes reveal wasting in the supraspinatus and/or infraspinatus fossa when a cuff tear is present. ROM is generally within normal limits, but patients with impingement syndrome almost always have a 'painful arc' of shoulder abduction from about 60 to 120°. In chronic cases, capsular tightness and subacromial adhesions can develop and lead to stiffness.

Pillar 3: Special Tests

Two commonly used provocative tests that are used for diagnosing subacromial impingement are **Neer's sign** and the **Hawkins-Kennedy test** [6].

Neer's sign is positive when pain is produced with passive shoulder elevation and internal rotation while stabilising the scapula. (Fig. 5.2) The Hawkins-Kennedy test places the arm in 90° of forward flexion and then gently brought into internal rotation. The end point of internal rotation is either when the patient experiences pain or when a rotation of scapula is felt or observed by the examiner (Fig. 5.3). A positive Neer's Test is demonstrated by relief of symptoms and negative provocation tests following an injection of local anaesthetic in the subacromial space. Both tests have been evalu-

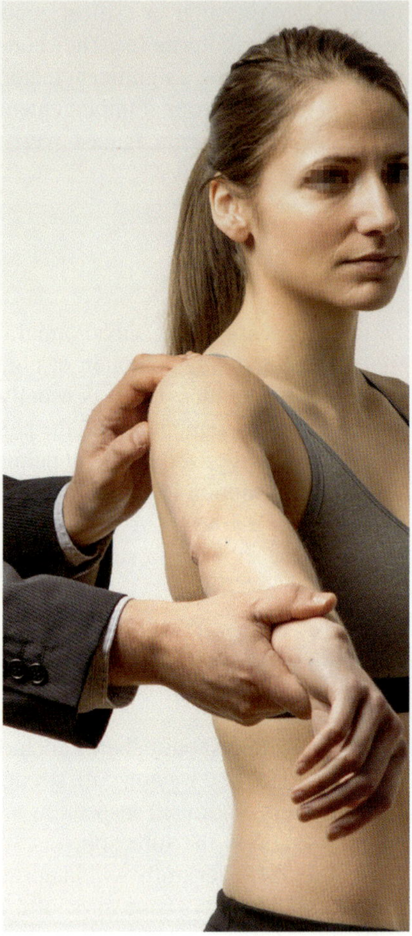

Fig. 5.2 Neer's sign. Image Published under License from www.shoulderdoc.co.uk and www.shoulderpedia.org

ated with MRI scanning—it was demonstrated that they could produce a significantly decreased distance from the supraspinatus insertion to the anterior acromion [7].

Another useful test to exclude the presence of a rotator cuff tear is Jobe's 'empty can' test, where supraspinatus strength is tested with the arm flexed and in maximum internal rotation (Fig. 5.4) [8].

Pillar 4: Imaging

Radiography: A standard series of radiographs should include AP, lateral (outlet) and axillary views to evaluate for any bony abnormalities of the coracoacromial arch. Acromial morphology can best be assessed on the lateral view. Typical

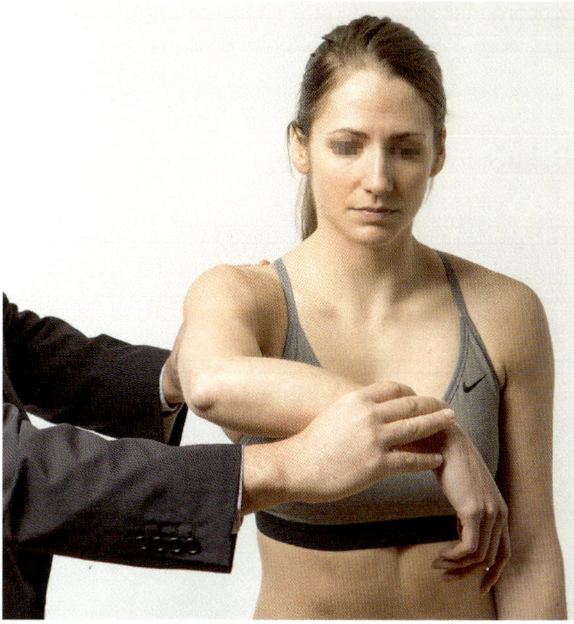

Fig. 5.3 Hawkins-Kennedy test. Image Published under License from www.shoulderdoc.co.uk and www.shoulderpedia.org

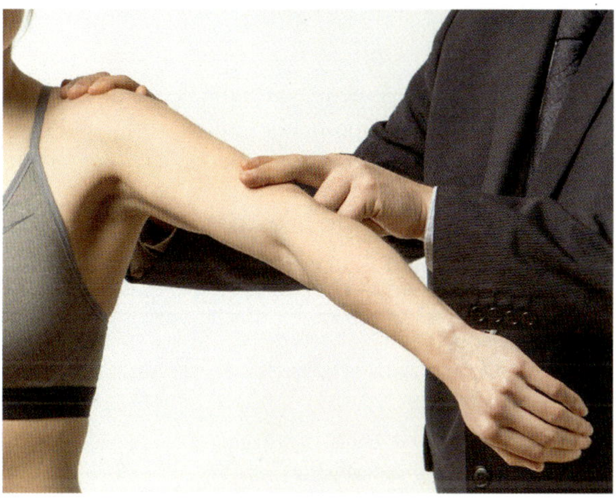

Fig. 5.4 Jobe's test. Image Published under License from www.shoulderdoc.co.uk and www.shoulderpedia.org

radiographic findings associated with impingement include AC joint arthritis with inferior osteophytes and sclerosis of the under surface of the acromion.

Ultrasound Scanning (USS): The main advantage of USS is that the rotator cuff can be assessed under dynamic conditions and that tears can be diagnosed with high accuracy.

Magnetic Resonance Imaging (MRI): Typical MRI findings in subacromial impingement include bursal thickening, fluid within the bursa and the presence of a subacromial spur. The size and location of rotator cuff tears can be assessed with high accuracy, and fatty atrophy of the rotator cuff muscles can be demonstrated.

Discussion of the Case

The patient described at the beginning of this chapter is very typical for someone with subacromial impingement syndrome. The gradual onset of symptoms without preceding trauma and the age of the patient make subacromial impingement a likely diagnosis. Examination shows no apparent wasting in the supra- and infraspinatus fossae and palpation demonstrates some tenderness anterior and lateral to the acromion. The patient has a painful arc of abduction from 60 to 120° and Neer's sign, as well as Hawkin's test, are positive. Radiographs show some degenerative changes of the AC joint, but no other bony abnormality. An ultrasound scan was performed and did not show any evidence of a cuff tear. The patient had a subacromial injection of local anaesthetic and steroid which significantly improved his symptoms. He was then referred to physiotherapy.

Summary

Subacromial impingement syndrome is one of the most common causes of shoulder pain. The aetiology is probably multifactorial and involves both intrinsic degeneration as well as extrinsic compression. Key diagnostic clusters are summarised in Table 5.2.

Making the diagnosis of impingement can usually be achieved by taking a detailed history and thorough physical examination. Conditions which may cause pain around the shoulder and which need to be differentiated from subacromial

Table 5.2 Summary of diagnostic clusters for subacromial impingement syndrome

Clinical history
1. Insidious onset of bursal distribution shoulder pain
2. Pain with overhead activities
3. Night pain
4. Late middle—to—early old age
Conventional examination
5. Painful 'impingement arc' in abduction—60°–120°
Special tests
6. Hawkins-Kennedy sign
7. Neer's Sign and test
8. Jobe's test
Investigations
9. X-Rays useful to rule out calcific tendonitis & assess ACJ
10. USS/MRI to exclude rotator cuff tear and confirm tendonosis/bursitis

impingement include glenohumeral instability, cervical radiculopathy, calcific tendinopathy, adhesive capsulitis, degenerative joint disease and isolated acromioclavicular joint arthritis.

Imaging is not essential to diagnose subacromial impingement syndrome but can be useful to exclude other pathologies and to rule out rotator cuff tears. The accurate diagnosis of subacromial impingement syndrome is important to initiate appropriate conservative measures. The majority of patients will make a full recovery with physiotherapy, simple analgesia and subacromial steroid injections. When conservative measures fail, arthroscopic subacromial decompression can lead to excellent results with high patient satisfaction.

References

1. de Witte PB, Nagels J, van Arkel ER, Visser CP, Nelissen RG, de Groot JH. Study protocol subacromial impingement syndrome: the identification of pathophysiologic mechanisms (SISTIM). BMC Musculoskelet Disord. 2011;12:282. doi:10.1186/1471-2474-12-282.
2. Neer CS 2nd. Anterior acromioplasty for the chronic impingement syndrome in the shoulder: a preliminary report. J Bone Joint Surg Am. 1972;54(1):41–50.
3. Bigliani LU, Morrison ES. The morphology of acromion and its relation to rotator cuff tears. Orthop Trans. 1968;10:216.
4. Harrison AK, Flatow EL. Subacromial impingement syndrome. J Am Acad Orthop Surg. 2011;19(11):701–8.
5. Lohr JF, Uhthoff HK. The microvascular pattern of the supraspinatus tendon. Clin Orthop Relat Res. 1990;9(5):35–8.
6. Park HB, Yokota A, Gill HS, El Rassi G, McFarland EG. Diagnostic accuracy of clinical tests for the different degrees of subacromial impingement syndrome. J Bone Joint Surg Am. 2005;87(7):1446–55.
7. Pappas GP, Blemker SS, Beaulieu CF, McAdams TR, Whalen ST, Gold GE. In vivo anatomy of the Neer and Hawkins sign positions for shoulder impingement. J Shoulder Elb Surg. 2006;15(1):40–9.
8. Jobe FW, Moynes DR. Delineation of diagnostic criteria and a rehabilitation program for rotator cuff injuries. Am J Sports Med. 1982;10(6):336–9.

Chapter 6
Biceps Tendinopathy

Suresh Srinivasan

Case Example

A 32-year-old self-employed plumber presents with anterior right shoulder pain for six months. He now presents with increasing pain in front of right shoulder radiating towards the elbow. He is unable to carry on working and points towards the bicipital groove as the area with worst pain. Examination reveals tenderness over the bicipital groove and a positive Speed's and Yergason's test.

Introduction

Long head of biceps (LHB) pathology is a well-recognised cause of shoulder pain and impairment. It can occur in isolation or more frequently with rotator cuff disease. LHB Tendinopathy encompasses a spectrum of pathophysiologies including intra-tendinous degeneration, synovitis of the sheath, partial tearing and complete rupture. Aetiology is multifactorial including rotator cuff disease with degeneration, degenerate osteophyte spurs and stenosis of the groove, traumatic injury, subscapularis or pulley complex lesions and SLAP tears (Chap. 7). While the natural history is not clear, patients with high-grade tendinopathy, with or without associated cuff tears, are at risk of tendon rupture.

S. Srinivasan
Leicester General Hospital, University Hospitals of Leicester NHS Trust, Leicester, UK
e-mail: susri75@yahoo.co.uk

© Springer International Publishing AG 2017

P. Monga, L. Funk (eds.), *Diagnostic Clusters in Shoulder Conditions*,
DOI 10.1007/978-3-319-57334-2_6

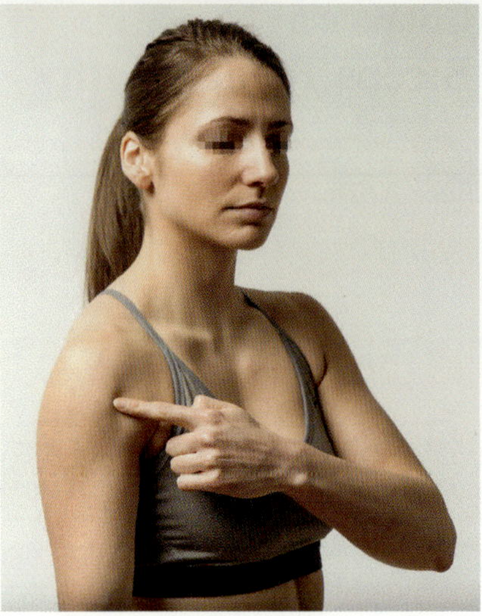

Fig. 6.1 Pain over bicipital groove. Image Published under License from www.shoulderdoc.co.uk and www.shoulderpedia.org

Pillar 1 History

The patient is typically either young person, under 35 years, in cases of isolated biceps tendinopathy or an older individual, aged 50 years and above, where biceps pathology is associated with rotator cuff disease. They usually present with anterior shoulder pain radiating to the front of the arm, occasionally radiating to the elbow. This pain is located over the bicipital groove (Fig. 6.1). Pain could be exacerbated by lifting activities involving elevation of the shoulder. A history of playing overhead sports must be sought. Symptoms could mimic impingement and be coexistent with cuff disease. Repetitive rotatory movements of the shoulder related to work and sports may be associated with biceps tendinopathy.

Patients might report a sudden resolution of chronic biceps related pain if there is spontaneous rupture of the tendon due to attrition.

Pillar 2 The Conventional Examination

There is typically tenderness to palpation over the bicipital groove. This is easier to elicit in the elderly compared to a muscular individual. Such tenderness is best felt inferior to the acromion, over the bicipital groove. There may also be a painful reproduction of clicking or snapping of the tendon if there are tears within the groove. The range of shoulder joint movements is typically maintained in isolated long head of biceps tendinopathy. A rupture of the long head of biceps may be associated with the development of a "Popeye" sign.

It is important to consider the differential diagnosis of anterior shoulder pain (Table 6.1).

Table 6.1 Differential diagnosis of anterior shoulder pain

Biceps tendinopathy
SLAP tear
Acromion clavicular (AC) joint pathology
Subscapularis pathology
Subcoracoid impingement
Early adhesive capsulitis

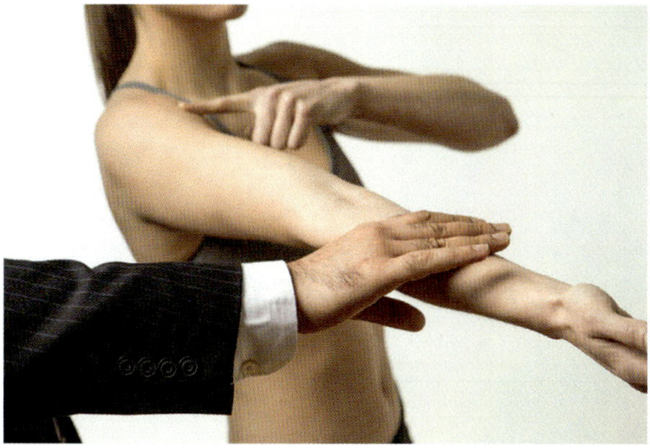

Fig. 6.2 Speed's test. Image Published under License from www.shoulderdoc.co.uk and www.shoulderpedia.org

Pillar 3 Special Tests

Speed test: The externally rotated (supinated) arm with an extended elbow is forward elevated. The examiner resists this forward elevation of the arm. The pain felt in the bicipital groove indicates biceps tendon pathology (Fig. 6.2).

Yergason test: A test for evaluation of biceps tendon pathology in which supination of the forearm is resisted. The elbow is flexed to 90° and the patient is asked to resist while externally rotating the arm. The test is considered positive if this resistance produces pain referred to the bicipital groove (Fig. 6.3).

Holtby and Razmjou [1] in their level I diagnostic study involving 50 subjects and arthroscopy as gold standard found sensitivity, specificity, positive and negative predictive values were 43, 79, 60, and 65% for Yergason's test and 32, 75, 50, and 58% for Speed's test, respectively. Kibler et al. [2] in their level II study of 101 patients used a binary logistic regression model to suggest a combination of newer with traditional tests (e.g., Speed's) were significantly better rather than tests in isolation. More recent evidence in the literature [3–5] recommends not using tests in isolation but in combination with history and examination. Suffice to say that the clinician must not rely on clinical examination tests alone due to variability in how they are performed and difference in patient populations and settings.

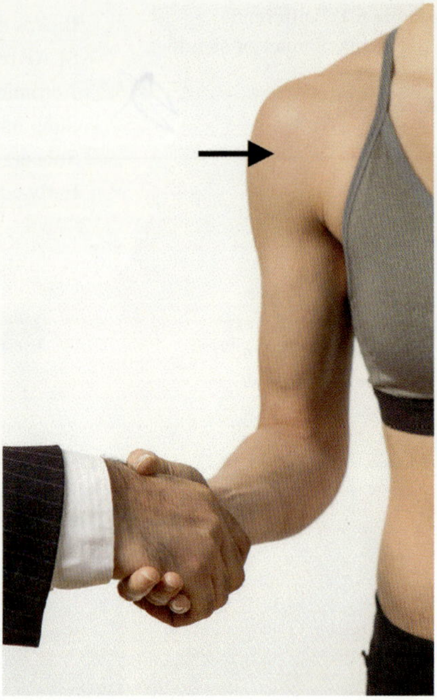

Fig. 6.3 Yergason's test. Image Published under License from www.shoulderdoc.co.uk and www.shoulderpedia.org

Pillar 4 Investigations

Plain radiographs are useful to rule out other causes of anterior shoulder pain such as AC Joint pathology. Ultrasound and MRI are often used to diagnose long head of Biceps tendinopathy. Management decisions are often based on the findings of radiological tests.

An ultrasound scan may reveal the presence of fluid around the biceps tendon (although this may be present in other conditions as well). Ultrasound may show spurs, bony irregularities or tendinopathy of the biceps. Ultrasound may also be used to give guided injection within the groove or tendon sheath for symptom relief and to aid diagnosis. The dynamic nature of this investigation, ability to inject simultaneously and easy availability makes it particularly appealing. One can also assess a subluxing or a dislocated LHB using an ultrasound scan.

MRI scan with or without arthrogram can identify intra-tendinous abnormality, bicipital sheath hypertrophy, coexisting superior labral, rotator cuff or subscapularis pathology, the intra-articular course of the tendon and its relationship to the structures of the annular pulley which stabilise it in the groove. However, the mere presence on MRI Scan of fluid in the biceps tendon sheath, which could be tracking from the gleno-humeral joint, must be interpreted with caution in the absence of other findings of inflammation around the tendon.

Literature regarding imaging diagnosis of LHB pathology [6–10] is very variable. It reveals sensitivity and specificity ranging from 49 &97% to 93&99% respectively for Ultrasound and 72 & 54% to 92 & 56% respectively for MR Imaging. Some of the reasons include small numbers of biceps pathologies, experience of person interpreting the result, various subgroups of biceps pathologies amongst others. None of the investigations on their own can provide a diagnosis. Hence the emphasis should be on importance of a cluster approach.

Discussion of the Case

The patient described earlier in the chapter has features typical of the long head of biceps tendinopathy. Anterior shoulder pain, anterior groove tenderness on palpation and a positive Speed's and Yergason's Test are classic features of this condition. An ultrasound scan confirmed fluid around the biceps tendon within the bicipital groove. The patient responded well to an ultrasound guided biceps tendon sheath injection.

Summary

Younger patients may develop long head of biceps tendinopathy related to overuse. In the older patients, it may be associated with rotator cuff disease. An overview of components forming a standard diagnostic cluster for biceps tendinopathy is listed in Table 6.2. Chronic biceps tendinopathy may lead to LHB rupture, resulting in a Popeye deformity. Such ruptures are frequently symptom-free, albeit leaving a cosmetic deformity. Other differential diagnoses of anterior shoulder pain such as AC joint pain, Subscapularis tears and subcoracoid impingement must be considered. Radiological confirmation of the diagnosis is helpful and is frequently combined

Table 6.2 Summary of diagnostic clusters for biceps tendinopathy

Clinical history: 1. Bimodal; 20–35 years sportspersons, 60+ years non-sports. 2. Pain over the anterior aspect of the shoulder—points to the LHB groove 3. Radiation to the biceps muscle belly 4. Worsening of pain on elevation of the shoulder 5. Commonly associated with Adhesive capsulitis and Rotator cuff disease
Conventional examination: 6. Tenderness over bicipital groove
Special tests: 7. Speed's test 8. Yergason test
Investigations: 9. Ultrasound scan to look for fluid around the biceps tendon sheath and symptom relief following Ultrasound guided injection into the biceps tendon sheath. 10. MRI findings of calibre changes and signal abnormalities

with guided injections into the tendon sheath. Failure of nonoperative management may be dealt with surgical biceps tenotomy or tenodesis of the tendon to the humerus.

References

1. Holtby R, Razmjou H. Accuracy of the Speed's and Yergason's tests in detecting biceps pathology and SLAP lesions: comparison with arthroscopic findings. Arthroscopy. 2004;20(3):231–6.
2. Kibler BW, Sciascia AD, Hester P, Dome D, Jacobs C. Clinical Utility of traditional and new tests in the diagnosis of biceps tendon injuries and superior labrum anterior and posterior lesions in the shoulder. Am J Sports Med. 2009;37(9):1840–7.
3. Hegedus EJ, Goode AP, Cook CE, Michener L, Myer CA, Myer DM, Wright AA. Which physical examination tests provide clinicians with the most value when examining the shoulder? Update of a systematic review with meta-analysis of individual tests. Br J Sports Med. 2012;46(14):964–78.
4. O'Kane JW, Toresdahl BG. The evidence-based shoulder evaluation. Curr Sports Med Rep. 2014;13(5):307–13.
5. Hanchard NC, Lenza M, Handoll HH, Takwoingi Y. Physical tests for shoulder impingements and local lesions of bursa, tendon or labrum that may accompany impingement. Cochrane Database Syst Rev. 2013;30(4):CD007427.
6. Teefey SA, Hasan SA, Middleton WD, Patel M, Wright RW, Yamaguchi K. Ultrasonography of the rotator cuff. A comparison of ultrasonographic and arthroscopic findings in one hundred consecutive cases. J Bone Joint Surg Am. 2000;82:498–504.
7. Armstrong A, Teefey SA, Wu T, et al. The efficacy of ultrasound in the diagnosis of long head of the biceps tendon pathology. J Shoulder Elb Surg. 2006;15:7–11.
8. Le Corroller T, Cohen M, Aswad R, Pauly V, Champsaur P. Sonography of the painful shoulder: role of the operator's experience. Skelet Radiol. 2008;37:979–86.
9. Mohtadi NG, Vellet AD, Clark ML, et al. A prospective, double- blind comparison of magnetic resonance imaging and arthroscopy in the evaluation of patients presenting with shoulder pain. J Shoulder Elb Surg. 2004;13:258–65.
10. Zanetti M, Weishaupt D, Gerber C, Hodler J. Tendinopathy and rupture of the tendon of the long head of the biceps brachii muscle: evaluation with MR arthrography. Am J Roentgenol. 1998;170(6):1557–61.

Chapter 7
SLAP Tears

P. Monga and L. Funk

Case Example

A 25-year-old volleyball player presents with a 3-month history of deep aching in the shoulder especially after training. There is also a reported loss of "power" during play, clicking and pseudo-locking. He reports that it started following a rather forceful spike. On examination, there is a loss of internal rotation, especially when tested in abducted position. The O'Brien's test, Labral shear test and the biceps load test are positive.

Introduction

The superior aspect of the labrum is loosely attached to the glenoid (in contrast to the inferior labrum, which is firmly attached) and provides attachment to the long head of the biceps. Also, the blood supply of the labrum is derived from the periphery towards the joint and hence predisposing the labrum to degenerative tears [1]. The injury was first described by Andrews et al. [2] and the term SLAP tear (Superior Labrum Anterior to Posterior) coined by Snyder et al. [3], following a review of 700 arthroscopies. SLAP tear represents pathological detachment of the superior labrum from the glenoid rim. Over the subsequent years, even though the diagnosis and surgical management of such tears have increased [4], it is well recognised that the clinical diagnosis of SLAP tears remains challenging.

P. Monga (✉)
Wrightington Hospital, Appley Bridge, Wigan, Lancashire WN6 9EP, UK
e-mail: trauma.orthopaedics@gmail.com

L. Funk
Wrightington Hospital, Wigan, UK

© Springer International Publishing AG 2017

P. Monga, L. Funk (eds.), *Diagnostic Clusters in Shoulder Conditions*,
DOI 10.1007/978-3-319-57334-2_7

Pillar 1: History

SLAP tears may be seen acutely after an injury or present with chronic pain in repetitive overhead activities.

An acute SLAP tear may occur following a deceleration injury, causing traction along the length of the biceps tendon, such as that seen during the follow-through phase of the throwing action [2]. Acute SLAP tears may also be caused by a superior compression mechanism, usually due to a fall on the outstretched arm, with the shoulder position in the abducted and slightly forward flexed position [3]. Sudden, traumatic inferior pull on the arm leading to inferior traction may also lead to a SLAP tear [3]. Finally, it is common to see acute SLAP tears associated with a shoulder dislocation or subluxation. Such injuries are commonly seen in patients participating in contact sports, such as rugby [5]. The SLAP tear in such a scenario commonly extends into either the anterior or posterior labrum.

Chronic SLAP tears from repetitive microtrauma may be seen in overhead sporting activities [6]. The mechanism of causation is centered around a repetitive overhead motion of hyperabduction and external rotation [7]. A throwing athlete may be predisposed to an injury to the labrum or the rotator cuff by alteration of the "kinetic chain," commonly associated with internal impingement.

Following an injury, patients with acute SLAP tears present with a deep ache commonly pointing anteriorly over the superior glenohumeral joint line. It is not uncommon for the pain to radiate along the biceps tendon anteriorly. It is also common for the patients to report a painful "click" during movements such as forward flexion and internal rotation.

In contrast, patients with chronic SLAP tears report a deep pain of an insidious onset. Such pain is felt in the posterosuperior aspect of the shoulder which is noted at the time of abduction and external rotation. In the Throwing athletes, pain is felt during the late cocking phase. They may report a "dead arm" with a loss of power in their throw [8], "loss of confidence" or a popping sensation. They frequently report that the shoulder "does not feel right". Patients may also present with rotator cuff insufficiency, especially in internal impingement, where rotator cuff tears are commonly associated with such SLAP tears.

Pillar 2 Physical Examination

There is usually no deformity, wasting or external sign of injury on clinical inspection in an isolated SLAP tear. Even though patients commonly complain of a "deep" pain, this does not usually correspond to any discreet areas of tenderness. The terminal range of abduction and forward flexion may be restricted due to pain. Such pain is often felt during abduction and external rotation. It is important to specifically look for glenohumeral internal rotation deficit (GIRD), which is commonly seen in Chronic SLAP tears from repetitive overhead sports. Such a restriction in internal rotation is best compared with the contralateral shoulder with the arm in 90° abduction. It is commonly noted in overhead athletes that the range of external rotation is increased and the internal rotation is correspondingly decreased, hence maintaining the overall "span" of rotation in this plane. Such adaptive changes are commonly seen in the dominant arm of throwing athletes [9].

Pillar 3 Special Tests

A wide variety of physical examination techniques has been described to clinically diagnose SLAP tears. None of these tests, however, are diagnostic of SLAP tears, either as stand-alone or in combination [10]. The authors prefer to use a combination of the O'Brien's test, O'Driscoll's SLAP test and the Biceps load test in diagnosing such tears.

O'Brien's Test is performed with the patient's arm forward flexed 90°, adducted to 10° and maximally internally rotated with the elbow extended. The patient resists a downward force applied by the examiner. The test is then repeated in the supination position. The test is considered positive for a SLAP tear if the patient feels a deep pain and click with the first manoeuvre, but not when testing in the supinated position. This test may also provoke pain over the AC joint if the latter is a source of pain [11] (Fig. 7.1).

The Dynamic Labral shear test is performed with the arm in maximal abduction and external rotation. The arm is then adducted while maintaining external rotation, and pain is considered as a positive response [12] (Fig. 7.2).

The biceps load test is especially useful when a SLAP tear is associated with an anterior labral tear. It is performed with the arm abducted and externally rotated to the point of apprehension. The elbow is flexed to 90° and supinated. Relief of apprehension during resisted elbow flexion is suggestive of an intact biceps anchor in the presence of a torn anterior labrum [13]. In the presence of an isolated SLAP tear, a similar manoeuvre produces pain on resisted elbow flexion [14] (Fig. 7.3).

Pillar 4: Investigations

As the clinical diagnosis of SLAP tears can be challenging, investigations are often used to conclude a diagnosis [15]. MRI Arthrography is the recommended investigation for a suspected SLAP tear. A radiographic dye is injected into the glenohumeral joint under ultrasound or X-ray control to distend the joint. The presence of the dye under the superior labrum is confirmatory of a SLAP tear. One needs to be aware of false negative MR Arthrography, which may be seen in subtle tears or due to under distension of the of the joint. Also, the superior labrum frequently has a physiological recess and is loosely attached, in contrast to the inferior labrum, and this may lead to false positive results. It is, therefore, crucial that the findings an MR arthrogram

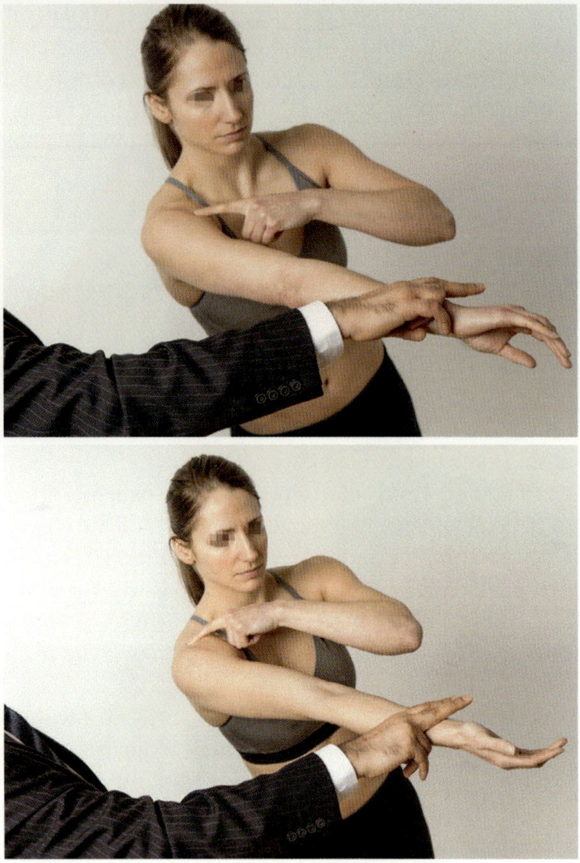

Fig. 7.1 O'Brien's test in pronation (**a**) and supination (**b**). Image Published under License from www.shoulderdoc.co.uk and www.shoulderpedia.org

are interpreted and actioned with caution. In isolation, MRI and MR Arthrography does not have a high accuracy, sensitivity or positive predictive value [16].

Arthroscopic assessment is confirmatory and is considered the "gold standard".

Case Discussion

The patient described earlier in the chapter is suspected to have a SLAP tear. He underwent an MR arthrogram, which confirmed the clinical suspicion with the injected dye undercutting the superior labrum and extending within the body of the biceps anchor. As in this case, it is frequently the situation that the clinical suspicion needs to be confirmed by appropriate investigations such as an MR Arthrogram. The patient underwent arthroscopic assessment and a SLAP repair after a trial of non-operative management.

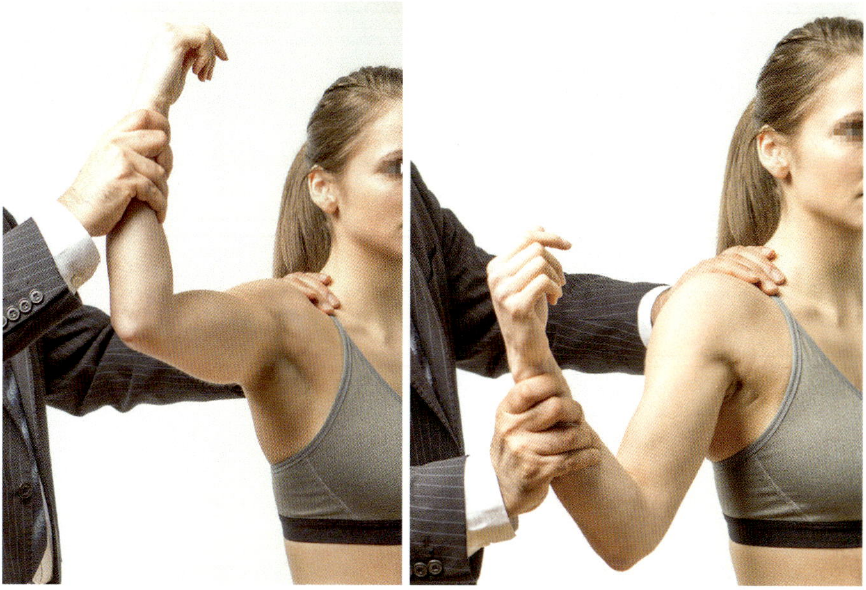

Fig. 7.2 Labral shear test starting position (**a**) and provocative action (**b**). Image Published under License from www.shoulderdoc.co.uk and www.shoulderpedia.org

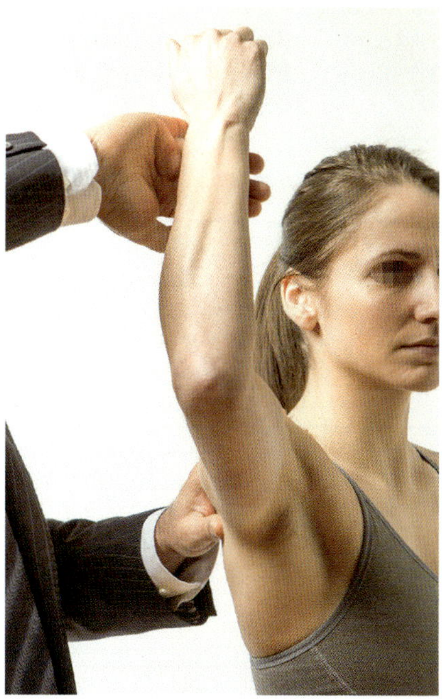

Fig. 7.3 Biceps load test. Image Published under License from www.shoulderdoc.co.uk and www.shoulderpedia.org

Table 7.1 Summary of diagnostic clusters for a SLAP tear

Clinical history
1. Sudden deceleration following throwing action.
2. Fall on the outstretched arm, with the shoulder position in abduction and slight forward flexion.
3. Repetitive overhead abduction and external rotation—Chronic SLAP tears
4. Deep anterior pain
Physical examination
5. GIRD—Glenohumeral Internal Rotation Deficit (Chronic tears)
Special tests
6. O'Brien's test
7. Dynamic labral shear test
8. Biceps load test
Investigations
9. MR Arthrogram—Seepage of dye under the superior labrum.
10. Arthroscopy is gold standard

Summary

The diagnosis of SLAP tear can be challenging when based purely on clinical examination. Even MR Arthrogram on its' own has a little accuracy and sensitivity. Hence neither clinical assessment nor radiological investigations are highly sensitive or entirely accurate, in isolation. A cluster approach to diagnosing a SLAP tear is recommended. A summary of cluster component is listed in Table 7.1. A combination of high index of suspicion, a cluster of positive special tests and suggestive MRA are sufficient to proceed to arthroscopy for confirmation of diagnosis and simultaneous repair. Concomitant Long Head of Biceps (LHB) pathology, patient profession, expectations, previous treatment and surgeon preference determines the appropriateness of either SLAP repair or biceps tenodesis for SLAP tears.

References

1. Cooper DE, Arnoczky SP, O'Brien SJ, Warren RF, DiCarlo E, Allen AA. Anatomy, histology, and vascularity of the glenoid labrum: an anatomical study. J Bone Joint Surg Am. 1992;74:46–52.
2. Andrews JR, Carson WG Jr, McLeod WD. Glenoid labrum tears related to the long head of the biceps. Am J Sports Med. 1985;13:337–41.
3. Snyder SJ, Karzel RP, Del Pizzo W, Ferkel RD, Friedman MJ. SLAP lesions of the shoulder. Arthroscopy. 1990;6:274–9.
4. Zhang AL, Kreulen C, Ngo SS, Hame SL, Wang JC, Gamradt SC. Demographic trends in arthroscopic SLAP repair in the United States. Am J Sports Med. 2012;40:1144–7.
5. Funk L, Snow M. SLAP tears of the glenoid labrum in contact athletes. Clin J Sports Med. 2007;17:1–4.
6. D'Alessandro DF, Fleischli JE, Connor PM. Superior Labral lesions: diagnosis and management. J Athl Train. 2000;35:286–92.

7. Burkhart SS, Morgan CD. The peel-back mechanism: its role in producing and extending posterior type II SLAP lesions and its effect on SLAP repair rehabilitation. Arthroscopy. 1998;14:637–40.
8. Kibler WB. The role of the scapula in athletic shoulder function. Am J Sports Med. 1998;26:325–37.
9. Bigliani LU, Codd TP, Connor PM, Levine WN, Littlefield MA, Hershon SJ. Shoulder motion and laxity in the professional baseball player. Am J Sports Med. 1997;25:609–13.
10. Knesek M, Skendzel JG, Dines JS, Altchek DW, Allen AA, Bedi A. Diagnosis and management of superior labral anterior posterior tears in throwing athletes. Am J Sports Med. 2013;41:444–60.
11. O'Brien SJ, Pagnani MJ, Fealy S, McGlynn SR, Wilson JB. The active compression test: a new and effective test for diagnosing labral tears and acromioclavicular joint abnormality. Am J Sports Med. 1998;26:610–3.
12. Hegedus EJ, Goode AP, Cook CE, Michener L, Myer CA, Myer DM, Wright AA. Which physical examination tests provide clinicians with the most value when examining the shoulder? Update of a systematic review with meta-analysis of individual tests. Br J Sports Med. 2012;46:964–78.
13. Kim SH, et al. Biceps load test: a clinical test for superior labrum anterior and posterior lesions in shoulders with recurrent anterior dislocations. Am J Sports Med. 1999;27(3):300.
14. Kim S-H, Ha K-I, Ahn J-H, Kim S-H, Choi H-J. Biceps load test II: a clinical test for SLAP lesions of the shoulder. Arthroscopy. 2001;17:160–4.
15. Michener LA, Doukas WC, Murphy KP, Walsworth MK. Diagnostic accuracy of history and physical examination of superior labrum anterior-posterior lesions. J Athl Train. 2011;46:343–8.
16. Sheridan K, Kreulen C, Kim S, Mak W, Lewis K, Marder R. Accuracy of magnetic resonance imaging to diagnose superior labrum anterior-posterior tears. Knee Surg Sports Traumatol Arthrosc. 2015;23:2645–50.

Chapter 8
AC Joint Pain

Pradyumna Raval and Arpit Jariwala

Case Example

A 52-year-old male manual worker presents with pain over the superior aspect of the shoulder. He points towards the AC joint as the worst site of pain. Such pain is exacerbated during terminal elevation, and also when performing the "bench-press" action. He has trouble lying on his affected side. Examination reveals point tenderness over the AC joint, pain during terminal elevation and a positive cross arm adduction test.

Introduction

The acromioclavicular (AC) joint is a diarthrodial joint which is formed by the articulation of the distal lateral clavicle and medial acromion. A fibrocartilaginous disc exists within the articulation which has a role similar to the meniscus in the knee. However, this fibrocartilaginous disc serves little purpose when one reaches the fourth decade and is more or less rudimentary at that age. Degenerative change in the fibrocartilage is a primary cause of age-related AC joint pain [1, 2].

Pillar 1: Clinical History

Patients with degenerative AC joint pain present with an insidious onset pain, over the superior and/or anterior aspect of the shoulder. Such pain commonly gets worse on cross body activities and weight lifting. Patient with AC joint pain may also

P. Raval • A. Jariwala (✉)
Ninewells Hospital and Medical School, Dundee, UK
e-mail: ajariwala01@gmail.com

© Springer International Publishing AG 2017

P. Monga, L. Funk (eds.), *Diagnostic Clusters in Shoulder Conditions*,
DOI 10.1007/978-3-319-57334-2_8

present with pain along the trapezius area. The most common presenting symptom is a pain on overhead activities. Pain at night while lying on the extremity is also common with underlying AC joint pathology. There may be features of pain exacerbated by 'grinding' [2, 3].

Patients may also present with AC joint pain following injuries such as fall on the outstretched hand, and seatbelt injuries which may indeed reflect a low-grade ligamentous disruption of the AC joint. The other causes of AC joint pain are septic arthritis, inflammatory arthropathy and distal clavicular osteolysis, which are relatively rare [4].

Pillar 2: Conventional examination

Inspection may reveal swelling over the AC joint with a prominent distal end of the clavicle. The joint is usually tender on palpation, mainly over the superior aspect. The terminal range of elevation may be restricted due to pain, with the patient pointing to the AC joint as the "worst" site of pain during extreme elevation [2, 3].

Pillar 3: Special Tests

Various clinical tests are described in the literature for the examination of AC joint; however, there is no single test with a high sensitivity and specificity. Cross-body adduction (Scarf) test is perhaps the most popular test and is considered positive if AC joint pain reproduced on 90° forward flexion and maximal shoulder adduction (77% sensitive) (Fig. 8.1). It is useful to perform this test in varying degrees of shoulder flexion [2].

The AC joint resisted extension test is performed with the patient actively extending against resistance when the shoulder is in 90° of forward flexion, resulting in pain at AC joint (Fig. 8.2). O'Brien active compression test is performed with the shoulder at 90° of forward flexion and 10° of adduction (Fig. 7.1). This test is considered positive for AC joint pain when a resisted shoulder flexion with the arm in maximal supination reproduces pain at the AC joint. In contrast, when the pain is elicited with the arm in maximal pronation in a patient with a SLAP tear [2, 5].

When performing the Paxinos test, the patient sits on a couch with the affected arm by his side. The examiner places his hand with his thumb on the posterolateral acromion and his index and long fingers on the superior and middle part of the clavicle. Pressure is then applied in an anterosuperior direction by the thumb on the acromion and in an inferior direction by the index and long fingers on the clavicle (Fig. 8.3). The test is considered positive when pain is reproduced at the AC joint [5].

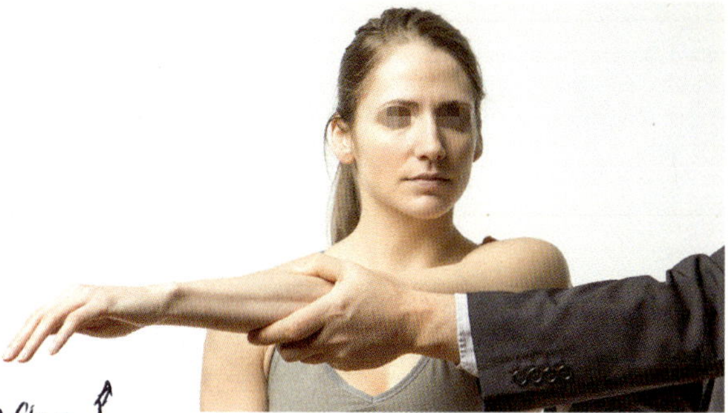

Fig. 8.1 Cross body adduction test. Image Published under License from www.shoulderdoc.co.uk and www.shoulderpedia.org

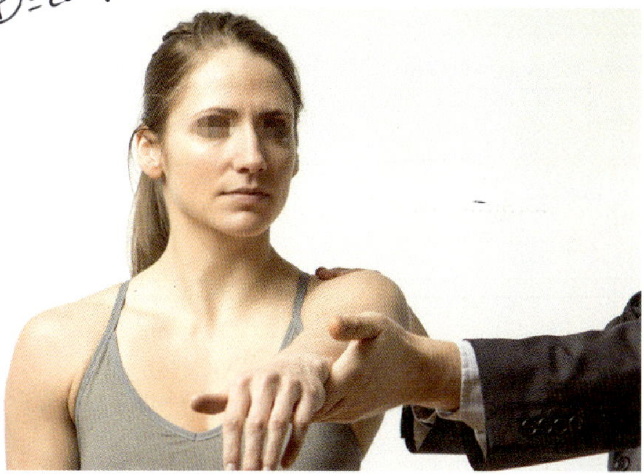

Fig. 8.2 AC resisted extension test. Image Published under License from www.shoulderdoc.co.uk and www.shoulderpedia.org

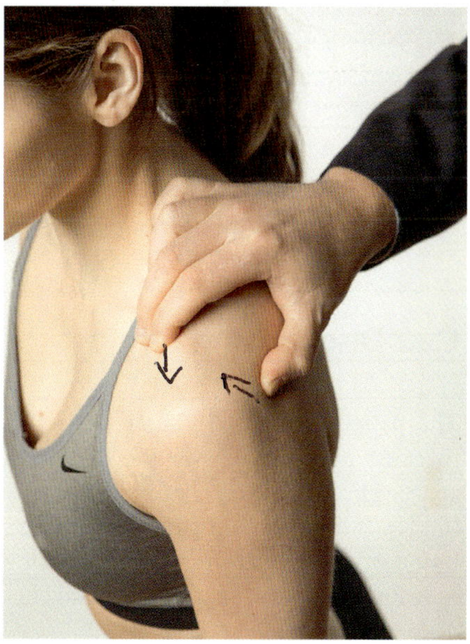

Fig. 8.3 Paxinos test. Image Published under License from www.shoulderdoc.co.uk and www.shoulderpedia.org

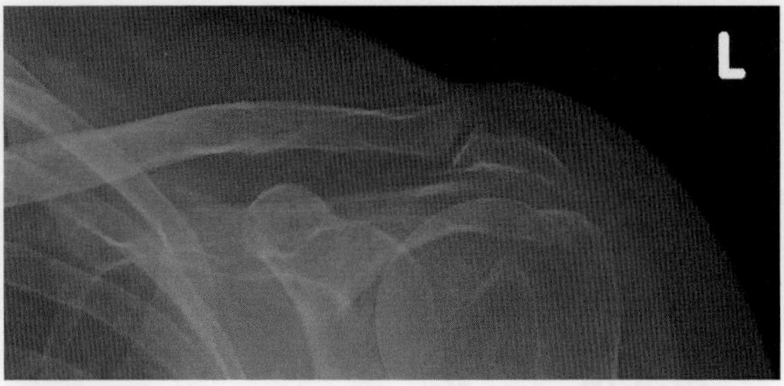

Fig. 8.4 Xray of AC joint arthritis Zanca view. Image Published under License from www.shoulderdoc.co.uk

Pillar 4: Investigations

An X-ray of the shoulder is the "initial" investigation for diagnosing AC joint pain (Fig. 8.4). The presence of arthritic changes in the AC joint on X-rays, however, is extremely common even in asymptomatic individuals. Such changes are seen on over 50% people beyond middle age, and one needs to exercise caution when attributing shoulder pain to the AC joint, purely on the basis of X-rays. A Zanca view performed with 10°–15° of cephalic tilt to the beam, and 50% exposure penetration on anteroposterior view of the shoulder provides superior visualisation of the AC joint [4].

MR Scans provide better visualisation of soft tissue lesions and joint. Bone oedema seen on fat suppression MRI scan can help to localise the zone of injury. Such changes, however, may again be seen in asymptomatic individuals and hence need to be correlated with the clinical findings [2, 4].

An Ultrasound scan provides limited visualisation of the AC joint. It is useful in guiding accurate needle placement for AC joint injections, which can be used for diagnostic purposes. The anterosuperior aspect of the AC joint is the widest area of joint penetration and ultrasound guided intra-articular injection is 96% accurate at the first attempt [6].

A CT scan provides superior osseous visualisation and is particularly helpful in evaluating residual bony spurs in patients with persistent pain following previous AC joint resection [2].

Case Discussion

The patient described earlier has a "typical" AC joint related pain. His X-rays revealed irregularity over the lateral end of the clavicle with narrowing of joint space. His MR scan confirmed increased signal (hyperintense) on Fat saturated images. An ultrasound guided injection into the AC joint led to near complete resolution of symptoms after local anaesthetic instillation. In cases of failure of non-operative management, he would be a candidate for arthroscopic AC joint decompression.

Table 8.1 Summary of diagnostic clusters for Acromio-clavicular joint pain

Clinical history	
1.	Traumatic—Repetitive microtrauma seen in weightlifters, basketball players & swimmers.
2.	Degenerative—Age-related degeneration, inflammatory arthritis.
3.	Presentation—Pain localised on the superior and anterior aspect of the shoulder joint.
Conventional examination	
4.	Tenderness elicited on palpation over AC joint
5.	Pain over AC joint on terminal elevation
Special tests	
6.	Cross-body adduction test
7.	AC resisted extension test.
8.	Paxinos test.
Radiological investigations	
9.	X-ray—AP and Zanca view
10.	MRI—Highly sensitive, however, changes do not always correlate with clinical findings

Summary

AC joint pain may be traumatic or degenerative in origin. As an isolated presentation, it may be seen in younger patients after trauma/micro trauma. More often, however, it is associated with rotator cuff disorders. A cluster approach to diagnosing AC joint is mandatory as radiological investigations frequently "over-diagnose" AC joint pathology in asymptomatic individuals. A summary of diagnostic clusters for the AC joint are presented in Table 8.1.

References

1. Keener JD. Acromioclavicular joint anatomy and biomechanics. Oper Tech Sports Med. 2014;22(3):210–3.
2. Mall NA, Foley E, Chalmers PN, Cole BJ, Romeo AA, Bach BR. Degenerative joint disease of the acromioclavicular joint a review. Am J Sports Med. 2013;41(11):2684–92.
3. Menge TJ, Boykin RE, Bushnell BD, Byram IR. Acromioclavicular osteoarthritis: a common cause of shoulder pain. South Med J. 2014;107(5):324–9.
4. Shaffer BS. Painful conditions of the acromioclavicular joint. J Am Acad Orthop Surg. 1999;7(3):176–88.
5. Walton J, Mahajan S, Paxinos A, Marshall J, Bryant C, Shnier R, Quinn R, Murrell GA. Diagnostic values of tests for acromioclavicular joint pain. J Bone Joint Surg Am. 2004;86(4):807–12.
6. Edelson G, Saffuri H, Obid E, Lipovsky E, Ben-David D. Successful injection of the acromioclavicular joint with use of ultrasound: anatomy, technique, and follow-up. J Shoulder Elb Surg. 2014;23(10):e243–50.

Chapter 9
Shoulder Arthritis

Jeremy Granville-Chapman

Case Example

A sixty-eight-year-old lady presents with pain in her right shoulder for the past 18 months. She describes an insidious onset pain, which has gradually been getting worse. She is unable to sleep at night due to pain, which is felt as a deep ache. She has noted a progressive loss of movement, which is affecting her activities of daily living. Examination reveals restriction of range of motion in all planes associated with pain and crepitus. External rotation is barely 10°. Rotator cuff strength is hard to assess due to pain related inhibition.

Introduction

The term arthritis describes a gradual, progressive biomechanical and chemical breakdown of the articular cartilage in a joint. Shoulder arthritis is the third most common large joint arthritis [1] and up to 17% of shoulders undergoing arthroscopy show signs of arthritis [2]. Sixty percent of all arthritis affects over 65 year-olds. In cases of young-onset arthritis, patients may give a history of injury, or they may have an inflammatory arthropathy (e.g. rheumatoid arthritis).

As arthritis progresses, the classic features of arthritis become evident on radiographs: loss of joint space, osteophytes, cysts and sclerosis. In the shoulder, progressive deformity of the humeral head and glenoid erosion also occurs.

J. Granville-Chapman
Frimley Health NHS Foundation Trust, Heatherwood and Wexham Park Hospitals, Slough SL2 4HL, UK
e-mail: Jeremy.Granville-Chapman@fhft.nhs.uk

© Springer International Publishing AG 2017
P. Monga, L. Funk (eds.), *Diagnostic Clusters in Shoulder Conditions*,
DOI 10.1007/978-3-319-57334-2_9

Accompanying these structural changes are symptoms of pain, grinding, loss of function and stiffness in the shoulder.

Pillar 1: Clinical History

Patients cannot generally remember when their symptoms began. Initially, pain is likely to be activity-related. Movements with the arm held away from the body increase joint forces and will be particularly painful. Initially, pain may be controlled by simple analgesics, such as Paracetamol or Naproxen. As the process progresses, patients begin to experience constant pain, including pain at night. The pain is typically felt deep within the joint or posteriorly, but it may also be felt over the upper outer arm. The pain and loss of function can be debilitating [3].

Patients may report a grinding sensation on movement of the shoulder and stiffness, which results in an inability to perform daily tasks such as donning clothes (bra strap, shirt sleeves) or reaching for items in a cupboard. If there is rotator cuff failure, there will be significant weakness as well as pain when using the arm held away from the body.

Pillar 2: The Conventional Examination

The conventional examination should reveal the signs of an arthritic shoulder. Special tests in shoulder arthritis focus on establishing the integrity of the rotator cuff, as this helps to determine what type of replacement is suitable.

Inspection may reveal a visible effusion, and this is seen commonly in cuff tear arthropathy. In cases of cuff arthropathy, one should look for muscle wasting in the supra and infraspinatus fossae due to chronic massive rotator cuff tear. One might also observe a high riding humeral head in cuff arthropathy, although this may be subtle.

Tenderness can be felt over the glenohumeral joint and crepitus or grinding is often felt over the joint when moving the shoulder, as the arthritic bearing surfaces rub over each other.

Movement assessment can reveal a globally restricted range of movement, particularly loss of external rotation. One might also observe abnormal scapulothoracic motion to compensate for a stiff glenohumeral joint. Such loss of scapulothoracic rhythm may also be seen due to loss of rotator cuff integrity ('pseudoparalysis' of massive cuff tear and cuff arthropathy). Here the patient relies on scapulothoracic motion to elevate the arm (Fig. 9.1). This makes it appear that they are shrugging the affected shoulder as they try to swing their arm up.

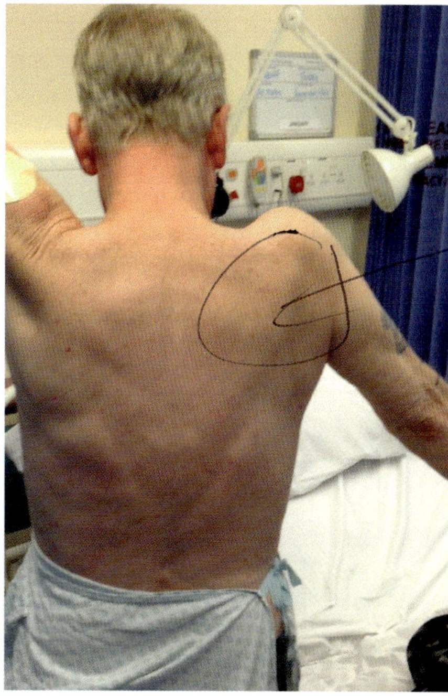

Fig. 9.1 Psudoparalysis. Image Published under License from www.shoulderdoc.co.uk

Pillar 3: Special Tests

For an arthritic shoulder, where replacement may be required, it is important to determine the function and integrity of the rotator cuff. Clinical assessment of the rotator cuff may be challenging due to the presence of pain, and hence, imaging is frequently needed to support clinical evaluation of the rotator cuff. Below a 'lag sign' (i.e. gross weakness) for each of the muscles of the cuff is presented. The respective chapters cover the specific tests for examining the rotator cuff in more detail.

- **Supraspinatus**—Codman arm drop test [4]

The arm is passively abducted to 90° with the palm facing the floor. The patient is asked to lower the arm slowly to their side. If the arm suddenly drops, this suggests a supraspinatus tear.

- **Infraspinatus**—External rotation lag test [5]

With the patient's elbow flexed to 90° and the shoulder elevated in the scapula plane by 20°, the arm is passively externally rotated to the limit of range and then taken back by 5°. The examiner supports the elbow. The patient is then asked to maintain that position of external rotation. If the arm collapses back towards internal rotation, this suggests a full-thickness tear of the infraspinatus (Fig. 17.2).

- **Teres Minor**—Patte's test [6]

With cuff arthropathy or massive cuff tears, the teres minor tendon can also fail. Teres minor is an external rotator, most important when the shoulder is abducted. Some surgeons advocate a tendon transfer as part of a reverse geometry shoulder replacement if the teres minor muscle has failed to improve rotational control. The patient's arm is abducted in the scapula plane to 90°. The elbow is flexed to 90°, and the arm externally rotated to limit of range. The patient is asked to hold the position against resistance as their elbow is supported in abduction. If the arm collapses into internal rotation, then there is a full thickness tear of teres minor (Fig. 17.3).

- **Subscapularis**—Bear hug test [7] lift-off test [8] and belly off tests [9]

The integrity of the repaired subscapularis tendon after anatomic total shoulder replacement is crucial for function and stability.

- Bear hug—The examiner places their hand on the patient's contralateral clavicle and asks the patient to clamp their hand over it. The patient is requested to maintain the pressure as examiner pulls their hand away from the patient's chest (Fig. 16.2).
- Belly Off test—the patient clamps their hands against their stomach at the level of the umbilicus. While pressing into their stomach, their elbows are passively pushed forwards (internally rotating their shoulder). They must maintain the contact with their stomach (Fig. 16.3).

The lift-off test (Fig. 16.1) is often too painful or impossible to complete in arthritis. A positive belly off test suggests at least 50% of the tendon is torn. The bear hug test will reveal tears as small as 30% of the tendon.

Pillar 4: Investigations

The initial investigation of a painful shoulder is shoulder radiographs. An oblique ('glenoid') AP view (Grashey view [10]), and an axillary lateral view. The Grashey view removes overlap of the glenoid and humeral head and affords a good indication of the features of arthritis, including osteophytes, loss of joint space, humeral head migration and cysts. The axillary lateral illustrates glenoid erosion, osteophytes and loss of joint space and demonstrates any joint incongruity; Plain radiography will also exclude rare but significant metastases or primary bone tumours. The acromiohumeral interval is preserved in glenohumeral arthritis (Fig. 4.2) in contrast to being lost in cuff tear arthropathy (Fig. 4.1).

If planning a total shoulder replacement, a CT scan of the affected shoulder is extremely useful. A fine cut CT provides excellent detail on bone stock, bony erosion patterns, subchondral cysts and osteophytes. CT is helpful when templating and planning arthroplasty, particularly on the glenoid side where orientation and positioning of the glenoid component are critical, and the bone stock can be compromised by disease. A CT Scan is also useful in assessment of wasting and atrophy of the rotator cuff muscles, best visualised in the sagittal reconstructions of the CT scan.

An ultrasound scan (US) is reliable in determining the integrity of the rotator cuff tendons. A meta-analysis demonstrated equivalent sensitivity and specificity between US and non-contrast Magnetic resonance imaging (MRI) in the determination of cuff tears [11]. In cases of clinical doubt about the rotator cuff, an ultrasound or MR scan can assist in the decision whether to perform anatomic or reverse-geometry arthroplasty. An MRI scan may be better to look at cuff integrity in arthritis as stiffness of the shoulder may prevent the arm from being positioned satisfactorily during an ultrasound scan. An MRI, however, is inferior to CT scan in assessing bone stock due to a higher slice thickness.

Discussion of the Case

The patient described earlier in the chapter underwent X-rays which revealed loss of joint space, subchondral sclerosis and cyst formation. The surgeon requested a CT scan to assess the glenoid bone stock, glenoid wear and also to assess rotator cuff wasting and fatty atrophy. In the absence of rotator cuff tears, an anatomical total shoulder replacement was offered.

Summary

Patients with shoulder arthritis typically present with progressively worsening pain associated with loss of range of motion in all planes. X-rays are useful for confirming the diagnosing and cross-sectional imaging, especially CT scans are useful in pre-operative planning. A summary of diagnostic clusters for shoulder arthritis is presented in Table 9.1.

Table 9.1 Summary of diagnostic clusters for Shoulder arthritis

Clinical history
1. Insidious onset of pain felt deep within shoulder joint
2. Pain and grinding which is worse on movement of the shoulder
3. Progressive stiffness and weakness of the shoulder
4. Pain at night and rest as condition deteriorates
5. Typically over 60 years of age (if younger, suspect a history of inflammatory arthritis or trauma)
Conventional examination
6. Global reduction in range of motion with crepitus
Special tests
7. Lag signs (e.g. Drop arm, External rotation lag, Hornblower) (cuff arthropathy)
Investigations
8. Xray—loss of joint space, cysts and osteophytes and sclerosis
9. CT scan aids surgical planning
10. Ultrasound or MR scan to assess rotator cuff integrity

References

1. Hutchinson M. The burden of musculoskeletal diseases in the United States: prevalence, societal and economic cost. J Am Coll Surg. 2009;208(1):e5–6. Available from: http://linkinghub.elsevier.com/retrieve/pii/S1072751508007357
2. Paley KJ, Jobe FW, Pink MM, Kvitne RS, ElAttrache NS. Arthroscopic findings in the overhand throwing athlete: evidence for posterior internal impingement of the rotator cuff. Arthroscopy. 2000;16(1):35–40.
3. Memel DS, Kirwan JR, Sharp DJ, Hehir M. General practitioners miss disability and anxiety as well as depression in their patients with osteoarthritis. Br J Gen Pract. 2000;50(457):645.
4. Codman E. The shoulder: ruptures of the supraspinatus tendon and other lesions in or about the subacromial bursa. Boston: Thomas Todd Co.; 1934. p. 216–24.
5. Hertel R, Ballmer FT, Lombert SM, Gerber C. Lag signs in the diagnosis of rotator cuff rupture. J Shoulder Elb Surg. 1996;5(4):307–13.
6. Walch G, Boulahia A, Calderone S, Robinson AHN. The Journal of Bone and Joint Surgery The 'dropping' and 'hornblower's' signs in evaluation of rotator-cuff tears. J Bone Joint Surg. 1998;80:624–8.
7. Barth JRH, Burkhart SS, De Beer JF. The Bear-Hug test: a new and sensitive test for diagnosing a subscapularis tear. J Arthrosc Relat Surg. 2006;22(10):1076–84.
8. Gerber C, Krushell RJ. Isolated rupture of the tendon of the subscapularis muscle. Clinical features in 16 cases. J Bone Joint Surg Br. 1991;73(3):389–94.
9. Scheibel M, Magosch P, Pritsch M, Lichtenberg S, Habermeyer P. The belly-off sign: a new clinical diagnostic sign for subscapularis lesions. J Arthrosc Relat Surg. 2005;21(10):1229–35.
10. Philip W, Ballinger EDF. Merrill's atlas of radiographic positions and radiologic procedures. Elsevier, Missouri, US; vol. 3; 1999; pp. 131–73.
11. De Jesus JO, Parker L, Frangos AJ, Nazarian LN. Accuracy of MRI, MR arthrography, and ultrasound in the diagnosis of rotator cuff tears: A meta-analysis. Am J Roentgenol. 2009;192(6):1701–7.

Chapter 10
Internal Impingement

Nicolas J. Dedy and Fraser J. Taylor

Case Example

A 25-year-old professional volleyball player presents with an insidious onset deep posterior shoulder pain and loss of power during play in his dominant arm. Examination reveals a protracted scapula, Glenohumeral Internal Rotation Deficit (GIRD) with an increase in external rotation of the shoulder in the abducted position and reduced internal rotation, a positive internal impingement test, and a positive relocation test.

Introduction

Internal impingement has been described as the contact between the articular side of the supraspinatus tendon and the posterior-superior glenoid rim with the shoulder in 90° of abduction and maximum external rotation (Fig. 10.1) [1]. Internal impingement was first described and demonstrated arthroscopically in the throwing and overhead athletes with posterior shoulder pain in the throwing position [1].

Evidence suggests, however, that contact between the rotator cuff insertion and the glenoid rim by itself may not be pathologic, but can occur in healthy, asymptomatic shoulders [2–5]. Symptomatic internal impingement leading to degenerative changes of the posterior labrum, posterior glenoid bone, and the articular side of the rotator cuff insertion is thought to be the result of repetitive and forceful contact

N.J. Dedy, Ph.D. (✉)
Krankenhaus Barmherzige Brüder Regensburg, Regensburg, Germany
e-mail: nicolas.dedy@gmx.de

F.J. Taylor
Gold Coast University Hospital, Gold Coast, Australia

© Springer International Publishing AG 2017

P. Monga, L. Funk (eds.), *Diagnostic Clusters in Shoulder Conditions*,
DOI 10.1007/978-3-319-57334-2_10

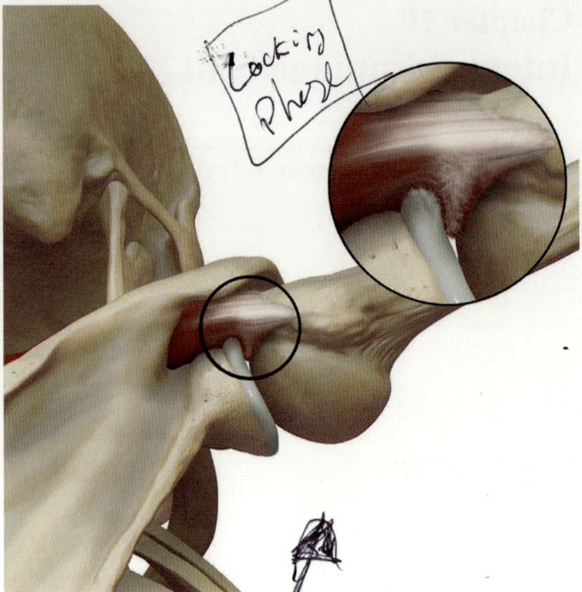

Fig. 10.1 Internal impingement—Pathomechanics. Image Published under License from www.shoulderdoc.co.uk

between these structures, as seen during the late cocking phase of throwing or in overhead athletes [5]. Internal impingement has been demonstrated in multiple arthroscopic studies visualising the contact between the posterosuperior glenoid and the rotator cuff insertion with the arm in 90° abduction and maximum external rotation [1, 3, 6–9]. Similarly, articular-sided partial rotator cuff tears and degenerative changes of the posterosuperior labrum and the superior glenoid cartilage have been consistently documented arthroscopically in patients with clinical signs of internal impingement [1, 6–10].

Different theories have been proposed as to the pathophysiology of internal impingement and the associated structural changes. Davidson et al. [11] and Jobe et al. [10] suspected anterior laxity of the throwing shoulder to play a role in what they termed superior glenoid impingement. Following these authors, recurrent stretching of anterior capsular structures, particularly the inferior glenohumeral ligament, in throwers leads to increased anterior translation of the humeral head during the throwing motion [10, 11]. This translation reduces the clearance between the supraspinatus insertion and the posterior superior glenoid rim and thereby allows for a pathologic contact between the involved structures [10, 11]. Mihata and co-workers [12] recently demonstrated increased glenohumeral contact pressures with the arm in the throwing position after stretching the anterior capsules of cadaveric shoulders, underpinning the theory of anterior laxity in the causation of pathologic internal impingement. Other authors, however, disagreed with the instability theory. Halbrecht and co-workers [4] did not find a relationship between clinical anterior instability and signs of internal impingement in MRI studies. McFarland and associates [3] failed to demonstrate a correlation between clinical instability and internal impingement in an arthroscopic study of 105 patients but did describe increased glenohumeral laxity in patients with an arthroscopic diagnosis of internal impingement when compared with patients without signs of impingement. Posterior capsular tightness has also been discussed as a cause of symptomatic internal impingement. Burkhart and associates [5] have introduced the concept of the glenohumeral internal rotation deficit (GIRD) describing an acquired hyper-external rotation and decreased internal rotation in the throwing arm when compared to the contralateral non-throwing arm. According to these authors, the GIRD is thought to be the result of a thickening and tightness of the posterior-inferior capsule in the throwing shoulder [5]. This posteroinferior capsular tightness causes a posterior-superior shift of the glenohumeral contact point during the cocking phase of throwing, resulting in increased shear forces on the posterosuperior labrum with concomitant labral tears [5]. Burkhart et al. [5] argued that it was the increase in external rotation seen in throwers that aggravated physiological internal impingement during the late cocking phase to become pathologic and to result in the previously described damage to the posterior-superior glenoid and the inside of the rotator cuff. The GIRD theory was recently supported by Mihata and colleagues [13] who artificially created excessive posterior capsular tightness in cadaveric shoulder specimens and demonstrated a posterior shift of the humeral head as well as significantly increased glenohumeral contact pressures in the throwing position with the arm in the maximum external rotation. The orientation of the scapula during the throwing motion has also been identified as a contributing factor in symptomatic internal impingement [14]. In a study of cadaveric shoulder specimens, Mihata et al. [14] recently demonstrated that an increase in the internal scapular rotation and a decrease in upward rotation significantly increased glenohumeral contact pressures between the greater tuberosity and the posterosuperior glenoid with the arm in throwing position. Although to date, no single theory has been definitively confirmed or refuted, the majority of authors appear to agree that internal impingement is most likely a physiologic phenomenon that occurs in a large percentage of asymptomatic shoulders [2, 5, 15]. Symptomatic internal impingement as seen in throwers is currently thought to be a multifactorial process involving hyper-external rotation and angulation, increased anterior translation, and posteroinferior capsular tightness with GIRD [15].

Pillar 1: Clinical History

A thorough clinical history is of paramount importance for the diagnosis of internal impingement, as symptoms may often be diffuse and nonspecific. Patients with symptomatic internal impingement are typically competitive throwing athletes complaining of poorly localised deep posterior or posterosuperior shoulder pain that is aggravated by maximum external rotation of the abducted arm, as seen in the late cocking and early acceleration phases of throwing [7, 15–20]. In the vast majority of cases, the dominant arm is affected [1, 6, 7, 9]. Patients are typically younger adults under the age of forty, with reported average ages between 23 and 27 years [6, 7, 9, 21]. The onset of symptoms is most commonly insidious, and athletes often also complain about a loss of throwing velocity and decreased overall performance [7, 15, 16, 18, 20, 22]. With regards to the type of sport, internal impingement has been most frequently described in baseball pitchers [7, 11, 15, 18], but other throwers such as javelin throwers, as well as overhead athletes including tennis, handball and volleyball players can also be affected [1, 9, 15]. While symptoms are most frequently experienced during the sporting activity, patients may also describe pain during activities of daily living with the arm in abduction and external rotation [9, 10]. Occupational factors should also be taken into consideration. Jobe [10] for instance described posterior superior impingement in a forklift driver, who spent most of his working day facing rear with his steering arm abducted and externally rotated.

Pillar 2: The Conventional Examination

Inspection of the undressed upper extremity does not typically reveal characteristic morphologic changes indicative of internal impingement. Asymmetry of the shoulder girdle with muscular hypertrophy of the dominant extremity is commonly seen in throwers. However, these changes are not characteristic of internal impingement [23]. The scapula may appear protracted (i.e., internally rotated) in throwing athletes, which has been associated with posterior capsular thickening [24]. Scapular internal rotation may indicate a predisposition for symptomatic internal impingement, as increased posterior-superior contact pressures have been demonstrated with increasing degrees of internal scapular rotation [14]. Palpation of the shoulder frequently produces pain over the posterior joint line, which may originate from the posterior capsule, posterior rotator cuff, or the glenoid-labral complex [5, 15–18]. Although active and passive shoulder range of motion may be normal in symptomatic internal impingement, throwers often exhibit a loss of internal rotation in abduction and a marked increase in external rotation in the throwing arm when compared with the contralateral shoulder [15, 17, 18]. It should be noted, however, that these findings are not diagnostic of pathologic internal impingement as they represent adaptive changes that are commonly found in asymptomatic throwing athletes [18, 25]. Wilk et al. [26] proposed a holistic concept of shoulder rotation by adding maximum internal and external rotation in 90° abduction to a total value termed *Total Shoulder Motion*. Total motion is thought to be equal bilaterally in asymptomatic throwers, with differences only in the degrees of internal and external rotation [18]. An increase in total motion in the dominant shoulder of a throwing or overhead athlete may indicate anterior laxity, which has been discussed as a cause of symptomatic internal impingement [18, 19].

Pillar 3: Special Tests

Few special tests are available to aid the clinician in the diagnosis of internal impingement. Jobe and co-workers described the relocation test for the diagnosis of superior glenoid impingement (i.e., internal impingement) [19]. The relocation test is performed with the patient in the supine position with the arm in 90° of abduction, slight extension and external rotation to create internal impingement (Fig. 10.2) [19].

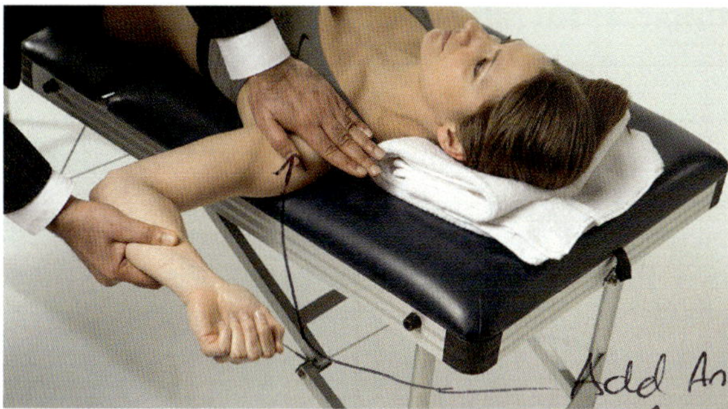

Fig. 10.2 Relocation test. Image Published under License from www.shoulderdoc.co.uk and www.shoulderpedia.org

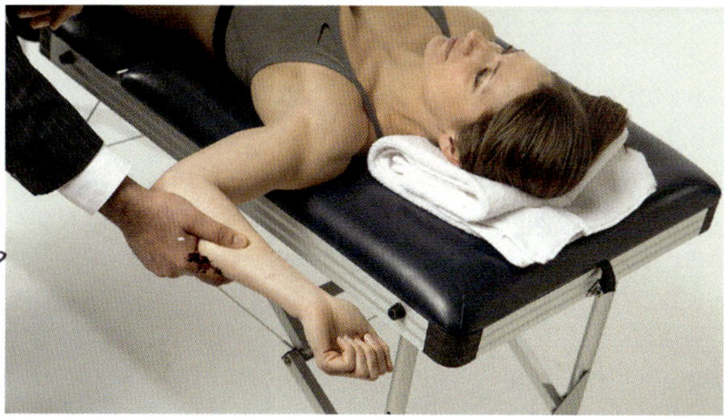

Fig. 10.3 Posterior impingement sign. Image Published under License from www.shoulderdoc.co.uk and www.shoulderpedia.org

Also, an anteriorly directed force may be applied by pulling the arm forward to increase anterior translation and internal impingement [19]. If posterior shoulder pain is elicited in this position, anterior to posterior pressure is applied to the shoulder [19]. The relocation test is positive if posteriorly directed pressure relieves the pain [19]. It should be noted that, in contrast to the relocation manoeuvre to assess for anterior instability, the marker of a positive test is pain and not apprehension. Paley and associates [7] found a strong association between a positive relocation test and arthroscopic signs of internal impingement. The authors performed the relocation test as described above on 41 male professional throwing athletes before arthroscopy and found posterior glenohumeral changes such as posterosuperior labral fraying and articular-sided rotator cuff fraying in all patients with a positive test [7].

Meister and colleagues [6] described the posterior impingement sign for the diagnosis of internal impingement (Fig. 10.3). This test is performed with the patient supine and the arm in the throwing position with 90–110° of abduction, 10–15° of extension, and maximum external rotation [6]. The test is positive if the patient's posterior shoulder pain is reproduced with the arm in the test position [6]. In a validation study, the authors correlated the test results of 69 young athletes with arthroscopic markers of internal impingement, demonstrating a sensitivity of 75.5%, and a specificity of 85% [6]. In the same study, the sensitivity was as high as 94.6%, and specificity was 100% when only data from patients with an insidious onset of pain and non-contact injuries were analysed [6]. Again it must be noted that in contrast to the apprehension test used to evaluate anterior instability the marker for the impingement sign is pain with the arm in the testing position, not apprehension.

Pillar 4: Investigations

Changes on conventional shoulder radiographs that have been described in patients with symptomatic internal impingement include cystic lesions on the humeral head, and posterior glenoid osteophytes [1, 7, 16]. Meister and associates [16] deemed the presence of a posterior glenoid osteophyte ("thrower's exostosis") demonstrated on the Stryker notch view of throwing athletes with symptomatic internal impingement predictive of undersurface tearing of the rotator cuff seen at arthroscopy. Computed tomography (CT) scanning has equally been reported to detect osteophytes on the posterior glenoid rim in patients with posterior shoulder pain and signs of internal impingement [1, 9].

Magnetic resonance imaging (MRI) represents the gold standard of imaging in the diagnosis of internal impingement as it allows for the simultaneous evaluation of rotator cuff and labral pathology, cartilage, as well as bony changes such as cysts [21]. Giaroli and co-workers [27] compared MRI scans of overhead athletes with clinical and arthroscopically confirmed internal impingement with scans of control patients. The authors found consistent changes in the MRI scans of the impingement patients and proposed the combination of articular-sided partial tears of the posterior rotator cuff, posterosuperior labral pathology, and cystic changes in the posterior aspect of the humeral head as confirmatory of internal impingement [27]. Similar results were reported by Kaplan et al. [8] who identified posterosuperior labral changes on MRI scans of nine throwing athletes with internal impingement that corresponded with findings at arthroscopy. Halbrecht and co-workers [4] on the other hand demonstrated MRI findings characteristic of internal impingement in the throwing shoulders of collegiate baseball players, but not in the non-throwing contralateral shoulders. Whereas an MRI is the most useful investigation to support the diagnosis of internal impingement, it has to be interpreted with caution. It should be noted that MRI findings of internal impingement were seen in both symptomatic and asymptomatic throwers, highlighting the importance of the clinical examination in the diagnostic process [4]. Conner et al. [28] conducted a longitudinal study of 20 asymptomatic throwing athletes with MRI changes characteristic of internal impingement. At the five-year follow-up, none of the athletes had developed symptoms of internal impingement, and none had required treatment [28]. Thus, the role of the cluster approach in the diagnosis of internal impingement cannot be over-emphasized.

Case Discussion

The athlete described in the chapter is an overhead athlete who repeatedly places their arm in maximal abduction and external rotation. Such position predisposes him to internal impingement. The examination findings of increased external rotation compared to the non-dominant arm may itself not be pathological, but represents a compensatory increase in response to his training needs. The sum of external and internal rotation is increased (*total shoulder motion*). The special tests such as relocation test and internal impingement test are useful adjuncts, along with an MR scan which confirms a partial articular surface tear of the rotator cuff along with a posterosuperior labral tear. The diagnosis of internal impingement was made, and a targeted physiotherapy programme was commenced. Failure of such a programme would be an indication to consider arthroscopic assessment and management.

Summary

Internal impingement of the shoulder is a phenomenon that is characterised by the contact between humeral head and posterosuperior glenoid with the arm in abduction and external rotation. Although internal impingement has been shown to occur in asymptomatic individuals, it is frequently associated with posterior shoulder pain with the arm in the critical position. Fraying and partial tears of the undersurface of the supra- and infraspinatus tendons, degenerative changes of the glenoid labrum, as well as SLAP lesions have consistently been documented in patients with symptomatic internal impingement. The diagnosis of internal impingement can be difficult and relies on the synopsis of multiple signs and symptoms in diagnostic clusters. A summary of diagnostic clusters for internal impingement is described in Table 10.1. A diagnosis of symptomatic internal impingement must be considered in young throwing or overhead athletes with an insidious onset of deep posterior shoulder pain in the dominant arm that is aggravated by the throwing motion, particularly the late cocking and early acceleration phases. A decrease in throwing performance and

Table 10.1 Summary of diagnostic clusters for internal impingement.

Clinical history
1. Insidious onset of diffuse posterior shoulder pain in overhead or throwing athletes
2. Pain aggravated by maximum external rotation of the abducted arm (e.g., late cocking phase of throwing)
3. Dominant (throwing) arm affected
4. Younger adults (under age 40)
5. Loss of throwing velocity or overall performance in throwing athletes
Conventional examination
6. Pain on palpation of posterior joint line
7. Loss of internal rotation and increased external rotation in abduction in throwing arm when compared with contralateral shoulder.
Special tests
8. Positive Relocation Test (test positive for internal impingement when posterior shoulder pain is elicited in test position)
9. Positive Posterior Impingement Sign
Investigations
10. Combination of articular-sided partial tears of the posterior rotator cuff, posterosuperior labral pathology on shoulder MRI

velocity is often noticed by athletes as well. Internal impingement should also be considered in non-athletes with occupational exposure to forced abduction and external rotation and poorly localised deep posterior shoulder pain. The clinical examination may reveal pain on palpation of the posterior joint line, corresponding with glenoid or posterior rotator cuff lesions. Radiological findings that support the diagnosis of pathological internal impingement in patients with a typical history and clinical presentation include tears and fraying of the undersurface of the rotator cuff and posterosuperior glenoid labrum seen on MRI, as well as cystic changes in the posterior humeral head and osteophytes on the posterior glenoid on conventional radiographs and CT. The apprehension sign is a highly sensitive and relatively specific test for internal impingement if the typical deep posterior shoulder pain is elicited in the testing position, particularly in patients with a history of gradual onset of the symptoms. The relocation test may further support the diagnosis of internal impingement if the testing position reproduces the patient's posterior shoulder pain, and the relocation manoeuvre results in pain relief. Before a diagnosis of internal impingement is made the clinician should make an effort to gather a comprehensive diagnostic overview of components and subcomponents of clinical history, examination, special tests, and imaging to recognise diagnostic clusters that are indicative of the condition.

References

1. Walch G, Boileau P, Noel E, Donell ST. Impingement of the deep surface of the supraspinatus tendon on the posterosuperior glenoid rim: an arthroscopic study. J Shoulder Elb Surg. 1992;1(5):238–45.
2. Gold GE, Pappas GP, Blemker SS, Whalen ST, Campbell G, McAdams TA, et al. Abduction and external rotation in shoulder impingement: an open MR study on healthy volunteers initial experience. Radiology. 2007;244(3):815–22.
3. McFarland EG, Hsu CY, Neira C, O'Neil O. Internal impingement of the shoulder: a clinical and arthroscopic analysis. J Shoulder Elb Surg. 1999;8(5):458–60.
4. Halbrecht JL, Tirman P, Atkin D. Internal impingement of the shoulder: comparison of findings between the throwing and nonthrowing shoulders of college baseball players. Arthroscopy. 1999;15(3):253–8.
5. Burkhart SS, Morgan CD, Kibler WB. The disabled throwing shoulder: spectrum of pathology Part I: Pathoanatomy and biomechanics. Arthroscopy. 2003;19(4):404–20.
6. Meister K, Buckley B, Batts J. The posterior impingement sign: diagnosis of rotator cuff and posterior labral tears secondary to internal impingement in overhand athletes. Am J Orthop (Belle Mead NJ). 2004;33(8):412–5.
7. Paley KJ, Jobe FW, Pink MM, Kvitne RS, ElAttrache NS. Arthroscopic findings in the overhand throwing athlete: evidence for posterior internal impingement of the rotator cuff. Arthroscopy. 2000;16(1):35–40.
8. Kaplan LD, McMahon PJ, Towers J, Irrgang JJ, Rodosky MW. Internal impingement: findings on magnetic resonance imaging and arthroscopic evaluation. Arthroscopy. 2004;20(7):701–4.
9. Levigne C, Garret J, Grosclaude S, Borel F, Walch G. Surgical technique arthroscopic posterior glenoidplasty for posterosuperior glenoid impingement in throwing athletes. Clin Orthop Relat Res. 2012;470(6):1571–8.

10. Jobe CM. Posterior superior glenoid impingement: expanded spectrum. Arthroscopy. 1995;11(5):530–6.
11. Davidson PA, Elattrache NS, Jobe CM, Jobe FW. Rotator cuff and posterior-superior glenoid labrum injury associated with increased glenohumeral motion: a new site of impingement. J Shoulder Elb Surg. 1995;4(5):384–90.
12. Mihata T, McGarry MH, Neo M, Ohue M, Lee TQ. Effect of anterior capsular laxity on horizontal abduction and forceful internal impingement in a cadaveric model of the throwing shoulder. Am J Sports Med. 2015;43(7):1758–63.
13. Mihata T, Gates J, McGarry MH, Neo M, Lee TQ. Effect of posterior shoulder tightness on internal impingement in a cadaveric model of throwing. Knee Surg Sports Traumatol Arthrosc. 2015;23(2):548–54.
14. Mihata T, Jun BJ, Bui CN, Hwang J, McGarry MH, Kinoshita M, et al. Effect of scapular orientation on shoulder internal impingement in a cadaveric model of the cocking phase of throwing. J Bone Joint Surg Am. 2012;94(17):1576–83.
15. Osbahr DC, Andrews JR. Arthroscopic treatment of internal impingement. In: Craig EV, editor. The shoulder. 3rd ed. Philadelphia: Wolter Kluwer Health/Lippincott Williams & Wilkins; 2013.
16. Meister K, Andrews JR, Batts J, Wilk K, Baumgarten T. Symptomatic thrower's exostosis. Arthroscopic evaluation and treatment. Am J Sports Med. 1999;27(2):133–6.
17. Winter SB, Hawkins RJ. Comprehensive history and physical examination of the throwing shoulder. Sports Med Arthrosc. 2014;22(2):94–100.
18. Reinold MM, Wilk KE, Dugas JR, Andrews JR. Internal Impingement. In: Wilk KE, Reinold MM, Andrews JR, editors. The Athlete's Shoulder. 2nd ed. Philadelphia: Churchill Livingstone/Elsevier; 2009. p. 123–41.
19. Jobe CM. Superior glenoid impingement. Current concepts. Clin Orthop Relat Res. 1996;330:98–107.
20. Laudner KG, Myers JB, Pasquale MR, Bradley JP, Lephart SM. Scapular dysfunction in throwers with pathologic internal impingement. J Orthop Sports Phys Ther. 2006;36(7):485–94.
21. Spiegl UJ, Warth RJ, Millett PJ. Symptomatic internal impingement of the shoulder in overhead athletes. Sports Med Arthrosc. 2014;22(2):120–9.
22. Malone TR. Standardised shoulder examination – clinical and functional approaches. In: Wilk KE, Reinold MM, Andrews JR, editors. The Athlete's shoulder. 2nd ed. Philadelphia: Churchill Livingstone/Elsevier; 2009. p. 45–53.
23. Drakos MC, Rudzki JR, Allen AA, Potter HG, Altchek DW. Internal impingement of the shoulder in the overhead athlete. J Bone Joint Surg Am. 2009;91(11):2719–28.
24. Thomas SJ, Swanik CB, Higginson JS, Kaminski TW, Swanik KA, Bartolozzi AR, et al. A bilateral comparison of posterior capsule thickness and its correlation with glenohumeral range of motion and scapular upward rotation in collegiate baseball players. J Shoulder Elb Surg. 2011;20(5):708–16.
25. Meister K. Injuries to the shoulder in the throwing athlete. Part one: biomechanics/pathophysiology/classification of injury. Am J Sports Med. 2000;28(2):265–75.
26. Wilk KE, Meister K, Andrews JR. Current concepts in the rehabilitation of the overhead throwing athlete. Am J Sports Med. 2002;30(1):136–51.
27. Giaroli EL, Major NM, Higgins LD. MRI of internal impingement of the shoulder. AJR Am J Roentgenol. 2005;185(4):925–9.
28. Connor PM, Banks DM, Tyson AB, Coumas JS, D'Alessandro DF. Magnetic resonance imaging of the asymptomatic shoulder of overhead athletes: a 5-year follow-up study. Am J Sports Med. 2003;31(5):724–7.

Chapter 11
Coracoid Impingement

Sedeek M. Mosaid and Charlie Talbot

Case Example

A 45-year-old taxi driver presents with a 6-month history of non-specific anterior shoulder pain. He does not describe any injury but finds that his symptoms are a lot worse after a busy day behind the wheel. Clinical examination reveals tenderness over the tip of the coracoid and a pain provocation over the coracoid area on adduction, forward flexion and internal rotation. Bear hug testing showed weakness of subscapularis along with associated pain.

Introduction

Coracoid impingement (CI) syndrome is an uncommon but recognised aetiology of anterior shoulder pain that can be overlooked. Subcoracoid pain can occur when the subscapularis tendon has impinged between the lesser tuberosity and coracoid process in certain shoulder movements, such as throwing. This can lead to degeneration and tendon tears of the subscapularis [1, 2].

The dynamic impingement of the coracoid with the lesser tuberosity and upper subscapularis was first recognised by Goldthwaith as early as 1909 [3] though in the modern era it was Gerber [4] who re-ignited the role of the coracoid in the chronic impingement syndrome. However, currently, a full and definite understanding of CI remains uncertain, perhaps due to its relative rarity.

Coracoid impingement has subsequently been associated with subcoracoid stenosis. This stenosis is characterised as a reduced interval between the under surface tip of

S.M. Mosaid • C. Talbot (✉)
Harrogate District NHS Foundation Trust, Harrogate, UK
e-mail: charlie.talbot@hdft.nhs.uk

© Springer International Publishing AG 2017

P. Monga, L. Funk (eds.), *Diagnostic Clusters in Shoulder Conditions*,
DOI 10.1007/978-3-319-57334-2_11

the coracoid and the humerus, otherwise known as the coracohumeral distance (CHD). This distance can be measured using magnetic resonance imaging (MRI), computerised tomography (CT) or even ultrasound scanning (USS) in experienced hands.

Idiopathic coracoid impingement results from a pre-existing reduced coracohumeral distance. It is assumed that the syndrome is more commonly encountered when there is a history of repetitive overuse, resulting in multiple episodes of microtrauma when the shoulder is in forward flexion, adduction and internal rotation.

Traumatic causes include malunion following fractures of the proximal humerus involving the lesser tuberosity, malunited glenoid or coracoid fractures, or displaced scapular neck fractures that lead to altered anatomical relationships. Iatrogenic impingement can arise from previous shoulder surgery. Certain procedures result in an abnormal orientation of the coracoid in relation to the humerus such as the Trillat procedure or posterior glenoid osteotomy [5, 6]. However, coracoid impingement has also been implicated in patients with on-going symptoms following failed rotator cuff repair or subacromial impingement surgery [7].

Secondary causes are due to space occupying lesions including subcoracoid bursal thickening, calcification within the subscapularis tendon, ganglion cysts or other soft tissue tumours. Other causes may be attributable to superior migration of the humeral head in the presence of a massive irreparable rotator cuff tear or possibly anterior translation of the humeral head in relation to the glenoid in subtle anterior instability of the joint [1].

The incidence of coracoid impingement is unknown, but the presence and significance of CI pain can be overlooked. An awareness of the condition, its clinical presentation, along with the physical examination and radiological findings are essential to ensure the diagnosis is not missed.

Pillar 1: Clinical History

Patients usually complain of a nonspecific dull pain in the anterior aspect of the shoulder region that can be referred to the upper arm and/or forearm [4, 6]. The differential diagnoses should be considered in an anatomical order and can be sequentially excluded. They include bicipital pain, ACJ pain, early capsulitis or frozen shoulder and labral or other joint pathology. CI can be present in some patients with subacromial impingement or rotator cuff pathology. The nature of pain may be useful in homing in on a diagnosis, and often coracoid impingement is a diagnosis of exclusion, given its rarity.

Patients complain about increases in pain with overhead activity particularly when a combined movement of forward flexion, internal rotation and adduction occurs [1]. There may be a history of chronic overhead arm use with gradual onset of symptoms, particularly in individuals who perform activities reproducing the combined shoulder movement described, such as driving, throwing or writing on a black/whiteboard.

A thorough history should include questioning about previous treatments or injuries, however many patients have vague or patchy recall of events that occurred many years, or even decades ago, unless specifically asked. Previous shoulder surgery may be evident when examining the patient, but injuries or fractures treated conservatively may have no outward signs obvious to the examiner. It is, therefore, important to specifically ask the patient about previous surgery or trauma to identify potential causes outlined previously.

Pillar 2: The Conventional Examination

Any history of anterior shoulder pain should ensure adequate palpation of structures that are known to cause anterior symptoms. Palpable tenderness of the soft tissues around the coracoid process and between the coracoid process and lesser tuberosity should lead the examiner to perform the coracoid impingement test. It should be noted, however, that the coracoid itself might be tender on palpation for unrelated reasons such as Pectoralis minor tightness. Such tenderness is not necessarily a reliable sign of coracoid impingement but should be taken in context with other signs [2, 6].

Pillar 3: Special Tests

The coracoid impingement test is performed with the patient's shoulder placed in forward elevation to around 90°, adduction and dynamic internal rotation to bring the tuberosity in contact with the coracoid (Fig. 11.1). The test is similar to the well-known Hawkins-Kennedy test, where impingement is elicited in the subacromial space with internal rotation of the abducted shoulder. However, bringing the arm into adduction, across the body, allows the lesser tuberosity to connect with the coracoid on internal rotation in symptomatic patients [8]. Pain is more consistently reproduced in the midrange of the forward elevation rather than in the full elevation [9]. The resulting position of the arm is also similar to that of the O'Brien's test for superior labral anteroposterior (SLAP) tears. However, the O'Brien's test requires active loading of the arm to reproduce pain [10]. The coracoid impingement test is, therefore, a passive test, while the active tests in the physical examination relate to the assessment of the integrity or involvement of the subscapularis.

It is thought that coracoid impingement may potentially lead to tears of the subscapularis. Even though subscapularis tears are not always present with coracoid impingement, but they may coexist. A clinical assessment of subscapularis function should be performed and is described in detail in the "subscapularis weakness" chapter. Other differential diagnoses of anterior shoulder pain should be carefully considered (Table 6.1).

Injections to the subcoracoid space have been advocated as both diagnostic and potentially therapeutic in the diagnosis and management of coracoid impingement. To avoid unintended injection into the subscapularis, or the biceps tendon or sheath, it is advisable to place the patient's arm at the side and in external rotation or to perform the injection under ultrasound guidance. Following the injection, the shoul-

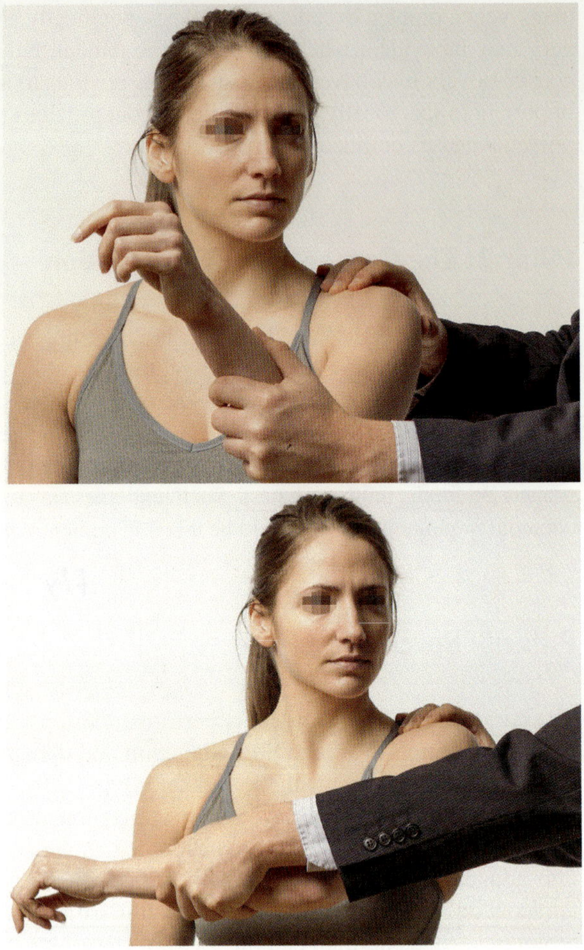

Fig. 11.1 Cocacoid impingement Test starting position (a) and provocative position (b). Image Published under License from www.shoulderdoc.co.uk and www.shoulderpedia.org

der can be re-examined to include the coracoid impingement test, as well as assessing the ACJ, biceps and rotator cuff, to determine the degree of symptoms relief [2, 10]. The proximity of multiple structures in the subcoracoid region, including the joint itself, makes the diagnostic accuracy of such injections doubtful and, as such, the validity or diagnostic accuracy of this test has not yet been determined [11].

Pillar 4: Investigations

Plain radiographs of the shoulder, particularly the anteroposterior and axillary views, can be used to detect bony elements that may contribute to the impingement. However, cross-sectional imaging such as magnetic resonance imaging (MRI) or computed tomography (CT) examinations is more precise.

CT can be used to assess the subcoracoid space and the coracohumeral distance. The coracohumeral distance is the minimum distance measured between the coracoid process and the lesser tuberosity. Gerber et al. [6] demonstrated an average distance with the shoulder in neutral of 8.7 mm and that this reduced to 6.8 mm with combined forward elevation. Perhaps unsurprisingly, they suggested a more likely risk of coracoid impingement with a coracoid that was close to the scapula neck and projecting far laterally.

The coracoid index, which is a measurement of the lateral projection of the coracoid process beyond a line tangential to the articular surface of the glenoid, is also determined by the axial CT view. Dines et al. [9] studied the coracoid index in 67 normal shoulders and found the average coracoid index to be 8.2 mm. A moderate correlation exists between the coracoid index and coracohumeral distance; whereby a higher coracoid index is most probably associated with a lower coracohumeral distance [12]. However, the coracoid index has not been validated, and values indicating coracoid impingement have yet to be determined.

In addition to measuring the coracohumeral distance, MRI offers greater sensitivity in identifying concomitant soft tissue lesions such as partial tears of the subscapularis, biceps tenosynovitis, and pulley lesions [2]. There may also be cystic changes seen in the lesser tuberosity and the coracoid tip. Bone oedema in the coracoid tip and reciprocally on the lesser tuberosity on fat suppression axial sequences may also be suggestive of coracoid impingement and is known as the 'kissing sign'. The CHD is best measured using an axial MRI scan with the humerus in the maximal internal rotation. In asymptomatic patients, the average coracohumeral distance has been measured at 11 mm, whereas symptomatic patients have a mean coracohumeral distance of 5.5 mm or less (Fig. 11.2) [13]. The sensitivity and specificity,

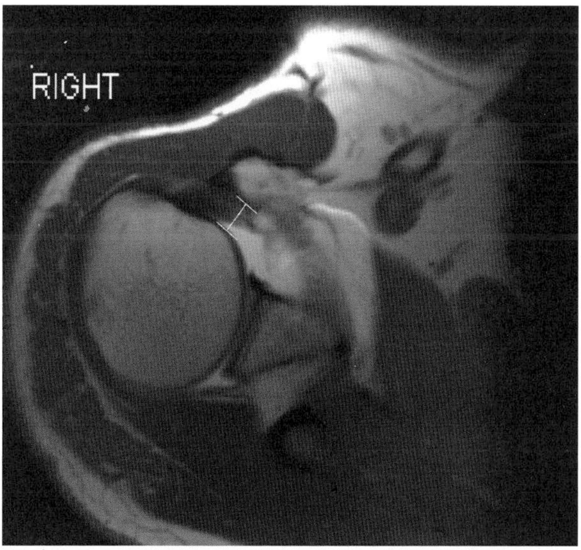

Fig. 11.2 Coraco humeral distance—MRI scan axial image. Image Published under License from www.shoulderdoc.co.uk

however, are 5.3% and 97.6% respectively. Therefore, imaging can support the diagnosis but fails to establish it [14].

Ultrasound scan (USS) has also been proposed for the evaluation of CI, providing the advantages of dynamic evaluation and ease of image guided injection [15]. USS imaging is clearly user dependent, but studies have shown its versatility and ability to assess the subscapularis tendon, transverse ligament, proximal biceps and the subcoracoid bursa as well as the coracohumeral distance [16].

Diagnostic arthroscopy allows dynamic assessment of possible coracoid impingement if non-surgical treatments have failed. By viewing from the posterior portal, impingement of the coracoid process against the subscapularis tendon and lesser tuberosity can be observed by manipulating the arm in a position simulating that used to elicit signs of coracoid impingement [17, 18]. Alternatively, a probe of known diameter can be used to calculate the CHD under direct vision.

Arthroscopy can clearly define the intra-articular pathology, particularly the articular surface of the subscapularis for partial tears while assessing the integrity of the remaining rotator cuff and the biceps. Dynamic arthroscopy can, therefore, be undertaken to establish the diagnosis and to proceed to definitive treatment of coracoplasty and subcoracoid decompression, as appropriate.

Case Discussion

The presentation of the patient described earlier in the chapter raises the suspicion of coracoid impingement. Clinical examination is directed, not only at confirming the suspicion of coracoid impingement but also ruling out differential diagnoses such as AC joint pain, biceps tendinopathy, and early adhesive capsulitis. MR Scan of this patient confirmed a reduced coraco-humeral distance to 4 mm. The patient underwent an ultrasound guided diagnostic subcoracoid injection. The injection gave excellent pain relief. In the case of recurrence of pain, this patient would be a candidate for arthroscopic assessment and coracoplasty.

Summary

The diagnosis of coracoid impingement can be challenging due to its relative rarity and the proximity of numerous other shoulder structures. The diagnosis is achieved by combining a thorough clinical history with the examination, special tests and appropriate imaging. The physical examination is just as important, as it excludes other causes of anterior shoulder pain, while it confirms coracoid tenderness and a positive coracoid impingement test. Additionally, relief of symptoms with a subcoracoid injection and imaging to show reduced CHD and possible concomitant lesions of the subscapularis really brings the puzzle pieces together. If there are doubts that justify the use of arthroscopy further direct visualisation can confirm the

Table 11.1 Summary of diagnostic clusters for Coracoid impingement

Clinical history
1. Anterior shoulder pain
2. Chronic overhead activity
3. Previous surgery/trauma
4. Setting; Idiopathic/Post-traumatic/Iatrogenic
Physical examination
5. Tender palpation of coracoid and anterior soft tissues
Special tests
6. Coracoid Impingement Test: Cross arm adduction, forward elevation, and internal rotation
7. Subscapularis tests (Belly press, Bear Hug, Lift off)
8. Sub-coracoid local anaesthetic injection
Investigations
9. Axial radiograph or CT—coraco-humeral distance (CHD)
10. MRI—CHD and soft tissue lesions—Subscapularis tears

diagnosis and lead directly to the treatment of the condition. A summary of diagnostic clusters helpful in achieving a diagnosis are listed in Table 11.1.

References

1. Garofalo R, Conti M, Massazza G, Cesari E, Vinci E, Castagna A. Subcoracoid impingement syndrome: A painful shoulder condition related to different pathological factors. Musculoskelet Surg. 2011;95(Suppl 1):S25–9.
2. Freehill MQ. Coracoid impingement: diagnosis and treatment. J Am Acad Orthop Surg. 2011;19(4):191–7.
3. Goldthwaite JE. An anatomic and mechanical study of the shoulder joint, explaining many cases of painful shoulder, many of the recurrent dislocations and many of the cases of brachial neuralgias or neuritis. Am J Orthop Surg. 1909;6:579–606.
4. Gerber C, Terrier F, Ganz R. The role of the coracoid process in the chronic impingement syndrome. J Bone Joint Surg Br. 1985;67(5):703–8.
5. Russo R, Togo F. The subcoracoid impingement syndrome: clinical, semeiologic and therapeutic considerations. Ital J Orthop Traumatol. 1991;17(3):351–8.
6. Gerber C, Terrier F, Zehnder R, Ganz R. The subcoracoid space. An anatomic study. Clin Orthop Relat Res. 1987;(215):132–8.
7. Suenaga N, Minami A, Kaneda K. Postoperative subcoracoid impingement syndrome in patients with rotator cuff tear. J Shoulder Elb Surg. 2000;9(4):275–8.
8. Osti L, Soldati F, Del Buono A, Massari L. Subcoracoid impingement and subscapularis tendon: is there any truth? Muscles Ligaments Tendons J. 2013;3(2):101–5.
9. Dines DM, Warren RF, Inglis AE, Pavlov H. The coracoid impingement syndrome. J Bone Joint Surg Br. 1990;72(2):314–6.
10. O'Brien SJ, Pagnani MJ, Fealy S, McGlynn SR, Wilson JB. The active compression test: a new and effective test for diagnosing labral tears and acromioclavicular joint abnormality. Am J Sports Med. 1998;26(5):610–3.
11. McFarland EG, Selhi HS, Keyurapan E. Clinical evaluation of impingement: what to do and what works. Instr Course Lect. 2006;55:3–16.

12. Brunkhorst JP, Giphart JE, RF LP, Millett PJ. Coracohumeral distances and correlation to arm rotation: an in vivo 3-dimensional biplane fluoroscopy study. Orthop J Sports Med. 2013;1(2):23.
13. Friedman RJ, Bonutti PM, Genez B. Cine magnetic resonance imaging of the subcoracoid region. Orthopedics. 1998;21(5):545–8.
14. Giaroli EL, Major NM, Lemley DE, Lee J. Coracohumeral interval imaging in subcoracoid impingement syndrome on MRI. AJR Am J Roentgenol. 2006;186(1):242–6.
15. Drakes S, Thomas S, Kim S, Guerrero L, Lee SW. Ultrasonography of Subcoracoid Bursal Impingement Syndrome. PM&R. 2015;7(3):329–33.
16. Tracy MR, Trella TA, Nazarian LN, Tuohy CJ, Williams GR. Sonography of the coracohumeral interval a potential technique for diagnosing coracoid impingement. J Ultrasound Med. 2010;29(3):337–41.
17. Okoro T, Reddy VR, Pimpelnarkar A. Coracoid impingement syndrome: a literature review. Curr Rev Musculoskelet Med. 2009;2(1):51–5.
18. Lo IK, Burkhart SS. Arthroscopic coracoplasty through the rotator interval. Arthroscopy. 2003;19(6):667–71.

Chapter 12
Adhesive Capsulitis

Marlis Sabo

Case Example

A 50-year-old woman presents to the clinic after a 6 month history of shoulder pain and loss of range of motion. She had a minor injury to her shoulder around the time this started, followed by insidiously increasing pain after that. She has pain at rest and with motion. She is unable to sleep due to the pain and is losing the ability to reach overhead or behind her back. She is in reasonable health but does have type 2 diabetes controlled on oral medications.

Introduction

Adhesive capsulitis is a diagnosis often shrouded with confusion. Many shoulder complaints can result in an active range of motion deficit with or without pain. Being able to differentiate between true adhesive capsulitis and other causes of painful loss of motion is critical to achieving effective treatment.

Adhesive capsulitis is a fibrosing condition of the capsular tissue of the shoulder that results in loss of intra-articular volume through thickening and adhesion of the capsule to the neck of the humerus [1]. It may occasionally be associated with certain conditions (Table 12.1). There is some evidence that early on, inflammation plays a role before fibrosis becomes dominant. The condition passes through four stages [2]. The first is pre-adhesive, with pain but no loss of motion. The second stage has acute adhesive synovitis, mostly in the axillary fold. Pain is prominent with mild loss of movement. The third stage (called the maturation stage) is characterised by more fibrosis than synovitis. There is much more stiffness than stage two.

M. Sabo
Clinical Assistant Professor, Section of Orthopaedic Surgery, Calgary, AB, Canada
e-mail: marlis.sabo@gmail.com

© Springer International Publishing AG 2017

P. Monga, L. Funk (eds.), *Diagnostic Clusters in Shoulder Conditions*,
DOI 10.1007/978-3-319-57334-2_12

Table 12.1 Conditions associated with adhesive capsulitis

• Antecedent Trauma: up to 22% have injury before symptoms
• Diabetes: up to 10 times the general population rate, more symptomatic, more often bilateral
• Dupuytren's: up to 50% crossover between conditions
• Thyroid disease
• Cerebrovascular disease

The final stage is marked by generally painless stiffness unless the patient attempts to push past the end-range of their motion.

Diagnosis of primary adhesive capsulitis is sometimes difficult. It is also a diagnosis that is applied inappropriately to nearly all people with painful and/or stiff shoulders. The term "frozen shoulder" should be avoided because it's imprecise and can lead to poor communication between primary care providers and specialists. Furthermore, misidentification of the aetiology of the pain and stiffness can direct an inappropriate treatment pathway. There are two components to successful diagnosis: determination of the features associated with adhesive capsulitis, and elimination of other potential causes of pain and/or stiffness of the shoulder.

Pillar 1: History

Especially early in the clinical presentation, the features of adhesive capsulitis are non-specific. Pain and loss of active motion are the most common clinical features. Adhesive capsulitis also appears in association with other medical and clinical conditions (Table 12.1) [3–6]. While these conditions are associated, they are not necessarily helpful diagnostically. Demographically, the condition typically manifests in middle age, and more commonly in females [1]. The onset of the pain is often insidious but may occur after a trauma [5]. The pain is experienced diffusely around the shoulder including a "deltoid," anterior and axillary pain distribution. Pain is present at rest and with motion depending on the stage of the condition [2].

Other important factors to consider relate to the history are a previous fracture (proximal humerus, glenoid rim, etc.) or dislocation, previous surgery (such as rotator cuff repair, stabilisation, fracture fixation, etc.). The differential diagnoses for pain and stiffness of the shoulder are listed in Table 12.2.

Pillar 2: Physical Examination

The hallmark examination feature of adhesive capsulitis is the global reduction in glenohumeral joint motion. A formal assessment of the range of motion in all planes should be made and recorded (Figs. 2.4–2.7) The active and passive range of motion is essentially the same and is reproducible. A patient may display substantial

Table 12.2 Differential diagnosis for pain and stiffness of the shoulder

	Normal AROM Normal PROM	Reduced AROM Normal PROM	Reduced AROM Reduced PROM
Subacromial bursitis	Y	Y	Y
Rotator cuff tear	Y	Y	Y
SLAP tear	Y	Y	Y
Calcific tendinitis	Y	Y	Y
Adhesive capsulitis	N	N	Y
Acromioclavicular arthrosis	Y	Y	Y
Early glenohumeral osteoarthritis	Y	Y	Y
Advanced glenohumeral osteoarthritis	N	N	Y
Rotator cuff arthropathy	N	Y	Y
Inflammatory arthropathy[a]	Y	Y	Y
Infection	N	N	Y
Neoplasm	Y	Y	Y
Post-traumatic contracture	N	N	Y
Missed glenohumeral dislocation	N	N	Y
Cervicogenic pain	Y	Y	N
Other pain syndromes[a]	Y	Y	N

[a]Most common scenario presented. Exceptions may be observed

forward elevation even without a contribution from the glenohumeral joint–the scapulothoracic joint contributes 1/3 of the arc of forward elevation and extension [7] of the lumbar spine can add to the apparent forward elevation of the shoulder. External and internal rotation at waist level is often dramatically reduced [2, 8]. Stabilising the scapulothoracic joint while applying passive motion to the arm will reveal that nearly all observed motion is arising from the scapula moving on the chest wall rather than movement arising from the glenohumeral joint (Fig. 2.7). A firm endpoint of the range of motion is also an associated finding [2]. Further features of the examination include that rotator cuff strength is typically conserved [2].

Pillar 3: Special Tests

There are no specific special tests for diagnosis of adhesive capsulitis in the clinic. Impingement testing is often not fruitful because the range of motion may be insufficient to achieve the required position for testing, or because the testing produces pain at end range of motion in any direction. **Special tests may be used to exclude other diagnoses**.

If one is uncertain about whether the apparent lack of motion is due to pain inhibition versus a fixed contracture, an examination under regional or general anaesthesia can provide substantial information. With pain taken out of the picture, any motion deficit is contracture-based. Examination of the range of motion still requires palpation of the scapula to determine the motion arising from the scapulothoracic articulation versus the glenohumeral joint.

Pillar 4: Imaging

The first role of imaging is to exclude other causes of a painful, stiff shoulder. Radiographs should be the first imaging undertaken. They will eliminate glenohumeral osteoarthritis, a common competing diagnosis, as well as other arthritic processes including rotator cuff arthropathy, calcific tendinopathy and (rarely) metastatic disease. Adhesive capsulitis by definition has normal radiographs, excluding asymptomatic ACJ pathology or some disuse osteopenia [1].

The next role of imaging is to provide supporting evidence in times of clinical equipoise. For the most part, excluding competing diagnoses is sufficient. One option is to determine if the intra-articular volume is reduced. This can be done with a plain arthrogram, or as part of advanced imaging. Adhesive capsulitis is associated with a reduction in the axillary pouch volume [8], and the amount of fluid that can be instilled into the glenohumeral joint is reduced compared to a normal shoulder with substantial pressure required at time of injection compared to a normal joint.

Finally, MRI scanning has been explored as a diagnostic tool for adhesive capsulitis. Obtaining advanced imaging is not necessary as a primary investigation, but may be available as part of the workup to exclude other diagnoses [2]. As always, findings on MR scanning need to be correlated with the clinical scenario for correct interpretation. Among the findings noted on MRI include obliteration of the axillary pouch, thickening (Fig. 12.1) [9] or scarring of the rotator interval, and changes to the coracohumeral ligament (less consistent). If gadolinium is used, hyperemia of the capsule can be noted as well [2].

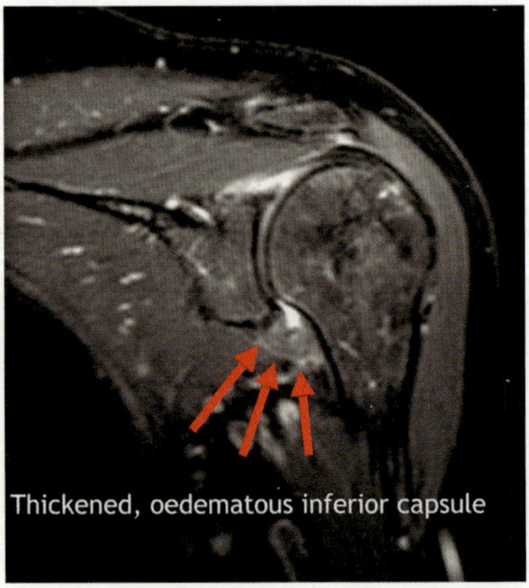

Fig. 12.1 MR of adhesive capsulitis—obliteration of axillary pouch. Image Published under License from www.shoulderdoc.co.uk

Discussion of the Case

Our patient is a classic example of a person presenting with adhesive capsulitis. Demographic associations include middle-aged, female, and suffering from type 2 diabetes. Other than that, her presentation is relatively non-specific, and the differential is broad (Table 1). On exam, she is capable of 90° of apparent forward elevation, external rotation to 0° at waist level, and internal rotation to her greater trochanter. Palpation of her scapula during examination demonstrates that all movement arises from the scapulothoracic articulation. Finally, she comes with an X-ray showing a normal glenohumeral joint and a mild amount of acromioclavicular arthrosis, and an ultrasound was demonstrating low-grade bursal-sided rotator cuff tearing and minimal bursitis. As shown in Table 12.2, the closest mimics of adhesive capsulitis can all be determined by history, physical, and basic diagnostic imaging (previous surgery or trauma, advanced arthropathy, missed dislocation). Based on these findings, a provisional diagnosis of adhesive capsulitis can be given, and appropriate treatment initiated.

Summary

The diagnosis of primary adhesive capsulitis can be challenging but is primarily a diagnosis arrived at through a careful history and physical examination. Exclusion of other diagnoses manifesting with pain and reduced range of motion is the primary goal. There are some key features positively associated with a diagnosis of primary adhesive capsulitis. Table 12.3 lists these. It should be emphasised that advanced imaging is not required to achieve a diagnosis of adhesive capsulitis, but may be obtained in an attempt to exclude other diagnostic entities. Advantages of

Table 12.3 Summary of diagnostic clusters for adhesive capsulitis

Clinical history
1. Insidious onset of pain and stiffness
2. Progressive decrease in range of motion
3. Sudden, unanticipated movements are exceptionally painful
4. Presence of associated medical conditions (Table 12.1)
5. Absence of other known shoulder pathology, injury, or recent surgery
6. Middle Aged Women
Conventional examination
7. Global reduction in active and passive range of motion (esp external rotation)
8. Observed motion is scapulothoracic
Special tests
9. Rotator cuff strength is maintained
Investigations
10. Normal glenohumeral joint on radiographs

the correct identification of primary adhesive capsulitis include appropriately targeted treatment and clearer communication between primary and specialist care providers.

References

1. Neviaser AS, Hannafin JA. Adhesive capsulitis: a review of current treatment. Am J Sports Med. 2010;38(11):2346–56.
2. Neviaser AS, Neviaser RJ. Adhesive capsulitis of the shoulder. J Am Acad Orthop Surg. 2011;19(9):536–42.
3. Waldburger M, Meier JL, Gobelet C. The frozen shoulder: diagnosis and treatment. Prospective study of 50 cases of adhesive capsulitis. Clin Rheumatol. 1992;11(3):364–8.
4. Arkkila PE, Kantola IM, Viikari JS, Ronnemaa T. Shoulder capsulitis in type I and II diabetic patients: association with diabetic complications and related diseases. Ann Rheum Dis. 1996;55(12):907–14.
5. Hand GC, Athanasou NA, Matthews T, Carr AJ. The pathology of frozen shoulder. J Bone Joint Surg. 2007;89(7):928–32.
6. Degreef I, Steeno P, De Smet L. A survey of clinical manifestations and risk factors in women with Dupuytren's disease. Acta Orthop Belg. 2008;74(4):456–60.
7. Itoi E, Morrey BF, An K. Biomechanics of the shoulder. In: Rockwood Jr CA, Matsen III FA, Wirth MA, Lippitt SB, editors. The shoulder, vol. 1. 4th ed. Philadelphia, PA: Saunders Elsevier; 2009. p. 213–65.
8. Robinson CM, Seah KT, Chee YH, Hindle P, Murray IR. Frozen shoulder. J Bone Joint Surg. 2012;94(1):1–9.
9. Kim KC, Rhee KJ, Shin HD. Adhesive capsulitis of the shoulder: dimensions of the rotator interval measured with magnetic resonance arthrography. J Shoulder Elb Surg. 2009;18(3):437–42.

Chapter 13
Cervical Spine Disorders Mimicking Shoulder Pathology

R. Verma

Case Examples

Case Study 1

44-year-old office worker complains of spontaneous onset pain in the left trapezius, medial border of the left scapula and left shoulder. This is accompanied by suboccipital headaches but no radiation of pain into the forearm or the hand. Pain is not affected by movements of the shoulder. There are no other medical co-morbidities.

Case Study 2

44-year-old office worker complains of spontaneous onset neck pain for 3–4 months followed by severe pain in the left upper arm and associated paraesthesia in the arm and forearm. Pain keeps the patient awake at night. Pain is not exacerbated by movements of the shoulder and is relieved by placing their hand on the head.

Introduction

Pain experienced in the shoulder, upper, and lower arm can be as a result of various medical conditions [1], including mechanical pain from nearby musculoskeletal structures such as the shoulder or the cervical spine [2]. Neck pain is the fourth

R. Verma
Salford Royal Hospital NHS Foundation Trust, Salford, UK
e-mail: backsurgeon@gmail.com

© Springer International Publishing AG 2017

P. Monga, L. Funk (eds.), *Diagnostic Clusters in Shoulder Conditions*,
DOI 10.1007/978-3-319-57334-2_13

leading cause of disability worldwide [3]. Cervical spondylosis is a general and nonspecific term that refers to the degenerative changes that develop with age or secondary to trauma or other pathological condition.

The initial change is the dysfunction of the disc secondary to decreased water content leading to altered biomechanics due loss of the shock absorber-like action of the discs. This leads to secondary changes in other component tissues like the facet joints and ligaments—thickening of the ligaments and formation of bridging bony deposits called marginal osteophytes called 'spurs'.

Kirkaldy-Willis [4] conceived of this process as passing through three phases; (a) Dysfunction, (b) Instability and (c) Stabilisation.

The instability phase may result in painful micro-motion or frank subluxation. Occasionally this chronic course can be complicated by acute disc herniation or a more gradual development of a posterior marginal osteophyte called a 'hard' disc-osteophyte complex. By the age of 60–65, 95% of asymptomatic men and 70% of asymptomatic women show degenerative change on plain films of the cervical spine [5].

Differentiating neck dominant pain from arm dominant pain means distinguishing referred pain from radicular pain. Radicular pain is usually secondary to direct involvement of a cervical nerve root by an acute disc prolapse. Referred pain originates from a structure within the cervical spine but hurts in a distant location.

Pillar 1: Clinical History

Spontaneous onset pain, commonly without any history of significant trauma. Neck pain is also more likely to develop in individuals with high job demands, low social support at work, job insecurity, low physical capacity and sedentary work positions with poor work posture accentuated by poor ergonomic work conditions [5].

Axial neck pain can be severe along the trapezius ridge and can be confused with shoulder pain. It can spread along the medial border of the scapula; this can be mistaken for thoracic spine pain. Referred cervical pain can be felt as a suboccipital or retro-orbital headache. When pain is referred to the left anterior chest wall—it is labelled as 'cervical angina' as it may lead to unnecessary anxiety and cardiac investigations.

There may be a vague aching referred to the proximal upper extremity but pain referred below the elbow suggests nerve root involvement. Depending on the nerve root involved there may be symptoms of paraesthesia affecting the fingers or the hand. Symptoms of radiculopathy may be exacerbated by coughing, sneezing or laughing as these actions increase the intraspinal pressure.

Pillar 2: The Conventional Examination

Examination of the cervical spine in patients with cervical spondylosis will reveal restricted movements of the cervical spine. Neurological examination is mandatory when a cervicogenic source of pain is being suspected. Patients who have radiculopathy usually will have unilateral symptoms and dermatomal pattern of sensory loss. It is

Table 13.1 Table showing clinically relevant cervical root distribution

Level	Muscle weakness	Sensory deficits/location of pain	Reflex
C5	Deltoid	Lateral arm	Biceps
C6	Biceps, wrist extension	Radial forearm, radial two digits	Brachioradialis
C7	Triceps, wrist flexion	Middle finger	Triceps
C8	Finger flexors	Ulnar two digits	
T1	Hand intrinsics	Ulnar forearm	

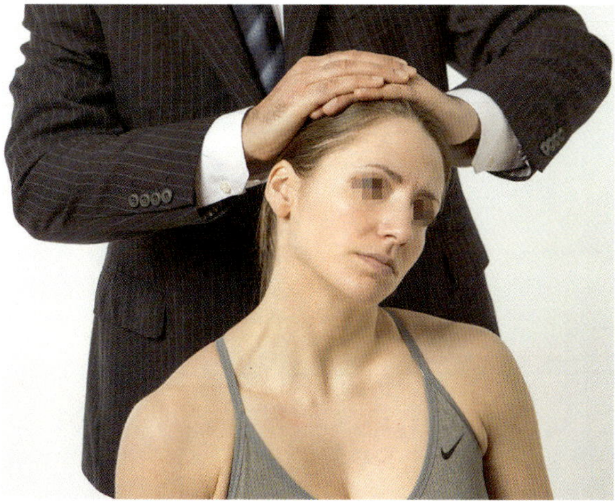

Fig. 13.1 Spurling test. Image Published under License from www.shoulderdoc.co.uk and www.shoulderpedia.org

important to look for wasting of muscles and motor weakness that generally follows myotomal patterns depending on the root affected (Table 13.1). Shoulder joint movements will not exacerbate pain, and the shoulder impingement tests are all negative.

Pillar 3: Special Tests

Spurling's test is used to assess cervical nerve roots for stenosis as they exit the foramen. The patient's neck is extended and rotated toward the side of the pathology. Once the patient is in this position, an axial load is applied (Fig. 13.1). If radicular symptoms are worsened by this manoeuvre, the test is said to be positive. It is thought that the extended and rotated position of the neck decreases the size of the foramen through which the nerve roots exit, thereby exacerbating symptoms when an axial load is applied.

Shoulder abduction test primarily tests relief of symptoms in patients with cervical radiculopathy as they place their hand on their head while holding their shoulder abducted (Fig. 13.2).

Hoffmann's sign is performed on the patient's pronated hand while the examiner grasps the patient's middle finger. The distal phalanx is forcefully and quickly extend (almost a flicking motion) while the examiner observes the other fingers and thumb. The test is termed positive if flexion is seen in the thumb and/or index finger.

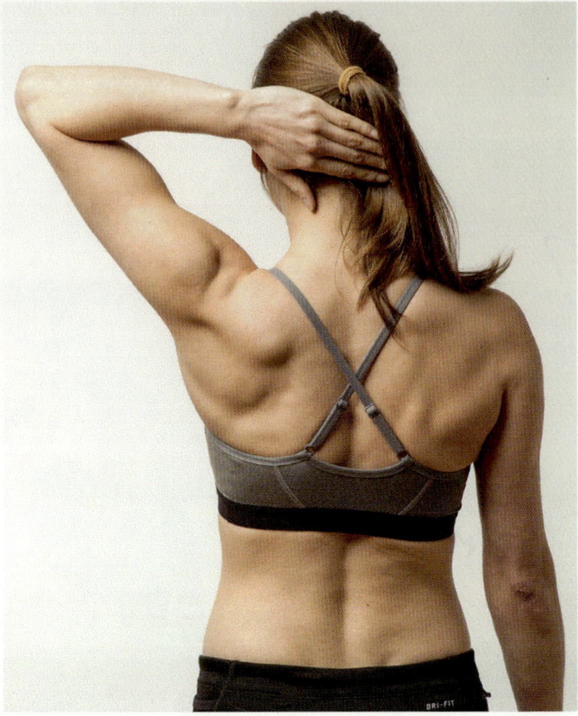

Fig. 13.2 Shoulder abduction test Image Published under License from www.shoulderdoc.co.uk and www.shoulderpedia.org

Hoffmann's sign implies and upper motor neurone lesion in the cervical spine region and it is an upper extremity reflex.

Inverted radial reflex is elicited by tapping the distal brachioradialis tendon. The reflex is present when the tapping produces spastic contraction of the finger flexors and suggests cord compression at the C5–C6 level.

Babinski's test is performed by stroking the lateral plantar surface of the foot from the heel to the ball of the foot and curving medially across the heads of the metatarsals. It is termed positive if there is dorsiflexion of the big toe and fanning of the other toes. This test is positive in cervical myelopathy.

Selective image guided root blocks may help to differentiate between shoulder pain and cervical radicular pain.

Pillar 4: Investigations

Plain X-rays will demonstrate overall alignment of the spine but are not very useful in patients with cervical radiculopathy. There is a high prevalence of degenerative changes in X-rays and MRI in asymptomatic individuals, and hence caution needs to be exhibited in attributing symptoms to these radiographic findings.

MRI scan of the cervical spine will demonstrate disc pathology including disc prolapse and nerve root compression secondary to disc-osteophyte complex. MRI scan is ideal to evaluate the condition of the spinal cord in patients with cervical myelopathy. MRI is the investigation of choice when a cervical source of pain is suspected in causation of shoulder pain and/or weakness.

In cases of diagnostic conflict or dual pathology, local anaesthetic injection into the subacromial space (Neer's Test) helps differentiate subacromial impingement pain from cervicogenic pain. Even a partial response to an accurately placed injection would determine if the source of pain is from the shoulder and if potential surgical treatment may be beneficial.

Discussion of the Cases

The first case described at the beginning of the chapter has features of referred pain from the cervical spine. Clinical examination is likely to reveal a reduced range of motion of the cervical spine and an MR scan was confirmatory of degenerative and disc related changes in the cervical spine. Physiotherapy, postural advice and workplace modification are likely to help in the management of symptoms for this office worker.

The second case presents with radicular symptoms from the cervical spine. The diagnosis is predominantly made from the clinical history and presentation. Clinical examination revealed markedly reduced range of motion of the cervical spine, paraspinal spasm and a positive Spurling's test. An MRI scan is the investigation of choice to confirm the clinical findings. An initial trial of non-operative management is successful in a majority of patients with surgical treatment reserved for those failing non-operative treatment, cervical myelopathy, acute disc prolapse with cord compromise or neurological compromise.

Summary

Shoulder joint pathology and cervical radiculopathy are frequently confused, perhaps because patients with shoulder problems often describe the pain in a way that can sound like radicular radiation. Differentiation is relatively easy with careful history and examination. A summary of diagnostic clusters is described in Table 13.2. Radicular pain generally radiates onto the scapular area and then down the arm, while shoulder pain is usually maximal anteriorly or laterally over the deltoid area of the shoulder. Movements of the arm at the shoulder exacerbate joint, but not radicular pain. Head turning or compression testing (pushing down firmly on the vertex of the head to see if the radicular pain is worsened) reproduces radicular pain. The most common differential diagnosis is subacromial impingement syndrome

Table 13.2 Summary of diagnostic clusters for cervical disc disease

Clinical history
1. Axial neck pain with referred pain along trapezius ridge and medial border of scapula
2. Pain in neck radiates down the arm below elbow
3. Altered sensation in digits with tingling
4. Pain improves by placing hand on head
Conventional examination
5. ROM of cervical spine limited
6. Dermatomal sensory loss
7. Motor weakness follows myotomal patterns depending on the root affected
Special tests
8. Spurling's Test-provokes pain
9. Shoulder abduction relieves pain
Investigations
10. MRI scan of cervical spine—disc prolapse, disc osteophyte complex, spinal cord signal, foraminal compression

and biceps tendinopathy with relevant clusters detailed in their respective chapters. Occasionally local anaesthetic and steroid injections in the shoulder are used to identify which area is most symptomatic in patients with a clinical picture that suggests both cervical osteoarthritis and shoulder pathology.

References

1. Pateder DB, Berg JH, Thal R. Neck and shoulder pain: differentiating cervical spine pathology from shoulder pathology. J Surg Orthop Adv. 2009;18:170–4.
2. Tyler TF, Nicholas SJ, Lee SJ, Mullaney M, McHugh MP. Correction of posterior shoulder tightness is associated with symptom resolution in patients with internal impingement. Am J Sports Med. 2010;38:114–9.
3. Vos T, Flaxman AD, Naghavi M, Lozano R, Michaud C, Ezzati M, et al. Years lived with disability (YLD's) for 1160 sequelae of 289 diseases and injuries 1990–2010: a systematic analysis for the Global Burden of Disease Study 2010. Lancet. 2012;380:2163–96.
4. Yong-Hing K, Kirkaldy-Willis WH. The three-joint complex. In: Weinstein JN, Wiesel SW, editors. The lumbar spine. Philadelphia: International Society for the Study of Lumbar Spine; 1990. p. 80–7.
5. Gore DR, Sepic SB, Gardner GM. Roentgenographic findings of the cervical spine in asymptomatic people. Spine. 1986;11:521–4.

Part III
Weakness Clusters

Chapter 14
Supraspinatus

A. Kapoor

Case Examples

Case 1: A 68-year-old man comes to clinic with pain and weakness in the left shoulder for 18-month presents. Such discomfort is especially worse following overhead work.

Case 2: A 55-year-old man complains of shoulder pain and weakness after a fall on his outstretched hand. He is unable to elevate his arm above the shoulder level. The pain is progressively getting worse, and the patient is unable to raise his arm on examination actively. The passive range of motion, however, is normal, albeit painful. A plain X-ray does not reveal any bony injuries.

Case 3: A 22-year-old baseball pitcher presents with a history of vague posterior shoulder pain and weakness in the throwing arm with no preceding history of trauma.

Introduction

The rotator cuff complex comprises of four tendons together with the underlined joint capsule. These are the supraspinatus, infraspinatus and teres minor, which originate from the posterior scapula and insert into the greater tuberosity of the proximal humerus, and the subscapularis that originates from the anterior scapula and inserts into the lesser tuberosity (Fig. 14.1). The RC moves and stabilises the humeral head in the centre of the glenoid by the principle of coupling forces. The subacromial bursa is related to the RC below and the acromion with the coracoacromial ligament (CAL) above. The normal separation between the glenohumeral and subacromial spaces is violated when there is a full-thickness tear of the RC. A

A. Kapoor
Royal Oldham Hospital, Manchester, UK
e-mail: amitorth@gmail.com

© Springer International Publishing AG 2017

P. Monga, L. Funk (eds.), *Diagnostic Clusters in Shoulder Conditions*,
DOI 10.1007/978-3-319-57334-2_14

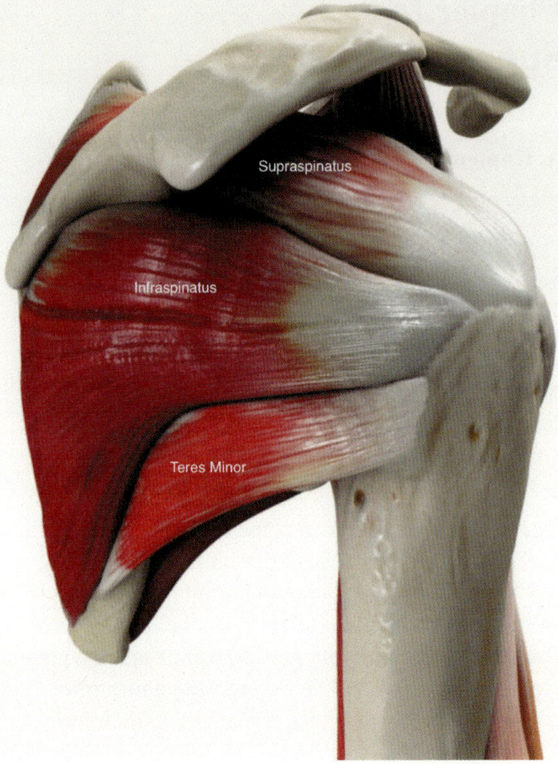

Fig. 14.1 Supraspinatus, infraspinatus and teres minor anatomy. Image Published under License from www.shoulderdoc.co.uk

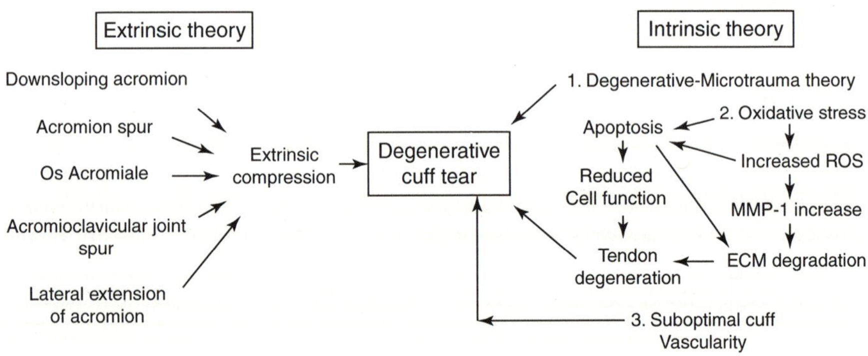

Fig. 14.2 Causation of rotator cuff tears as per Pandey and Willems [4]

majority of rotator cuff tears commence at the supraspinatus and hence, in other words, this is the most common rotator cuff tendon to tear [1].

By far the most common setting for supraspinatus weakness is rotator cuff disease or subacromial impingement syndrome. The rotator cuff is weakened by both extrinsic and intrinsic factors (Fig. 14.2), leading to a progressive failure of the tendon with or without superimposed acute injury, which eventually results in a full-thickness tear [2, 3]. Supraspinatus tears hence are either traumatic or degenerative or a combination [4].

Table 14.1 Differential diagnoses of supraspinatus wasting

	Setting	Features	Investigations
Cuff tear	Acute/chronic	Painful Arc/impingement features	Ultrasound/MRI
Brachial neuritis	Acute	Neuropathic pain at outset/ profound wasting	EMG
Suprascapular neuropathy	Chronic	SST/IFT wasting	EMG/NCV
Cervical radiculopathy	Acute/chronic	Neck pain/radicular pain	MR Spine, EMG

Table 14.2 Differential diagnosis of supraspinatus weakness

Diagnosis	History	Examination	Investigations
Partial- thickness acute tear	Fall or sudden attempt to lift the arm, followed by pain	Pain on resisted elevation of the arm	Thinning of tendon at insertion, with a defect in the deep aspect of the tendon on MR/Ultrasound
Full Thickness Acute tear	Sudden loss of strength after a fall or sudden attempt to lift the arm	Weakness of the arm during elevation and/or external rotation, pseudoparalysis, a palpable defect in the tendon insertion	A full-thickness defect in cuff tendon on MR/ Ultrasound.
Acute fracture of tuberosity	Sudden loss of shoulder strength after a definite injury	Weakness of the arm during elevation and possibly during external rotation	Tuberosity fracture seen on X-ray
Degenerative rotator cuff failure	Insidious onset of shoulder weakness without major injury	Weakness of the arm during elevation And/or external rotation, palpable a defect in tendon insertion	Full-thickness defect in cuff tendon or tendons; atrophy, fatty degeneration, or both of cuff musculature on MR/ ultrasound
Acute calcific tendinitis	Severe pain at rest, difficulty moving the arm, +/− history of minor injury	Local tenderness over supraspinatus tendon insertion, pain on the elevation of the arm	Calcific density in supraspinatus tendon near insertion on X-ray/ ultrasound
Spinoglenoid Notch cyst (ganglion)	Onset of weakness in suprascapular nerve distribution	Weakness of supraspinatus, infraspinatus, or both	Ganglion on MR, Suprascapular nerve denervation on EMG

Failure of the supraspinatus due to either tear or wear is the most common clinical problem of the shoulder, accounting for more than 4.5 million physician visits per year in the United States [5]. The prevalence of rotator cuff tears in the general population is 20% [6]. Other causes for supraspinatus weakness may be in association with suprascapular nerve palsy and brachial plexus palsy, which are discussed in details in their respective chapters. A comparison of various differential diagnosis for supraspinatus wasting are presented in Table 14.1 and for supraspinatus weakness are provided in Table 14.2.

Pillar 1: Clinical History

The clinical manifestations of supraspinatus weakness vary widely among patients (Tables 14.1 and 14.2). Patients with acute, traumatic, full-thickness cuff tears may experience the sudden onset of weakness with elevation of the arm after an injury in which the arm has been forced to the side (e.g., during a fall while skiing with the arm out to the side or on catching a heavy falling object with the extended arm) [7]. Bruising around the arm and the shoulder after an injury in the setting of a normal X-ray in mid to late adulthood is to be considered as a rotator cuff tear unless proven otherwise.

Patients with chronic degenerative defects may notice a gradual onset of shoulder weakness, often accompanied by pain and crepitus on active movement; Pain is aggravated by shoulder elevation, internal rotation and at night.

Massive rotator cuff tears may lead to shoulder instability. As the patient attempts to raise the arm, the humeral head subluxes anteriorly. The deltoid muscle is unable to abduct the arm in this situation. Such a clinical presentation is called pseudoparalysis.

In cases of cervical nerve root compression, the patient presents with pain in the neck radiating to the shoulder region with paraesthesias in the distribution of nerve root affected. Patients with suprascapular nerve entrapment are typically young overhead athletes who present with dull aching pain in the posterior aspect of the shoulder but may present with painless atrophy and weakness of the supraspinatus or infraspinatus depending on the level of compression.

Pillar 2: Conventional Examination

The examination of the shoulder may reveal atrophy of the supraspinatus and wasting; hence a hollowed supraspinatus fossa. Palpation at the anterior greater tuberosity may reveal a defect in the cuff–tendon attachment. Palpation below the acromion as the arm is rotated may reveal crepitus from the edges of the supraspinatus. The patient with an uncompensated tear would be unable to elevate their arm actively above the shoulder level, although passive elevation would be possible. This manoeuvre primarily differentiates weakness of the rotator cuff versus stiffness of the joint. Both active and passive movements of the joint are restricted in a stiff shoulder. In chronic cases of supraspinatus tears, one might observe secondary capsular contraction, which in turn leads to restriction of the movements.

Acute supraspinatus tears following trauma may be associated with bruising and such a sign is precious in raising the suspicion of a tear.

Examination of the cervical spine and brachial plexus should be part of assessing a patient with a weak rotator cuff if suspected from the history. Further details and diagnostic clusters for cervical disc disease and suprascapular neuropathy are described in Chaps. 13 and 24 respectively.

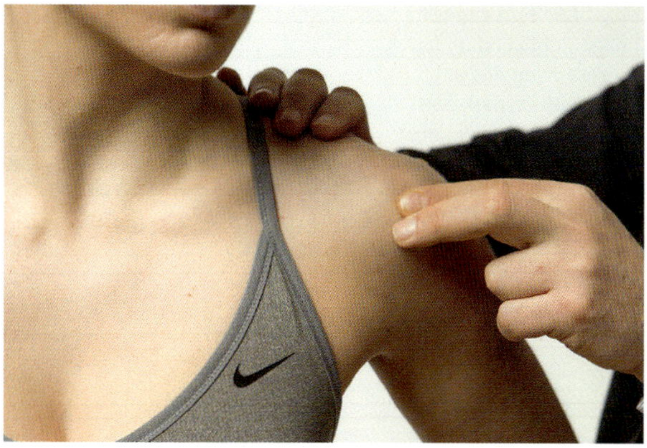

Fig. 14.3 Rent test. Image Published under License from www.shoulderdoc.co.uk and www.shoulderpedia.org

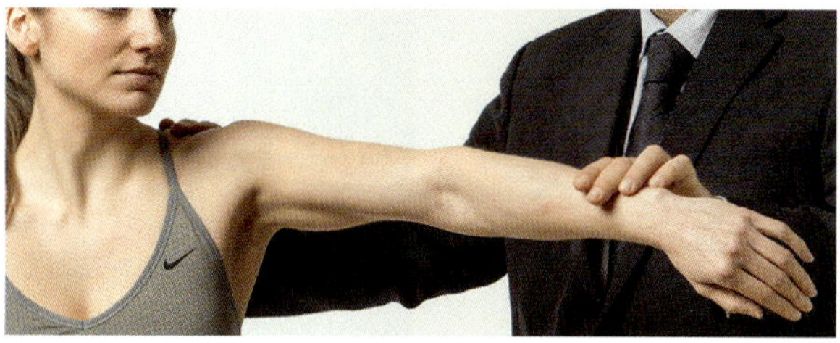

Fig. 14.4 Empty can test. Image Published under License from www.shoulderdoc.co.uk and www.shoulderpedia.org

Pillar 3: Special Tests

When performing the Codman's Sign (Drop Arm Sign) the arm is passively abducted, but when the external support is removed the patient is unable to maintain the arm in the elevated position. Palpation of a supraspinatus tear through the deltoid comprises the Rent Test (Codman). This is accomplished in a relaxed patient, just beyond the anterolateral border of the acromion (Fig. 14.3).

When performing the empty can/full can test: The patient is tested at 90° elevation in the scapula plane and full internal rotation (empty can) (Fig. 14.4) or 45°external rotation (full can) (Fig. 14.5) respectively. Patient resists downward pressure exerted by the examiner. It is important to apply reasonable resistance, as excessive force may lead to a false positive result by overcoming even a normal supraspinatus strength. A positive test is denoted by pain and/or muscle weakness.

Pillar 4: Investigations

Although the clinical history is invaluable in suspecting supraspinatus weakness, clinical examination is notoriously poor in diagnosing supraspinatus weakness on its own. It is hence, frequently necessary to complement clinical assessment with imaging.

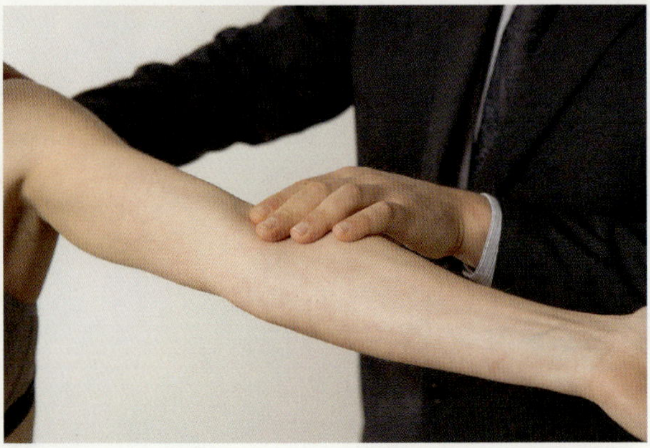

Fig. 14.5 Full can test. Image Published under License from www.shoulderdoc.co.uk and www.shoulderpedia.org

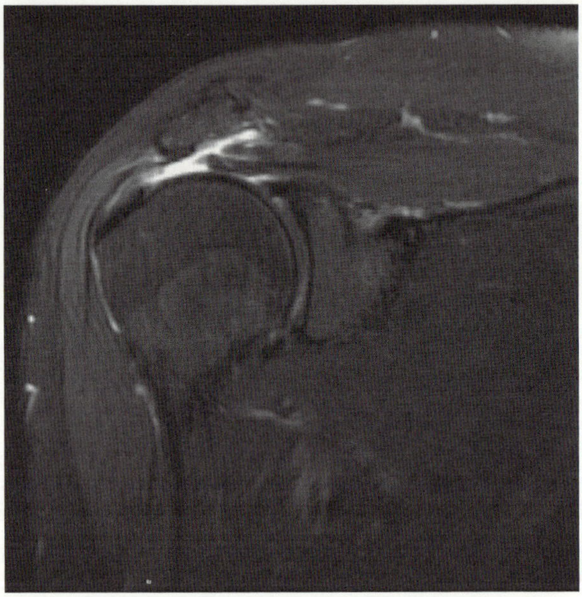

Fig. 14.6 MRI supraspinatus tear. Image Published under License from www.shoulderdoc.co.uk and www.shoulderpedia.org

Plain films of the shoulder may show proximal migration of the humeral head with narrowing of the acromio-humeral interval.

Both ultrasound (US) and MRI scans are useful in evaluating the supraspinatus integrity. Ultrasonography has the benefit of being a dynamic form of imaging as compared to the static MRI. Ultrasound is portable, quick, and a more cost-effective method, which is also better tolerated by the patient and allows interaction with the patient. The patient can also point out the symptomatic area. The advent of portable Ultrasound scanners has led the way to surgeon-performed ultrasound scans and provision of one-stop clinics.

MRI not only provides a diagnosis of rotator cuff tears but also allows for assessment of the muscle wasting and fatty atrophy (Fig. 14.6). Although it may be time-consuming, modern scanners allow examination of tendons in great detail and are invaluable in diagnosis, prognosis and surgical planning.

Electrophysiological tests are helpful and are gold standard in cases where suprascapular nerve entrapment is suspected.

With modern imaging techniques, it is rare for arthroscopy to be used solely as a diagnostic tool for rotator cuff tears. It, however, remains the gold standard for diagnosis in cases of diagnostic conflict or uncertainty regarding tendon integrity.

Discussion of the Case

The first case described in the chapter represents one of the most common scenarios in a shoulder clinic. This history is suggestive of a degenerate rotator cuff tear. Examination findings included a painful arc, positive impingement features and positive empty can sign. An ultrasound scan confirmed a full-thickness tear of the supraspinatus. Management usually involves an initial trial of non-operative management, before considering surgical repair.

The second case represents an acute rotator cuff tear. A fall on the arm, leading to pain, bruising and lack of elevation is highly suggestive of an acute rotator cuff tear. Pseudo-paralysis and a positive drop arm sign are indicative of an uncompensated tear. An ultrasound /MRI is confirmatory of the diagnosis. Early surgical repair of such an injury ought to be given consideration.

The third case is typical of a young athlete presenting with suprascapular nerve entrapment. Atrophy of muscle in suprascapular and infrascapular fossa with weakness of abduction and external rotation is evident on examination. Definitive diagnosis is based on MR and EMG studies. Treatment is conservative with physiotherapy initially however in certain cases surgical decompression of the nerve may be warranted.

Summary

By far the most common cause of supraspinatus weakness is seen in the setting of rotator cuff disease/subacromial impingement syndrome. Although the history is very useful in raising suspicions of a supraspinatus tear, clinical examination on its own is unreliable in diagnosing supraspinatus weakness. Plain radiography is required to rule out other pathologies and observe acromion morphology while Ultrasound and MRI are used to define the tear. Muscle wasting and fatty atrophy are best assessed using MR scanning. A summary of diagnostic clusters is presented in Table 14.3. The primary treatments involve activity modification, analgesia and exercises for a few months before considering surgical repair. Early repair is often regarded in traumatic tears in relatively young and/or active patients.

Table 14.3 Summary of diagnostic clusters for supraspinatus weakness

Clinical history
1. Chronic Tears: Deltoid region pain and weakness exacerbated by overhead activities
2. Acute Tears: History of fall
3. Night pain
Conventional examination
4. Wasting of supraspinous fossa/infraspinous fossa
5. Loss of active elevation, but passive elevation preserved
Special tests
6. Drop Arm (Codman) sign
7. Empty can/Full Can test
Investigations
8. Ultrasound—Easily available, sensitive, operator dependent
9. MR Scan—better for assessing muscle wasting/fatty atrophy, suprascapular notch encroachment
10. EMG in neurological causes of weakness

References

1. Clark J, Harryman D. Tendons, ligaments, and capsule of the rotator cuff. Gross and microscopic anatomy. J Bone Joint Surg Am. 1992;74(5):713–25.
2. Codman E. Complete rupture of the supraspinatus tendon; operative treatment with report of two successful cases. Boston Med Surg J. 1911;164(20):708–10.
3. Neer C. Anterior acromioplasty for the chronic impingement syndrome in the shoulder. J Bone Joint Surg Am. 1972;54(1):41–50.
4. Pandey V, Willems WJ. Rotator cuff tear: a detailed update. Acia Pac J Sports Med Anthrosc Rehabil Technol. 2015;2(1):1–14.4.
5. Oh L, Wolf B, Hall M, Levy B, Marx R. Indications for rotator cuff repair. Clin Orthop Relat Res. 2007;455:52–63.
6. Yamamoto A, Takagishi K, Osawa T, Yanagawa T, Nakajima D, Shitara H, et al. Prevalence and risk factors of a rotator cuff tear in the general population. J Shoulder Elb Surg. 2010;19(1):116–20.
7. Matsen F. Rotator-cuff failure. N Engl J Med. 2008;358(20):2138–47.

Chapter 15
Infraspinatus

P. Wright

Case Example

A 28-year-old male presents with pain over the posterior aspect of his dominant right shoulder. He does not report any acute injury. He likes to play cricket at amateur level and has been unable to bowl with his right arm due to "loss of power" and weakness for the last 4 months. Clinical examination reveals tenderness over the posterior glenohumeral joint line along with wasting over the infraspinatus fossa. There is marked weakness on objective testing of infraspinatus.

Introduction

The infraspinatus muscle arises from the infraspinous fossa of the scapula and inserts onto the greater tuberosity of the humerus (Fig. 14.1). It is supplied by the suprascapular nerve, which arises directly from the superior trunk of the brachial plexus (C5, C6). The nerve passes into the supraspinous fossa through the suprascapular notch, beneath the transverse scapular ligament to supply supraspinatus before entering the infraspinous fossa through the spinoglenoid notch, beneath the spinoglenoid ligament to supply infraspinatus.

Infraspinatus weakness is a relatively common finding in combination with other shoulder symptoms and signs but rare in isolation. The differential diagnosis for a patient exhibiting infraspinatus weakness in addition to other symptoms or signs is very broad but when isolated weakness is present the differential narrows considerably. Thus the most important distinction to be made is whether there are features

P. Wright
Bradford Teaching Hospitals Foundation Trust, Bradford Royal Infirmary, Duckworth Lane, Bradford, UK
e-mail: info@shouldersolutions.co.uk

© Springer International Publishing AG 2017

P. Monga, L. Funk (eds.), *Diagnostic Clusters in Shoulder Conditions*,
DOI 10.1007/978-3-319-57334-2_15

Table 15.1 Infraspinatus weakness clinical features matrix

	Onset	Trauma	Pain	Wasting
Cuff tear	Acute/chronic	Traumatic/atraumatic	Common subacromial pattern	Both
Brachial neuritis	Acute	Atraumatic	Common neck, shoulder, arm	Both
Spinoglenoid/para labral cyst	Chronic	Repetitive trauma	Uncommon	Infra only
SSN neuropathy	Chronic	Repetitive trauma	Common posterior shoulder	Both
Cervical radiculopathy	Acute/chronic	Atraumatic	Common cervical spine, lateral border of the forearm	Both

present in addition to infraspinatus weakness. Various differential diagnosis are compared in the clinical features matrix (Table 15.1).

Weakness may be due to an intrinsic disorder of the muscle-tendon unit, as in degenerate or traumatic rotator cuff tears, or due to an extrinsic condition affecting the nerve supply to the muscle. Muscle innervation may be compromised at the level of the suprascapular nerve, the brachial plexus or the nerve roots within the cervical spine.

Pillar 1: Clinical History

As with any other musculoskeletal condition, it is essential to determine the time course over which symptoms have occurred and whether there has been a history of trauma. Symptoms may be precipitated by a single traumatic episode or by the shoulder being subjected to repeated supra-physiologic loads over a period of time, as in the case of the overhead athlete.

Rapid onset of weakness occurring following an index episode of trauma should raise the suspicion of a traumatic rotator cuff tear. Although most commonly injured with the supraspinatus tendon, there are case reports of isolated traumatic tears of the infraspinatus tendon [1].

A more delayed onset of weakness over weeks or months may indicate progressive compression of the suprascapular nerve. This may be due to extrinsic compression of the nerve by the transverse scapular ligament [2] or due to compression from a para labral cyst at the spinoglenoid notch [3]. Such cysts are commonly associated with a tear of the glenoid labrum [4]. Such phenomena have frequently been reported to occur in athletes engaged in sports with repetitive overhead activity, such as volleyball, baseball and tennis [5–7].

The onset of weakness after a viral illness or vaccination should prompt consideration of the diagnosis of a post-viral brachial neuritis (neuralgic amyotrophy/ Parsonage-Turner Syndrome) [8]. This does not usually cause isolated weakness of supraspinatus but rather more widespread effects on shoulder girdle musculature.

With any of the aetiologies as mentioned earlier pain may be present. With infraspinatus weakness due to rotator cuff disease, pain may originate from the subacromial space and pain distribution is down the anterolateral aspect of the shoulder. Suprascapular nerve compression may cause deep, diffuse, posterolateral shoulder pain, on occasion radiating to the upper arm, neck or chest [9]. In many cases of entrapment of the nerve at the level of the spinoglenoid notch, there is no associated pain since the sensory nerve originates proximal to this level [10]. Pain is a prominent feature of brachial neuritis with 96% of patients reporting an acute, severe and relentless pain in the neck, shoulder girdle and arm [11].

The functional deficit due to infraspinatus weakness is variable and may be greatest when there are other muscles affected. Infraspinatus weakness may cause difficulty with lifting heavy loads above shoulder height, combing the back of the hair or throwing a ball [3, 12]. In the case of elite athletes, despite the presence of infraspinatus weakness and wasting, there may be little or no impact on shoulder function or sporting performance [6, 7].

It should not be forgotten that neuropathy proximal to the plexus and shoulder girdle may cause infraspinatus weakness and the presence of symptoms related to the cervical spine suggestive of a radicular problem should be sought.

Pillar 2: Conventional Examination

Inspection of the posterior aspect of the shoulder girdle may reveal wasting of the infraspinatus muscle belly within the infraspinous fossa [13]. Any associated loss of the bulk of the supraspinatus muscle should be noted. There may be evidence of scapulothoracic dyskinesia during attempted shoulder movements [14].

Tenderness to palpation may be a non-specific finding, being common in patients with many painful shoulder conditions. One case series records the prevalence of tenderness in patients with spinoglenoid notch cysts as 78%, with the most commonly localised area of tenderness the posterior aspect of the shoulder [4].

Although infraspinatus activity is similar during external rotation at all positions of abduction, the best position to isolate infraspinatus is external rotation at 0° abduction (Fig. 15.1) [15] or at 90° flexion [16]. Strength testing should be compared between symptomatic and non-symptomatic sides, noting the dominance of the patient. In an asymptomatic individual infraspinatus strength should be greater on the dominant side. In elite volleyball players it has been observed that, even in the absence of symptoms, the dominant infraspinatus may be weaker than the non-dominant [12].

Examination of the cervical spine should not be neglected and a thorough peripheral neurological examination performed. The presence of weakness in a myotome distribution should alert the examiner to the potential for weakness due to nerve root

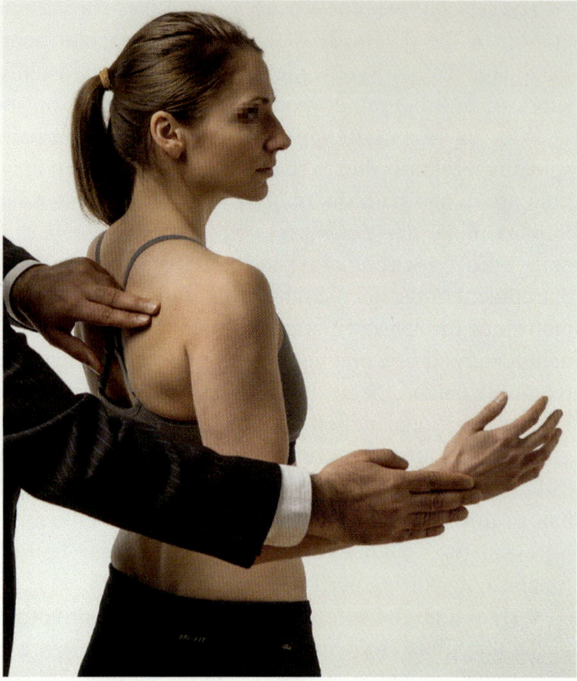

Fig. 15.1 Infraspinatus strength testing. Image Published under License from www.shoulderdoc.co.uk and www.shoulderpedia.org

compression. The suprascapular nerve is supplied by the C5 and C6 nerve roots which also supply the musculocutaneous nerve supplying the brachial and biceps brachii muscles.

Pillar 3: Special Tests

When performing the Dropping Sign [17], the arm is held at 0° abduction and placed into a position of 45° external rotation by the examiner. The patient is asked to externally rotate while being resisted by the examiner's arm (Fig. 15.2). A positive dropping sign is indicated by the patient's forearm falling back into a position of 0° rotation. A positive dropping sign is associated with an irreparable tear of infraspinatus.

The Infraspinatus Test [12] is performed with the patient lying with the arm to be tested uppermost with the shoulder at 0° abduction, and the elbow flexed to 90° with a 3 kg in hand. The patient is asked to externally rotate the shoulder until the weight is held above the horizontal level (Fig. 15.3). Inability to do this is an early sign of infraspinatus weakness and has been suggested as a screening test in overhead athletes to identify infraspinatus weakness, potentially before weakness impacts upon sports performance.

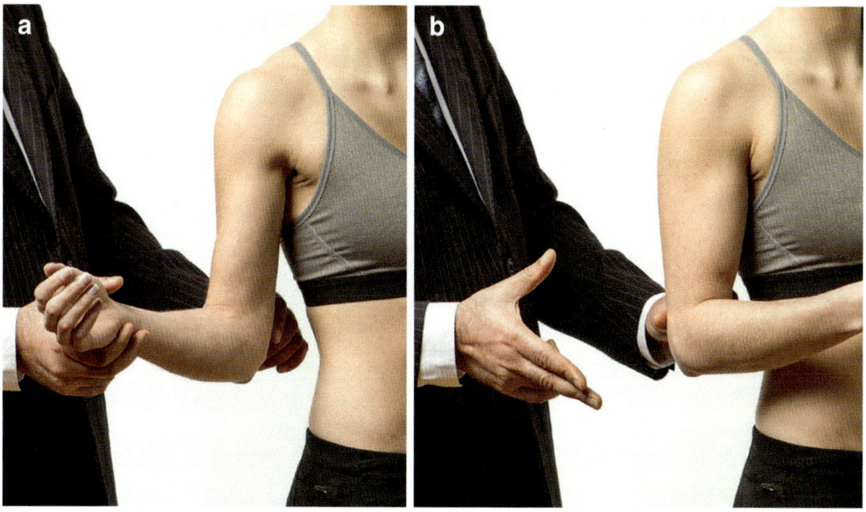

Fig. 15.2 The dropping sign starting position (**a**) and a positive test (**b**). Image Published under License from www.shoulderdoc.co.uk and www.shoulderpedia.org

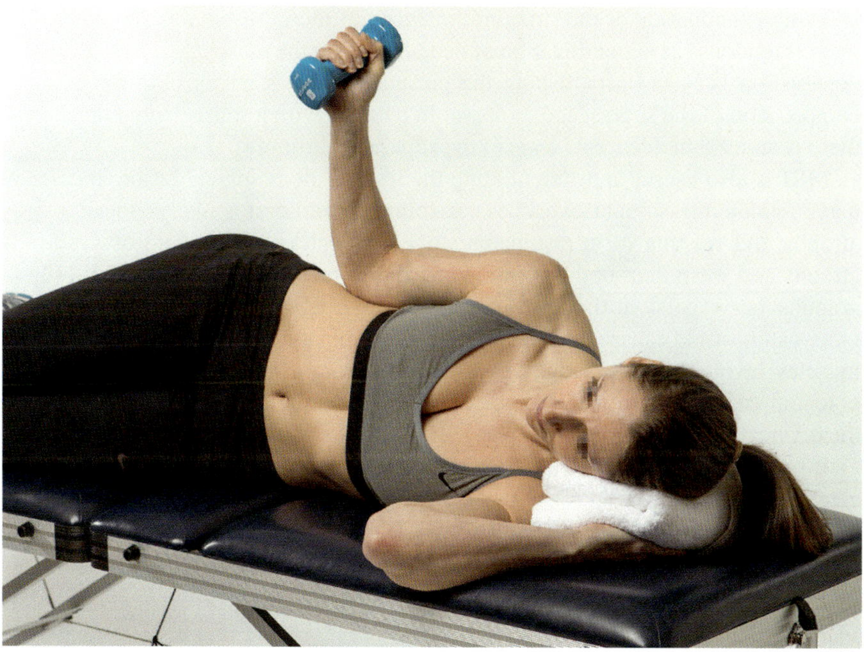

Fig. 15.3 The infraspinatus test. Image Published under License from www.shoulderdoc.co.uk and www.shoulderpedia.org

The External Rotation Lag Sign (Fig. 17.2) is also useful to detect Infraspinatus weakness and has been described in detail in Chap. 16.

Pillar 4: Investigations

Radiographs should be considered with symptoms occurring after significant trauma to the shoulder to exclude bony injury. Patients suffering from rotator cuff disease may exhibit changes to the bony anatomy of the subacromial space and, in cases of significant tears to the rotator cuff proximal humeral migration increase the likelihood of a rotator cuff tear extending into the infraspinatus tendon [18].

An Ultrasound is a useful imaging modality if a tear of the infraspinatus tendon is suspected. It's sensitivity and specificity matches that of magnetic resonance imaging and is only exceeded by MR arthrography [19]. Fatty atrophy of the rotator cuff muscle belly can be assessed by ultrasound although this has not been validated for infraspinatus, only supraspinatus [20]. While it is possible to identify spinoglenoid cysts on ultrasound [3], MRI is a better investigation.

Magnetic resonance imaging (MRI) is perhaps the most useful investigation, allowing examination of the structural integrity of the infraspinatus and other rotator cuff tendons [21], identification of oedema within the muscle belly suggestive of denervation [22] and establishing the presence of cysts responsible for extrinsic compression of the suprascapular nerve. In patients with a spinoglenoid notch cyst, there is an 89% incidence of tears to the superior labrum [4].

MRI is also useful in differentiating the level of neurological lesion in cases of nerve related infraspinatus weakness. A spinioglenoid cyst is likely to lead to fatty atrophy and wasting of infraspinatus alone. In contrast, one would observe fatty atrophy and wasting of both supraspinatus and infraspinatus in patients with suprascapular nerve palsy at the level of suprascapular notch. Brachial neuritis, on the other hand, would cause signal changes in supraspinatus, infraspinatus and all other muscles involved in the pathology as well (commonly deltoid). Where there is potential concern there may be radicular nerve root compression, an MRI scan of the cervical spine is worthwhile.

It has been demonstrated that electrophysiology (nerve conduction studies and electromyography) are more reliable than clinical examination in distinguishing brachial neuritis from suprascapular nerve compression [23]. In cases of nerve compression, nerve conduction velocity and motor nerve action potential amplitudes are reduced while latency is increased. Where established denervation is present electromyography demonstrates increased insertional activity (depolarization of muscle fibres on electrode insertion), fibrillation potentials and positive sharp waves (entrapment of the suprascapular nerve).

Discussion of the Case

The presentation of the patient described earlier in the chapter with an isolated infraspinatus weakness is highly suggestive of a compressive lesion of the suprascapular nerve at the level of the spinoglenoid notch. In a higher lesion of the suprascapular nerve at the level of suprascapular notch, both supraspinatus and infraspinatus are affected. When the lesion is present further proximally, in the brachial plexus/cervical spine, other muscles such as the deltoid are also involved. This patient underwent an MR arthrogram which confirmed the presence of a posterior labral tear and a para labral cyst encroaching the spinoglenoid notch. The MR also revealed isolated wasting and fatty atrophy of the infraspinatus muscle but no tendon tears. The patient underwent arthroscopic decompression of the cyst and a posterior labral repair.

Summary

Formulating a definitive diagnosis in patients with weakness of the infraspinatus muscle may be challenging. There is considerable overlap between the clinical features of differing pathologies and diagnosis may rely heavily on the fourth pillar (investigations). This should not undermine the value of a thorough history and clinical examination. A summary of diagnostic clusters for infraspinatus is listed in Table 15.2.

Table 15.2 Summary of diagnostic clusters for infraspinatus weakness

Clinical history
1. Trauma—direct blow from anterior to posterior or forced hyperabduction of shoulder in extension and external rotation
2. Overhead throwing athlete (volleyball, tennis, weightlifting)
3. Manual occupation involving repetitive overhead activity (painter and decorator, plasterer)
4. Prodromal viral illness or recent administration of vaccine
Conventional examination
5. Wasting of infraspinatus within infraspinous fossa
6. Loss of active external rotation with shoulder in either neutral position
Special tests
7. Dropping sign
8. The Infraspinatus test
Investigations
9. Magnetic resonance imaging findings of tendon tear, fatty atrophy, presence of para labral cyst
10. Electromyography and Nerve conduction studies

References

1. Lunn JV, Castellanos-Rosas J, Tavernier T, Barthélémy R, Walch G. A novel lesion of the infraspinatus characterized by musculotendinous disruption, edema, and late fatty infiltration. J Shoulder Elb Surg. 2008;17:546–53.
2. Rengachary SS, Neff JP, Singer PA, Brackett CE. Suprascapular entrapment neuropathy: a clinical, anatomical, and comparative study. Neurosurgery. 1979;5:441–6.
3. Skirving AP, Kozak TK, Davis SJ. Infraspinatus paralysis due to spinoglenoid notch ganglion. J Bone Joint Surg Br. 1994;76:588–91.
4. Piatt BE, Hawkins RJ, Fritz RC, Ho CP, Wolf E, Schickendantz M. Clinical evaluation and treatment of spinoglenoid notch ganglion cysts. J Shoulder Elb Surg. 2002;11:600–4.
5. Ferretti A, De Carli A, Fontana M. Injury of the suprascapular nerve at the spinoglenoid notch. The natural history of infraspinatus atrophy in volleyball players. Am J Sports Med. 1998;26:759–63.
6. Cummins CA, Messer TM, Schafer MF. Infraspinatus muscle atrophy in professional baseball players. Am J Sports Med. 2004;32:116–20.
7. Young SW, Dakic J, Stroia K, Nguyen ML, Harris AH, Safran MR. High Incidence of Infraspinatus Muscle Atrophy in Elite Professional Female Tennis Players. Am J Sports Med. 2015;43:1989–93.
8. Helms CA, Martinez S, Speer KP. Acute brachial neuritis (Parsonage-Turner syndrome): MR imaging appearance--report of three cases. Radiology. 1998;207:255–9.
9. Fabre T, Piton C, Leclouerec G, Gervais-Delion F, Durandeau A. Entrapment of the suprascapular nerve. J Bone Joint Surg Br. 1999;81:414–9.
10. Reeser JC, Fleisig GS, Cools AM, Yount D, Magnes SA. Biomechanical insights into the aetiology of infraspinatus syndrome. Br J Sports Med. 2013;47:239–44.
11. van Alfen N. The neuralgic amyotrophy consultation. J Neurol. 2007;254:695–704.
12. Hama H, Morinaga T, Suzuki K, Kuroki H, Sunami M, Yamamuro T. The infraspinatus test: an early diagnostic sign of muscle weakness during external rotation of the shoulder in athletes. J Shoulder Elb Surg. 1993;2:257–9.
13. Cordova CB, Owens BD. Infraspinatus muscle atrophy from suprascapular nerve compression. JAAPA. 2014;27:33–5.
14. Pohlgeers KM, Becker JA. Infraspinatus atrophy in a volleyball player: a case of a Bennett lesion causing nerve impingement. Curr Sports Med Rep. 2014;13:358–60.
15. Escamilla RF, Yamashiro K, Paulos L, Andrews JR. Shoulder muscle activity and function in common shoulder rehabilitation exercises. Sports Med. 2009;39:663–85.
16. Hughes PC, Green RA, Taylor NF. Isolation of infraspinatus in clinical test positions. J Sci Med Sport. 2014;17:256–60.
17. Walch G, Boulahia A, Calderone S, Robinson AH. The 'dropping' and 'hornblower's' signs in evaluation of rotator-cuff tears. J Bone Joint Surg Br. 1998;80:624–8.
18. Keener JD, Wei AS, Kim HM, Steger-May K, Yamaguchi K. Proximal humeral migration in shoulders with symptomatic and asymptomatic rotator cuff tears. J Bone Joint Surg Am. 2009;91:1405–13.
19. de Jesus JO, Parker L, Frangos AJ, Nazarian LN. Accuracy of MRI, MR arthrography, and ultrasound in the diagnosis of rotator cuff tears: a meta-analysis. AJR Am J Roentgenol. 2009;192:1701–7.
20. Khoury V, Cardinal E, Brassard P. Atrophy and fatty infiltration of the supraspinatus muscle: sonography versus MRI. Am J Roentgenol. 2008;190:1105–11.
21. Evancho AM, Stiles RG, Fajman WA, Flower SP, Macha T, Brunner MC, Fleming L. MR imaging diagnosis of rotator cuff tears. Am J Roentgenol. 1988;151:751–4.
22. Fleckenstein JL, Watumull D, Conner KE, Ezaki M, Greenlee RG Jr, Bryan WW, Chason DP, Parkey RW, Peshock RM, Purdy PD. Denervated human skeletal muscle: MR imaging evaluation. Radiology. 1993;187:213–8.
23. Clarke CJ, Torrance E, McIntosh J, Funk L. Neuralgic amyotrophy is not the most common neurologic disorder of the shoulder: a 78-month prospective study of 60 neurologic shoulder patients in a specialist shoulder clinic. J Shoulder Elb Surg. 2016;25:1997–2004.

Chapter 16
Subscapularis

Santosh Venkatachalam

Case Example

A 68-year-old female presents to clinic with residual anterior shoulder pain and weakness 6 months following an anterior shoulder dislocation which was manipulated successfully in casualty. Clinical examination reveals a flexion lag of 20°. The external rotation is increased compared to the opposite side. The bear hug, lift off, and belly press tests are positive.

Introduction

The subscapularis is the largest of the rotator cuff muscles, and its insertion is onto the lesser tuberosity providing almost 50% of the rotator cuff strength. It functions as an internal rotator and dynamic stabiliser of the humeral head. The nerve supply is from the upper and lower subscapular nerves, which arise from the posterior cord of the brachial plexus. Prevalence of subscapularis tears is around 30% of chronic rotator cuff tears.

Pillar 1: Clinical History

Acute tears of the subscapularis are most commonly seen following anterior shoulder dislocations occurring in mid to late adulthood. Lesser tuberosity avulsion fracture is a possibility with an anterior shoulder dislocation, and this tends to occur in

S. Venkatachalam
Northumbria Healthcare, North Shields, UK
e-mail: santakshi@gmail.com

© Springer International Publishing AG 2017

P. Monga, L. Funk (eds.), *Diagnostic Clusters in Shoulder Conditions*,
DOI 10.1007/978-3-319-57334-2_16

individuals less than 40 years of age. The pain is present in the front of the shoulder, and there may be no apparent bruising. The patients complain of weakness of the arm on forward lifting, twisting the arm inwards and some sporting activities. Beware of subscapularis deficiency in patients who have undergone a previous shoulder arthroplasty. The deltopectoral arthroplasty approach commonly involves a subscapularis tenotomy or lesser tuberosity osteotomy, and failure of this to heal may lead to a clinical picture of a deficient subscapularis.

Diagnosis can be challenging and needs a high index of suspicion with a correlation of mechanism of injury, presenting complaints and examination findings.

Pillar 2: Conventional Examination

As the subscapularis muscle belly is a deep structure, wasting is not clinically evident. One would see features of associated pathology such as supraspinatus weakness, biceps pain and subacromial and/or subcoracoid impingement. There may be tenderness in the anterior aspect of the shoulder over the lesser tuberosity, in acute cases. There may be a weakness of glenohumeral internal rotation and a passive increase in external rotation in comparison to the opposite side.

Pillar 3: Special Tests

Despite numerous clinical tests being described to identify these tears, clinical diagnosis of partial subscapularis tears remains challenging. On the other hand, full-thickness subscapularis tears are relatively easily diagnosed, if one maintains a high index of suspicion. Sometimes a combination of these tests along with investigations may be required to diagnose subscapularis tears [1]. In fact, a combination of bear hug, Napoleon belly-press and lift-off test can improve the sensitivity of clinical diagnosis to over 80%.

When performing the Gerber's lift-off test, The patient is examined in standing position and is asked to place their hand behind their back with the dorsum of the hand resting in the region of the mid- lumbar spine. The dorsum of the hand is raised off the back by maintaining or increasing the internal rotation of the humerus and extension at the shoulder. To perform this test, the patient must have a full passive internal rotation so that it is physically possible to place the arm in the desired position and pain cannot be a limiting factor during the manoeuvre. The examiner needs to ensure that the patient does not use elbow extension as a trick movement to "mimic" shoulder internal rotation. Positive test: The ability to actively lift the dorsum of the hand off the back constitutes a normal lift-off test. Inability to move the dorsum of the wrist off the back represents an abnormal lift-off test and indicates subscapularis rupture or dysfunction [2] (Fig. 16.1).

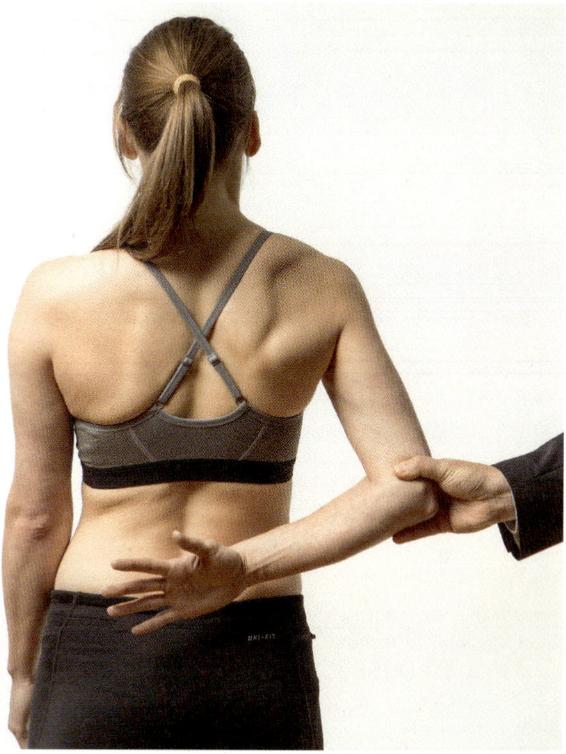

Fig. 16.1 Gerber's lift-off test. Image Published under License from www.shoulderdoc.co.uk and www.shoulderpedia.org

Greis et al. [3] used EMG analysis to determine the muscle activity of the shoulder muscles during the lift-off test and during resisted internal rotation. The activity in the subscapularis in the upper and lower fibres during a lift-off test from the region of the mid-lumbar spine was approximately 70% of maximum voluntary contraction. The level was significantly ($p < 0.05$) higher than all the other muscles tested. The lift-off test with the hand placed in the region of the mid-lumbar spine resulted in one-third more EMG activity in the subscapularis than when the test was modified and performed with the hand at the buttock area. They concluded that if a patient has a full range of passive internal rotation and if the active internal rotation is not limited by pain then an abnormal lift-off test reliably diagnoses subscapularis dysfunction.

In the Bear Hug Test test, the patient is instructed to hold arm across the chest, and the examiner tries to pull arm away from the chest wall. In patients with subscapularis tear, the patient will demonstrate weakness in resisting this manoeuvre [4] (Fig. 16.2).

The patient can be seated or standing when performing the Belly press test/Napoleon test. The examiner stands in front of the patient while passively moving the affected upper extremity into flexion and maximal internal rotation with the elbow flexed at 90°. The examiner supports the patient's elbow while the other hand brings the arm into a maximal internal rotation and the patient is instructed to press the palm of their neutral wrist against their abdomen. The examiner pushes on the

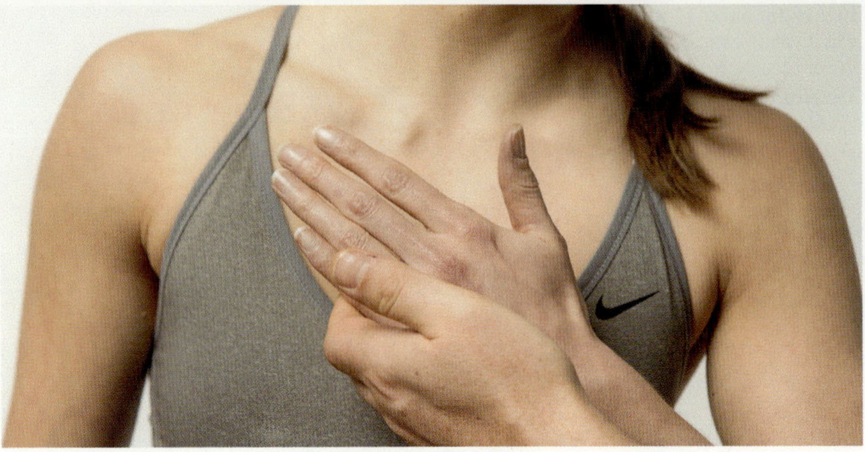

Fig. 16.2 Bear hug test. Image Published under License from www.shoulderdoc.co.uk and www.shoulderpedia.org

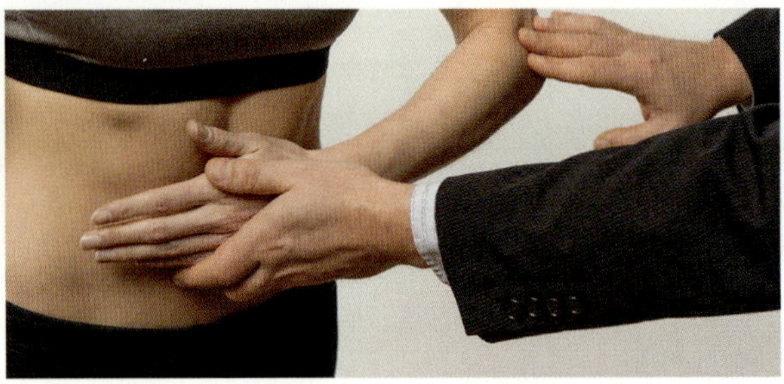

Fig. 16.3 Belly press/Napoleon test. Image Published under License from www.shoulderdoc.co.uk and www.shoulderpedia.org

elbow posteriorly on the affected side. In patients with subscapularis tear [5], they will be unable to press against the abdomen without volar flexion of the wrist or the elbow falling posteriorly (Fig. 16.3).

Lift off lag test/Internal rotation lag sign test: Examiner passively holds off the patients' hand away with the arm in internal rotation from the back at the level of the lumbar region and then lets go of the hand. The patient is asked to maintain this position. The patient will be unable to keep the hand away from the back in subscapularis tears/dysfunction.

Belly off sign: The examiner standing in front of the patient while passively moving the affected upper extremity into flexion and maximal internal rotation with the elbow flexed at 90°. The examiner supports the patient's elbow while the other hand brings the arm into maximal internal rotation placing the palm of the hand on the abdomen. The patient is asked to keep the wrist straight and actively maintain this position of internal rotation as the examiner releases the wrist (maintaining elbow support). Confirmatory findings: the patient is unable to maintain the position, the wrist flexes or lag occurs, and the hand is lifted off the abdomen. The integrity of the musculotendinous unit is evaluated in this test [6].

Pillar 4: Investigations

Plain Radiographs of the shoulder AP/axillary views are useful to identify lesser tuberosity avulsion in axillary views, which may suggest subscapularis deficiency. An anterosuperior escape of the humeral component can be present due to lack of anterior constraint of intact subscapularis in cases of subscapularis failure following arthroplasty.

Identifying tears of the subscapularis on ultrasound is possible. Medial subluxation of the long head of biceps should raise the suspicion of subscapularis tendon tear. This is due to the anatomical arrangement in this area where the biceps sling is formed by the combination of the coracohumeral ligament, superior glenohumeral ligament and superior fibres of the subscapularis. Partial tears of the subscapularis are more challenging to diagnose on an ultrasound scan. Ultrasound may, in fact, be a preferred investigation in cases when postoperative subscapularis insufficiency is suspected as an MRI is associated with significant metallic artefact.

In traumatic injuries, tears involving the upper portion of the subscapularis may be associated with medial biceps subluxation for reasons outlined under ultrasound. MRI can demonstrate fatty infiltration especially the upper portions of subscapularis on parasagittal scapular Y views sections on MRI in fat suppressed or T2 images. On the axial sections, there may be attenuated and medially subluxed biceps tendon into the upper fibres of the subscapularis. Fatty infiltration or muscle atrophy in the belly of subscapularis muscle can be appreciated on MRI. MRI can also suggest the possible aetiology for subscapularis tears [7] with reduced coracohumeral distance (space between the tip of coracoid process and lesser tuberosity in maximal internal rotation-average is 11 mm) and increased coracoid index (extension of the coracoid process beyond a line drawn in tangent to the articular surface of the glenoid-average is around 8 mm).

Diagnostic arthroscopy of the shoulder can demonstrate a tear in the subscapularis when visualised from the posterior portal. The biceps can be seen to be subluxed medially into the upper fibres of the subscapularis. Applying a posterior pressure on the proximal humerus can help in better visualisation of the tear. A 70-degree arthroscope visualises a subscapularis tear better than a 30-degree arthroscope.

Discussion of the Case

The index case in this chapter has features of a subscapularis related pain and weakness. Subscapularis tears are frequently underdiagnosed and hence notoriously undertreated. An MRI scan confirmed a full thickness tear of the subscapularis in this case. It revealed a degree of wasting and atrophy. The patient had significant persistent symptoms despite physiotherapy and underwent arthroscopic surgery for repairing the subscapularis.

Table 16.1 Summary of diagnostic clusters for subscapularis tears

Clinical history
1. Acute: Anterior shoulder dislocation >40 yrs
2. Chronic: Anterior shoulder pain/Part of subacromial impingement syndrome
3. Weakness following previous shoulder arthroplasty
Conventional examination
4. Increased passive external rotation
5. Weakness in internal rotation
Special tests
6. Gerber's lift off test
7. Bear hug test
8. Belly press test
Investigations
9. U/S—medially subluxed biceps tendon with subscapularis tear
10. MRI—medial subluxation of the long head of biceps tendon, fatty infiltration/atrophy of the subscapularis reduced coracohumeral distance on axial images

Summary

Rotator cuff disease is the most common cause of subscapularis tears and weakness. The tears typically start in the anterior aspect the supraspinatus and progress postero-superiorly (more common) or anteriorly (less common). Such anterior extension of cuff tears is in fact, the most common cause of subscapularis tears. Subscapularis tears are also very commonly seen following traumatic dislocations of the shoulder in mid to late life. The diagnosis of partial subscapularis tears remains challenging although full thickness tears of subscapularis are relatively easy to diagnose using described special tests. MRI is the investigation of choice for confirming the diagnosis. A cluster approach to diagnosing subscapularis tears is recommended, and a summary of such clusters is presented in Table 16.1.

References

1. Hegedus EJ, Goode A, Campbell S, et al. Physical examination tests of the shoulder: a systematic review with meta-analysis of individual tests. Br J Sports Med. 2008;42:80–92.
2. Gerber C, Krushell RJ. Isolated rupture of the tendon of the subscapularis muscle. Clinical features in 16 cases. J Bone Joint Surg Br. 1991;73:389–94.
3. Greis PE, Kuhn JE, Schultheis J, Hintermeister R, Hawkins R. Validation of the lift-off test and analysis of subscapularis activity during maximal internal rotation. Am J Sports Med. 1996;24:589–93.
4. Barth JR, Burkhart SS, De Beer JF. The bear-hug test: a new and sensitive test for diagnosing a subscapularis tear. Arthroscopy. 2006;22:1076–84.
5. Burkhart SS, Tehrany AM. Arthroscopic subscapularis tendon repair: technique and preliminary results. Arthroscopy. 2002;18:454–63.
6. Bartsch M, Greiner S, Haas NP, Scheibel M. Diagnostic values of clinical tests for subscapularis lesions. Knee Surg Sports Traumatol Arthrosc. 2010;18:1712–7.
7. Giaroli EL, Major NM, Lemley DE, Lee J. Coracohumeral interval imaging in subcoracoid impingement syndrome on MRI. Am J Roentgenol. 2006;186:242–6.

Chapter 17
Teres Minor

J.A. Baxter, G. Howell, and R. Heasley

Case Example

A 75-year-old lady presents with a 4-year history of progressive shoulder pain. She has now developed pain at night and hence seeks medical attention. She feels her shoulder has also become weaker. Clinical examination reveals pseudoparalysis with an inability to actively elevate her arm above the shoulder level, although her passive movements are preserved. Clinical examination reveals wasting of the supraspinatus and infraspinatus fossa and an inability to get her arm into the "combing" position. Patte's sign, drop arm sign and external rotation lag sign are positive.

Introduction

Teres minor is one of the four rotator cuff muscles and probably the one with the lowest profile. When the rest of the rotator cuff is healthy, it is of limited clinical interest, but in patients with a failing rotator cuff, it becomes increasingly important.

Teres derives from the Latin for rounded or cylindrical, and teres minor is a narrow muscle lying inferior to the infraspinatus muscle and superior to teres major. It originates from the dorsal surface of the lateral border of the scapula. Its fibres run

J.A. Baxter (✉)
St George's Hospital, London, UK
e-mail: jonabaxter@doctors.org.uk

G. Howell
Royal Preston Hospital, Preston, UK

R. Heasley
Pennine Acute Hospitals, Manchester, UK

© Springer International Publishing AG 2017

P. Monga, L. Funk (eds.), *Diagnostic Clusters in Shoulder Conditions*,
DOI 10.1007/978-3-319-57334-2_17

superolaterally in an oblique fashion, to insert into the inferior aspect of the greater tuberosity of the humerus. This tendon is the most inferior of the posterior rotator cuff, and often its fibres are difficult to differentiate from those of the adjacent infraspinatus tendon (Fig. 14.1). Deep to the tendon lies the glenohumeral joint capsule. The posterior branch of the axillary nerve innervates teres minor.

As part of the rotator cuff, teres minor has a role in stabilising the humeral head during glenohumeral joint abduction and forward flexion, maximising deltoid function across the joint. Along with infraspinatus, teres minor externally rotates the humerus.

Teres minor also forms the superior border of the quadrilateral (quadrangular) space through which the axillary nerve and posterior humeral circumflex artery pass. Teres major forms the inferior border, with the long head of triceps and the medial aspect of the humeral shaft acting as the medial and lateral borders respectively.

Teres minor dysfunction is usually only part of a wider pathology, which can be degenerative, traumatic or neurological. Degenerative and traumatic tears are almost always associated with tears of other tendons of the rotator cuff. Usually, the supraspinatus and infraspinatus are torn concomitantly, resulting in a massive cuff tear. The axillary nerve can be involved in neurological diseases such as Parsonage-Turner syndrome resulting in teres minor dysfunction. In these cases, the teres minor deficit is usually overshadowed by the deficit of the other muscles involved.

When teres minor dysfunction is not a part of wider pathology, a diagnosis of quadrilateral space syndrome should be considered. There are also case reports of congenital absence of teres minor [1, 2].

Pillar 1: Clinical History

Teres minor weakness is most commonly seen in the context of a loss of function (external rotation in abduction) in patients with massive rotator cuff tears. Most patients with massive rotator cuff tears do retain teres minor function. Only 3.2% of patients with a rotator cuff tear have been found to have an atrophic teres minor [2], although higher levels were observed with the combined supraspinatus and infraspinatus tears. Identifying the minority group of patients with a deficient teres minor is important, as they can be counselled preoperatively regarding poorer function following surgery. Involvement of teres minor in massive rotator cuff tears signifies a higher risk of irreparability. In reconstructive procedures such as lattisimus dorsi transfer, a concomitant teres minor tear is associated with an inferior outcome and is hence a relative contraindication.

Reverse total shoulder replacement (TSR) has become an important technique for the management of severe rotator cuff pathology, such as rotator cuff arthropathy. As such, there is increasing interest in factors that will optimise the function of patients receiving a reverse total shoulder replacement. External rotation, particularly in abduction is important. Patients losing this function may struggle with everyday activities such as feeding and hair brushing. Patients undergoing reverse

TSR who are teres minor deficient will have poorer function and worse outcome scores compared to patients who have a functioning teres minor [3]. Boileau et al. describe a technique of combined latissimus dorsi and teres major transfer, recommending it for patients requiring a reverse TSR who have a deficient teres minor and lack active elevation and external rotation [4].

Teres minor weakness may present as a rare cause of weakness and pain associated with compression of the axillary nerve. Known as Quadrilateral space syndrome, this is an uncommon, and often difficult to diagnose cause of pain and weakness in the shoulder [5]. Quadrilateral space syndrome is caused by the compression of the axillary nerve (or its branch to teres minor) and the posterior humeral circumflex artery as it passes through the quadrilateral space.

The clinical picture is usually that of a dull, diffuse pain over the posterolateral aspect of the shoulder often affecting young, sporty male patients. It generally affects the dominant arm, often in throwing athletes. Compression of the axillary nerve can cause atrophy with subsequent weakness, of both teres minor and deltoid. Compression can also cause paraesthesia in the sensory distribution of the axillary nerve (skin overlying the lateral deltoid).

Causes of quadrilateral space syndrome may include compression from teres minor, space occupying lesions in the quadrilateral space and trauma to the shoulder. Hypertrophy of teres minor and abnormal fascial bands within the quadrilateral space have been described, both of which have been implicated as the reason teres minor compresses the axillary nerve. Chafik et al. have investigated this on cadaveric specimens [6]. They found no abnormal fascial bands but postulated that a fascial sling formed by the combined fascia of the deltoid, infraspinatus, teres minor, and long head of the triceps compressed the nerve to teres minor. However, the main limitation of this study is that the cadavers were not known to have any pathology and did not match the demographics of patients with quadrilateral space syndrome.

Pillar 2: The Conventional Examination

External rotation of the shoulder is a movement produced by a combination of muscles. Teres minor is a contributor, but there is also substantial involvement of both infraspinatus and the posterior fibres of deltoid. It is not possible to isolate the functions of an intact teres minor and infraspinatus, but their combined function can be assessed independently of the deltoid by abducting the shoulder to 90° [7].

In a healthy rotator cuff only approximately 20% of external rotation strength is provided by teres minor [8]. However, in patients with a ruptured infraspinatus, isolated assessment of teres minor function can be made. In this situation, the teres minor can become hypertrophied preserving external rotation function. Even in patients with a ruptured teres minor (along with ruptured infraspinatus and supraspinatus) external rotation in abduction is often maintained, with 66% of patients retaining this function [9]. Repeated external rotation in abduction to test for fatiguability may unmask such a weakness.

Clinical findings for quadrilateral space syndrome are limited. Tenderness over the quadrilateral space at the site of the axillary nerve compression may be present. This is located on the posterior aspect of the shoulder, approximately 2–3 cm inferior to the typical posterior arthroscopy portal site. Other potential and usually subtle clinical findings for quadrilateral space syndrome include wasting of the teres minor and deltoid, as well as some mildly altered sensation over the regimental badge area (area innervated by the axillary nerve) [10].

Pillar 3: Special Tests

Testing of teres minor integrity and strength becomes relevant in the case of massive rotator cuff tears when one needs to identify any residual posterior cuff function. The following tests allow the surgeon to assess this. As with all tests of power in the shoulder, the examiner should be wary of pain inhibition, which can easily result in a falsely positive outcome.

The drop sign was described as a test for assessing infraspinatus [11]. The drop sign is a lag sign evaluated with the shoulder in 90° abduction in the scapular plane, and the elbow flexed to 90°. The shoulder is then externally rotated to 90°, and the patient is asked to maintain the position against gravity (Medical Research Council Grade 3). Failure to resist gravity and subsequent internal rotation of the shoulder is considered a positive drop sign (Fig. 17.1). When assessed by Collin et al. as a test for teres minor integrity in massive cuff tears, the drop sign had a sensitivity of 87% and a specificity of 88% [9].

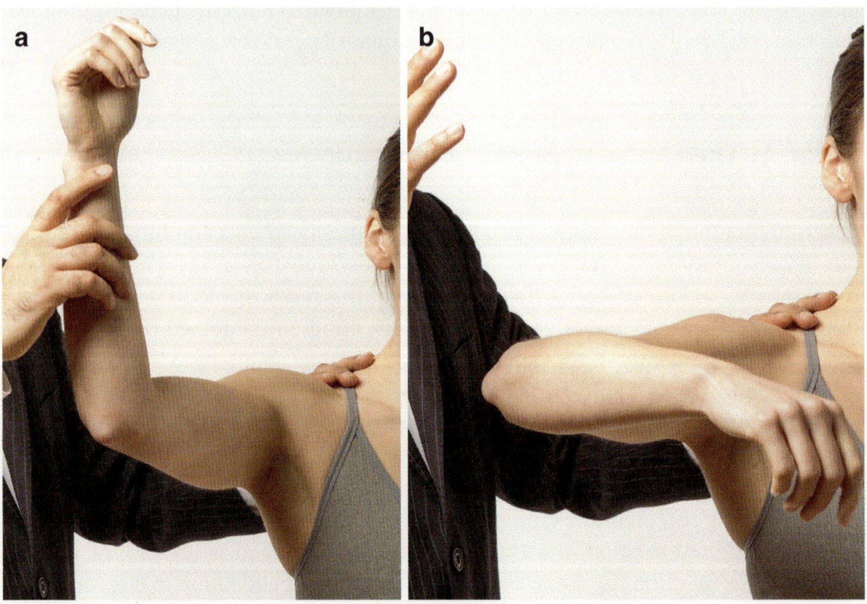

Fig. 17.1 Drop sign starting position (**a**) and a positive sign (**b**). Image Published under License from www.shoulderdoc.co.uk and www.shoulderpedia.org

External rotation lag sign greater than 40° was originally described by Hertel as a test for assessing the integrity of the supraspinatus and infraspinatus tendons [11]. The test is performed with the patient seated. The shoulder is abducted to 20° in the plane of the scapula, and the elbow is flexed to 90°. The examiner supports the elbow and externally rotates the shoulder to its maximal rotation (minus 5° to allow for elastic recoil). The forearm is then released, a positive result occurs when the forearm lags/drops more than 10° (Fig. 17.2). Collin et al. assessed this test for evaluating teres minor function in the presence of massive cuff tears [9]. They found a lag of greater than 40° to be the most accurate test for teres minor dysfunction. An external rotation lag sign (greater than 40°) was found to have a sensitivity of 100% and a specificity of 92%.

The Patte test/Hornblower sign is performed by passively moving the patient's arm into the following position [9]. The shoulder is abducted to 90° in the scapular plane, the elbow is flexed to 90°, and the shoulder is in neutral rota-

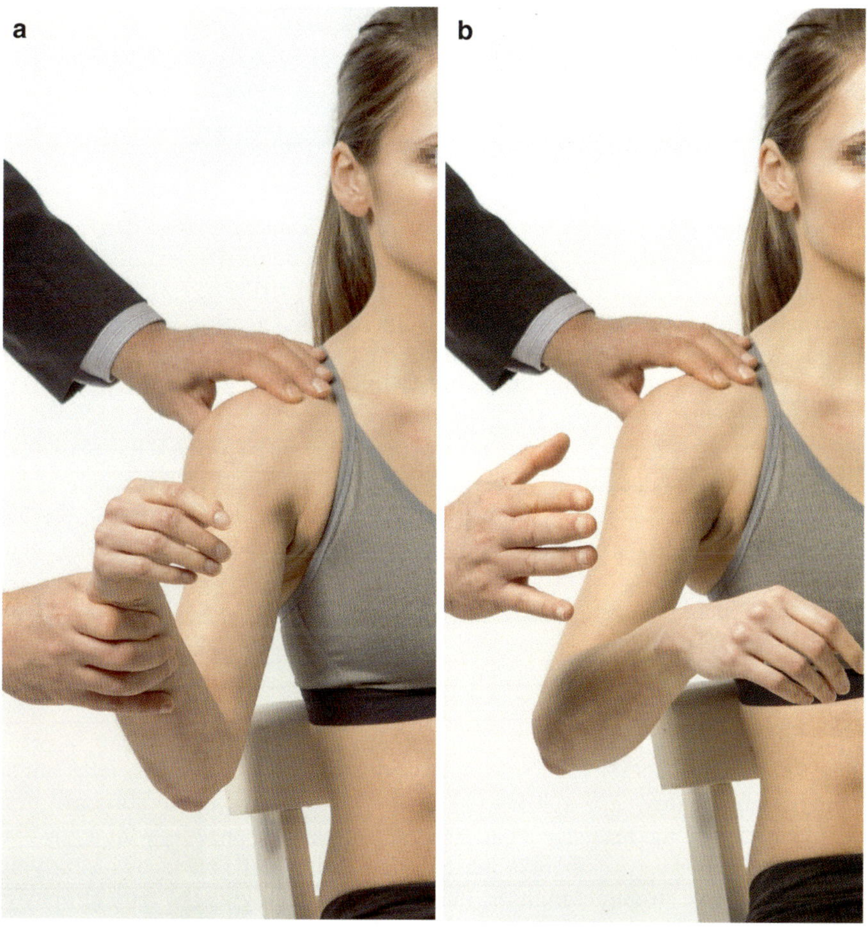

Fig. 17.2 External rotation lag sign starting position (**a**) and a positive sign (**b**). Image Published under License from www.shoulderdoc.co.uk and www.shoulderpedia.org

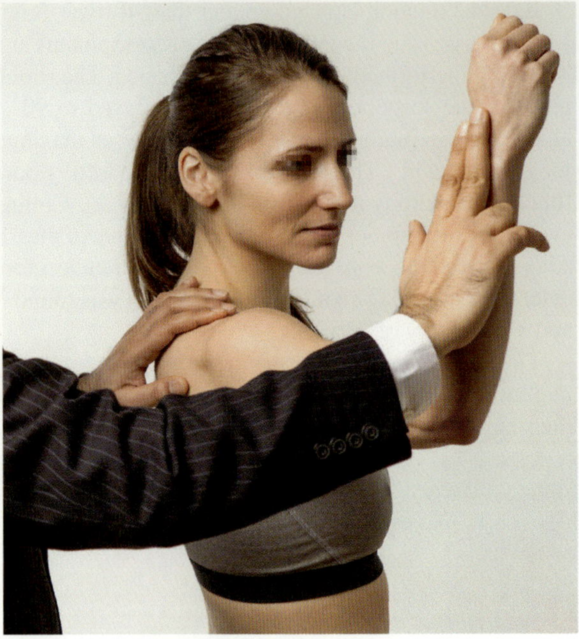

Fig. 17.3 Patte test. Image Published under License from www.shoulderdoc.co.uk and www.shoulderpedia.org

tion. The patient is then asked to actively external rotate the shoulder from this position against resistance. A positive Patte test is defined as external rotation power less than Medical Research Council Grade 4 (Fig. 17.3). Walch et al. reported 100% sensitivity and 93% specificity for detecting irreparable teres minor degeneration in patients with combined supraspinatus and infraspinatus tears [12]. Collin et al.'s study found the Patte test to have a sensitivity of 93% and a specificity of 72% [9].

A provocation test for quadrilateral space syndrome is to ask the patient to perform resisted abduction and external rotation of the shoulder, this recreates the position in which the contents of the quadrilateral space are compressed. A positive finding would be exacerbation of the patient's posterior shoulder pain (Fig. 17.4) [10].

Pillar 4: Investigations

Magnetic resonance (MR) imaging is the optimum modality to assess teres minor integrity and quality, although US [13] and CT may also pick up abnormalities. MR can identify the presence of an intact teres minor in patients with a massive rotator cuff tear. An assessment of muscle quality can also be made, by quantifying the level of fatty atrophy within the muscle [14]. A high grade of fatty atrophy is important in two situations. Firstly, patients with a massive cuff tear and a high

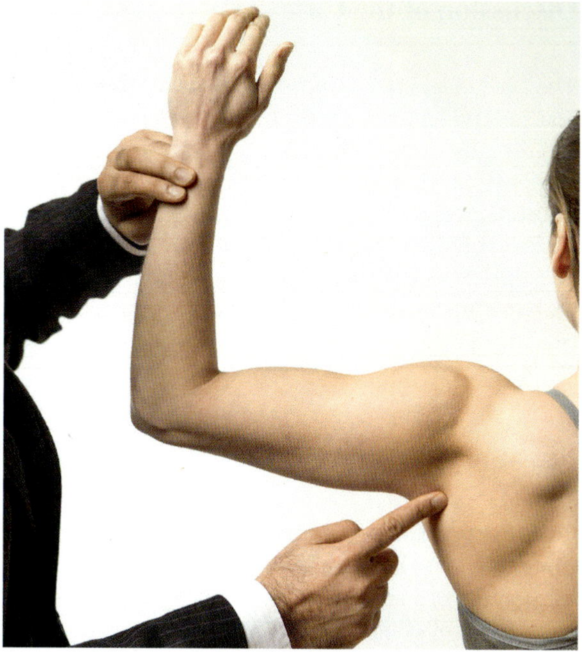

Fig. 17.4 Quad space syndrome provocation test. Image Published under License from www.shoulderdoc.co.uk and www.shoulderpedia.org

grade of fatty atrophy in their remaining posterior cuff (i.e., Goutallier grade 3 or 4) are unlikely to retain good external rotation power. Secondly, the finding of isolated teres minor atrophy with an otherwise healthy cuff. This in combination with the correct clinical picture would confirm a diagnosis of quadrilateral space syndrome [15, 16].

Imaging will also identify space-occupying lesions in the quadrilateral space, which can be a rare cause of quadrilateral space syndrome. Reported cases include para labral cysts [17], osteochondromas [18], and bone spikes [19]. In the presence of cysts, an MR arthrogram is helpful to assess any corresponding labral pathology.

As always radiological findings should be correlated with the clinical findings, as studies have shown an incidence of isolated teres minor atrophy in patients with no symptoms of quadrilateral space syndrome [20].

Arteriograms may also be used to assess for any related pathology to the posterior humeral circumflex artery, which also passes through the quadrilateral space.

Electrophysiological tests (EMG, NCV) are useful to assess axillary nerve function/entrapment in quadrilateral space. As well as investigating for teres minor pathology, electrophysiological testing can also exclude other neuromuscular causes of shoulder symptoms such as Parsonage-Turner syndrome.

Quadrilateral space syndrome can cause EMG abnormalities to both teres minor and deltoid, as well as delayed motor conduction time in the axillary nerve on NCS [21]. However, unlike other diagnostic tests, electrophysiological testing will not help identify the underlying pathological cause of dysfunction.

Discussion of the Case

The case discussed earlier in the chapter represents a patient with massive cuff tear involving teres minor. In the setting of an irreparable cuff tear or cuff tear arthropathy, treatment options include a reverse total shoulder replacement. A reverse total shoulder replacement does not restore external rotation strength in the abducted position, which is needed for activities such as hair combing. The patient should, therefore, be appropriately counselled preoperatively. It may be possible to restore active external rotation in the abducted position by augmenting the reverse total shoulder replacement with an appropriate tendon transfer.

Summary

Teres minor tears are rare in isolation but usually present with massive posterosuperior cuff tears. The presence of a teres minor tear is a negative prognostic factor for reparability of a massive cuff tear, and need special attention in cases of reverse total shoulder replacement performed for massive cuff tears/cuff arthropathy. Teres minor weakness in the presence of a normal supraspinatus and infraspinatus should raise the suspicion of quadrilateral space syndrome. A summary of diagnostic clusters for teres minor are presented in Table 17.1.

Table 17.1 Short list of diagnostic clusters teres minor

Clinical history
1. Loss of function (external rotation in abduction) in patients with massive rotator cuff tears
2. Rare cause of weakness and pain associated with compression of axillary nerve; Quadrilateral Space Syndrome(QSS)
Conventional examination
3. Loss of external rotation power—particularly in abduction
4. Tenderness over teres minor/quadrilateral space
Special tests
5. Drop sign
6. External rotation lag sign
7. Patte test
8. Pain on resisted abduction and external rotation of the shoulder (QSS)
Investigations
9. MRI to assess tendon integrity and atrophy of muscle belly
10. NCS to evaluate axillary nerve function/entrapment in quadrilateral space

References

1. Kruse LM, Yamaguchi K, Keener JD, Chamberlain AM. Clinical outcomes after decompression of the nerve to the teres minor in patients with idiopathic isolated teres minor fatty atrophy. J Shoulder Elb Surg. 2015;24:628–33.
2. Melis B, DeFranco MJ, Lädermann A, Barthelemy R, Walch G. The teres minor muscle in rotator cuff tendon tears. Skelet Radiol. 2011;40:1335–44.
3. Simovitch R, Helmy N, Zumstein M, Gerber C. Impact of fatty infiltration of the teres minor muscle on the outcome of reverse total shoulder arthroplasty. J Bone Joint Surg Am. 2007;89(5):934–9.
4. Boileau P, Rumian AP, Zumstein MA. Reversed shoulder arthroplasty with modified L'Episcopo for combined loss of active elevation and external rotation. J Shoulder Elb Surg. 2010;19:20–30.
5. Cahill BR, Palmer RE. Quadrilateral space syndrome. J Hand Surg Am. 1983;8:65–9.
6. Chafik D, Galatz LM, Keener JD, Kim HM, Yamaguchi K. Teres minor muscle and related anatomy. J Shoulder Elb Surg. 2013;22:108–14.
7. Jenp YN, Malanga GA, Growney ES, An KN. Activation of the rotator cuff in generating isometric shoulder rotation torque. Am J Sports Med. 1996;24(4):477–85.
8. Gerber C, Blumenthal S, Curt A, Werner CM. Effect of selective experimental suprascapular nerve block on abduction and external rotation strength of the shoulder. J Shoulder Elb Surg. 2007;16:815–20.
9. Collin P, Treseder T, Denard PJ, Neyton L, Walch G, Lädermann A. What is the best clinical test for assessment of the teres minor in massive rotator cuff tears. Clin Orthop Relat Res. 2015;473:2959–66.
10. Hoskins WT, Pollard HP, McDonald AJ. Quadrilateral space syndrome: a case study and review of the literature. Br J Sports Med. 2005;39(2):e9.
11. Hertel R, Ballmer FT, Lombert SM, Gerber C. Lag signs in the diagnosis of rotator cuff rupture. J Shoulder Elb Surg. 1996;5(4):307–13.
12. Walch G, Boulahia A, Calderone S, Robinson AH. The 'dropping' and 'hornblower's' signs in evaluation of rotator-cuff tears. J Bone Joint Surg Br. 1998;80:624–8.
13. Brestas PS, Tsouroulas M, Nikolakopoulou Z, Malagari K, Drossos C. Ultrasound findings of teres minor denervation in suspected quadrilateral space syndrome. J Clin Ultrasound. 2006;34(7):343–7.
14. Goutallier D, Postel JM, Bernageau J, Lavau L, Voisin MC. Fatty muscle degeneration in cuff ruptures. Pre- and postoperative evaluation by CT scan. Clin Orthop Relat Res. 1994;(304):78–83.
15. Linker CS, Helms CA, Fritz RC. Quadrilateral space syndrome: findings at MR imaging. Radiology. 1993;188(3):675–6.
16. Elsayes KM, Shariff A, Staveteig PT, Mukundan G, Khosla A, Rubin DA. Value of magnetic resonance imaging for muscle denervation syndromes of the shoulder girdle. J Comput Assist Tomogr. 2005;29(3):326–9.
17. Robinson P, White LM, Lax M, Salonen D, Bell RS. Quadrilateral space syndrome caused by glenoid labral cyst. AJR Am J Roentgenol. 2000;175(4):1103–5.
18. Cirpar M, Gudemez E, Cetik O, Uslu M, Eksioglu F. Quadrilateral space syndrome caused by a humeral osteochondroma: a case report and review of literature. HSS J. 2006;2(2):154–6.
19. Amin MF, Berst M, el-Khoury GY. An unusual cause of the quadrilateral space impingement syndrome by a bone spike. Skelet Radiol. 2006;35(12):956–8.
20. Sofka CM, Lin J, Feinberg J, Potter HG. Teres minor denervation on routine magnetic resonance imaging of the shoulder. Skelet Radiol. 2004;33(9):514–8.
21. Kallio MA, Kovala TT, Niemelä EN, Huuskonen UE, Tolonen EU. Shoulder pain and an isolated teres minor nerve lesion. J Clin Neurophysiol. 2011;28(5):524–7.

Chapter 18
Trapezius

S. Russell, J. Thomas, and J. Walton

Case History

A 45-year-old lady presents with burning pain over the trapezius and weakness of the shoulder girdle. She had a cervical lymph node biopsy 6 months ago, following which she had developed these symptoms. Examination reveals loss of trapezial contour, a lower shoulder level on the affected side, loss of active elevation beyond 120° and a well preserved passive elevation. Scapula winging, triangle test and active elevation lag sign were positive.

Introduction

The trapezius muscle is a large flat triangular muscle that extends from the skull to the shoulder girdle. It originates from the medial third of the superior nuchal line and external occipital protuberance of the occiput, the ligamentum nuchae and the spinous processes of C7–T12. The upper fibres run downwards and laterally attaching to the posterior border of the lateral third of the clavicle. The middle fibres run horizontally to the medial border of the acromion and upper border of the crest of the spine of the scapula. The lower fibres run upwardly converging into a tendon which attaches to the inferior edge of the medial edge of the scapula spine (Fig. 18.1). A bursa separates the middle fibres from the spine of the scapula [1].

The trapezius is innervated by the spinal part of the accessory nerve (XI) which enters it from the posterior triangle. It also receives sensory innervation from the ventral rami of C3 and C4 via the cervical plexus. The dermatome is supplied by the

S. Russell (✉) • J. Thomas • J. Walton
Wrightington Hospital, Wigan, UK
e-mail: Sarah.Russell@wwl.nhs.uk

© Springer International Publishing AG 2017

P. Monga, L. Funk (eds.), *Diagnostic Clusters in Shoulder Conditions*,
DOI 10.1007/978-3-319-57334-2_18

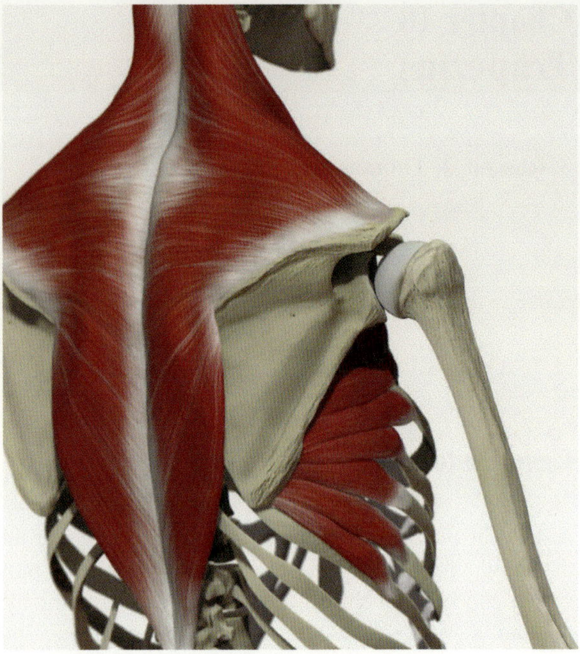

Fig. 18.1 Trapezius anatomy. Image Published under License from www.shoulderdoc.co.uk

Table 18.1 The three functional components of the trapezius

Component	Function
Upper fibres	The upper fibres elevate the shoulder girdle maintaining the shoulder position against gravity or upper limb load. When contracted bilaterally they can extend the neck, but unilaterally can produce side flexion of the cervical spine
Middle fibres	The middle horizontal fibres pull the scapula towards the midline resulting in retraction. When combined, the upper and middle fibres draw the scapula backwards
Lower fibres	The lower fibres depress the scapula and rotate the inferior angle laterally

dorsal rami of C3-T12. The relative functional importance of two sources of nerve supply is still a matter of controversy [2].

The trapezius is a vital scapula stabiliser, allowing upper limb movement and function, and increases the possible range of motion of the shoulder. It elevates, retracts and rotates the scapula [3]. The trapezius works with lower components of serratus anterior as a force couple to rotate the scapula on the thoracic wall positioning the glenoid fossa to face upwards. This enables a greater range of shoulder movement [4]. The upper, middle and lower trapezius are functionally distinct (Table 18.1).

As a force couple, the counteracting muscles demonstrate obvious action when a movement is loaded or performed quickly [5]. One muscle (agonist) acts concentrically, whereas the other, the antagonist, acts eccentrically in a controlled, harmonised fashion, to produce a smooth movement. Also, these muscles may work by co-contraction or co-activation to provide a stabilising effect and joint control [5]. The role of trapezius as a force couple with serratus anterior continues throughout shoulder range motion and is of particular importance in the overhead position [6, 7]. The weakness of the trapezius muscle can alter scapular mechanics resulting in anterior secondary impingement.

Pillar 1: Clinical History

A thorough, detailed history should be taken to determine the onset of symptoms. This history should include hand dominance, occupation, medical history, surgical history of the shoulder, cervical spine, and breast. The principal functional limitation is difficulty in forward elevation with an extended arm, for example when lifting overhead or throwing [8].

Identification of trauma or iatrogenic cause is particularly helpful in determining the appropriate method of management [8]. An iatrogenic injury to the spinal accessory nerve during surgery or trauma will result in trapezius weakness [3]. This diagnosis is frequently delayed [9].

The spinal accessory nerve lies particularly superficially along its course, thus making it susceptible to trauma [3]. A history of a direct blow to the area, wound or bite to the neck may cause injury to the spinal accessory nerve, resulting in trapezius weakness [3]. The nerve is also susceptible to indirect trauma, for example via prolonged heavy lifting, or during a motor vehicle accident [3]. Although uncommon, there have also been reports of idiopathic spinal accessory nerve palsy [10].

Pain is centred around the levator scapulae and rhomboid minor. Typically patients will complain of pain and weakness. The patient may describe a history of generalised shoulder or upper arm pain, which can worsen on elevation of the upper limb, fatigue or stiffness. Pain may also be present when sitting for extended periods of time, for example when driving, due to the prominent scapular border [8].

The trapezius can refer pain from the occiput to the lateral aspect of the head, superior to ear, tip of jaw, the spinous processes to medial border of scapula and along spine of scapula; may also refer to the lateral aspect of the upper arm. Traction of the unsupported shoulder on the brachial plexus or even a sensory element in the spinal accessory nerve have both been proposed as possible causes of pain [11].

Paralysis of the trapezius muscle is usually neurogenic, via an injury to the spinal accessory nerve, which results in a shoulder droop and difficulty in shoulder movement, in particular abduction. Some patients retain almost full movement. Paralysis of the upper parts of trapezius results in the downward rotation of the acromion, and a markedly angulated acromion process with a loss of the smooth curve of the upper border between the occiput and the acromion process [3]. It can also present with winging of the scapula, which occurs because trapezius paralysis allows the medial border of the scapula to lift off the chest wall. The patient may also describe numbness over the angle of the jaw and around the ear due to the associated injury of the transverse cervical and great auricular nerves [1].

Trapezius damage is rare and difficult to diagnose. The physical examination must assess muscle power and pain provocation which may indicate a muscle lesion. A direct blow to the scapula leading to scapular muscle detachment may rarely be seen [12].

Pillar 2: Conventional Examination

The function of trapezius should be fully assessed when a patient presents with weakness of the arm and/or shoulder girdle. Many people can manage with a loss of trapezius function, but some have weakness and difficulty with manual and overhead activities.

The examiner should observe for signs of asymmetry. Upper Trapezius weakness or damage will result in drooping of the shoulder as the scapula is translated laterally and rotated downwards; their neckline will be asymmetric due to the lateral end of the clavicle dropping resulting in a more prominent clavicle superior border. The middle and lower trapezius weakness or damage will result in a more prominent medial border and inferior angle [10]. Disruption in the muscle bulk contours of trapezius can arise from a tear from bony detachments from muscle insertions due to traction type injuries. Trapezius wasting can be caused by disuse or deneravtion.

To palpate all three parts of the trapezius muscle, the patient must be in combined abduction to 90°, full external rotation, and elbow flexion to 90°. In this position, each of the three components can be easily identified on palpation, and in a lean patient may also be visualised. A hollow may be palpable between C6 and T3 which correspond to the triangular aponeurosis [1]. The course of the muscle should be palpated and compared contra-laterally. Increased muscle tone/spasm or wasting should be noted. Wasting will occur unilaterally with pathology to the trapezius. Increase tone of levator scapulae may be present as a compensatory effort in the presence of a trapezius deficit, especially in the absence of the upper fibres of trapezius.

When assessing trapezius activity the ability to elevate the arm will be reduced, and the patient may present with other compensatory efforts [10]. The weakness of the trapezius may result in winging of the scapula similar to that of serratus weakness. However, there will be more of a lateral displacement of the scapula through range [13].

The examiner should exclude spinal pathology. Symptoms of which would include altered sensation, pins and needles in the C3–4 dermatome (lateral aspects of head and neck). Equally, the patient should have normal reflexes [5]. On testing upper limb sensation, a sensory alteration may be present due to brachial plexus symptoms resulting from traction forces caused by a downwardly rotated and depressed shoulder girdle.

Pillar 3: Special Tests

In patients who have a winging scapula at rest, the trapezius muscle's ability to maintain a neutral scapula can be assessed by asking the patient to retract their scapula to neutral and maintain this position. The arm should remain by their side.

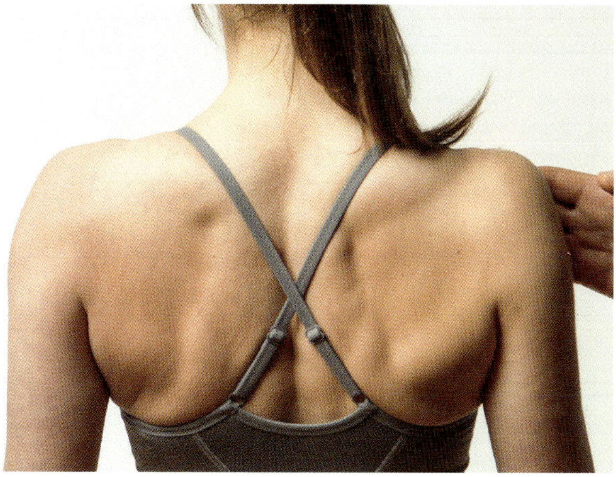

Fig. 18.2 Scapula retraction test. Image Published under License from www.shoulderdoc.co.uk and www.shoulderpedia.org

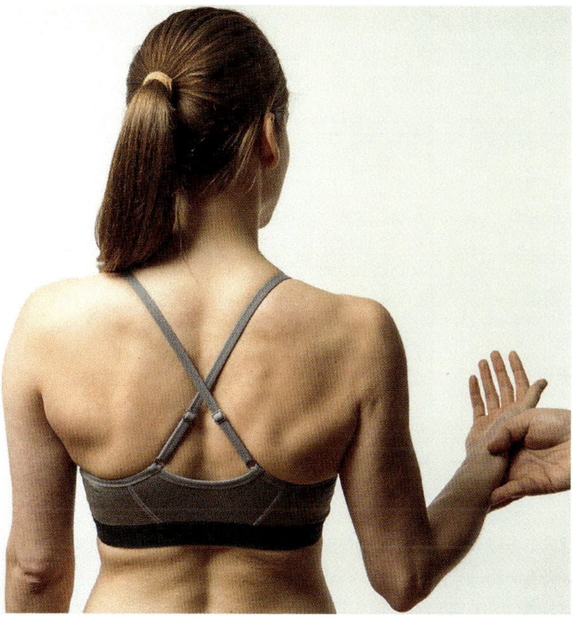

Fig. 18.3 Winging provocation test. Image Published under License from www.shoulderdoc.co.uk and www.shoulderpedia.org

A positive test is an inability to achieve a neutral scapula. In some cases, the patient may not have the proprioceptive awareness to be able to achieve this position. If the test is positive, the examiner may provide manual assistance to achieve neutral, and then ask the patient to actively maintain the position (Fig. 18.2). Chan et al. [14] suggest an additional test for accessory nerve palsy, requiring the patient to externally rotate the shoulder against a force provided by the examiner's hand. Any medial winging of the scapula is indicative of accessory nerve palsy (Fig. 18.3).

Triangle Test: The patient lies in prone with both arms elevated. As the patient is instructed to further elevate the arms to full elevation, in the presence of trapezius weakness, the patient is unable to elevate the arm in this plane, producing a lag. The

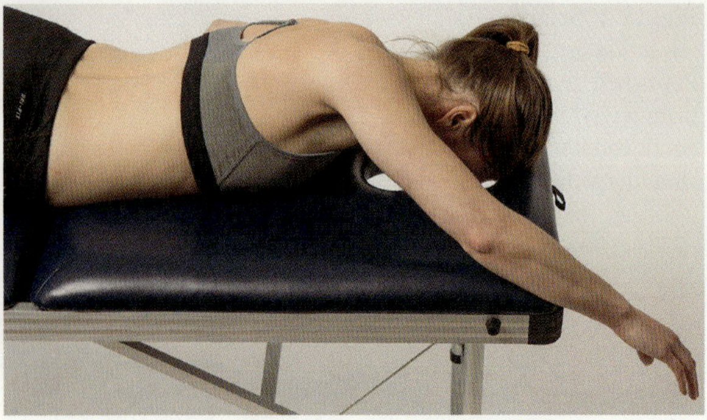

Fig. 18.4 A positive triangle test. Image Published under License from www.shoulderdoc.co.uk and www.shoulderpedia.org

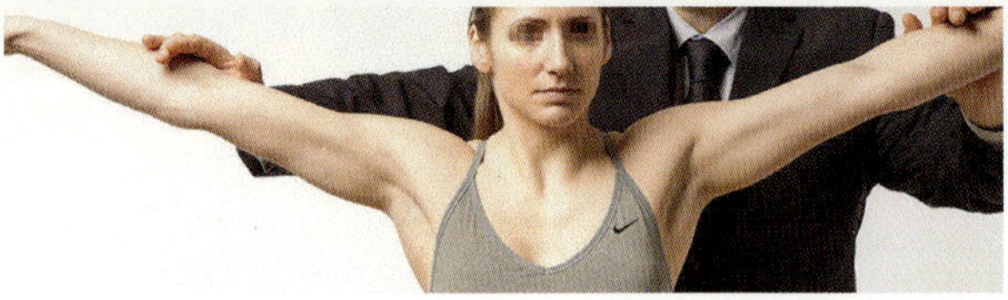

Fig. 18.5 Trapezius composite assessment. Image Published under License from www.shoulderdoc.co.uk and www.shoulderpedia.org

Table 18.2 Specific strength testing for trapezius weakness

Component	Test
Upper	Elevating the shoulder with the arm slightly abducted or by elevating the shoulder against resisted shoulder abduction and ipsilateral head side flexion simultaneously (Fig. 18.6)
Middle	In prone with arm abducted to 90° and externally rotated. The examiner retracts the shoulder then gives resistance over the scapula near the posterior glenoid. The examiner resists retraction of the shoulder by providing resistance over the scapula near the glenohumeral joint (Fig. 18.7)
Lower	In prone lying with the arm abducted to 120° and the shoulder externally rotated. The examiner retracts the shoulder then gives resistance to the patient retraction over the scapula near the posterior glenoid (Fig. 18.8)

patient compensates by hyperextending the lumbar spine to attempt to reach further resulting in a triangle sign (Fig. 18.4) [15].

When testing the trapezius, the patient is asked to abduct and extend the arm against resistance (Fig. 18.5). To accurately test the three different components of trapezius the following positions are tested see Table 18.2.

Pillar 4: Investigations

Gleno-humeral, scapular and thoracic plain radiographs can exclude bony pathology [8]. Nerve conduction studies and EMG are the gold standard diagnostic for trapezius weakness. Currently, electromyographic testing is the only definitive

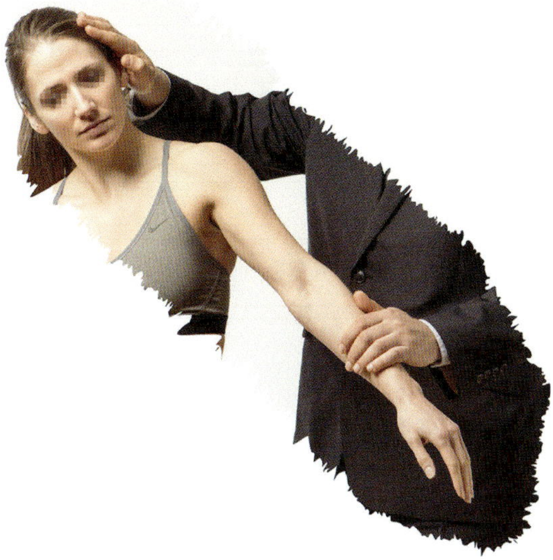

Fig. 18.6 Upper trapezius strength test. Image Published under License from www.shoulderdoc.co.uk and www.shoulderpedia.org

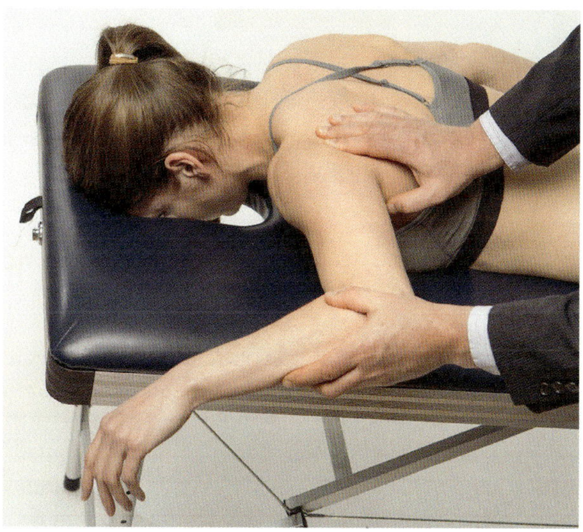

Fig. 18.7 Middle trapezius strength test. Image Published under License from www.shoulderdoc.co.uk and www.shoulderpedia.org

diagnostic test for trapezius weakness and is essential for determining which muscle is involved and to what degree of denervation. Although diagnostically helpful in determining muscle involvement and detecting improvement and reinnervation, the initial degree of denervation cannot be used to predict the extent of recovery [16].

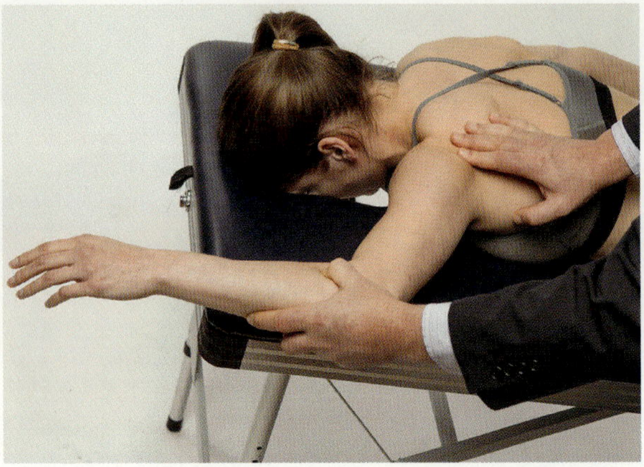

Fig. 18.8 Lower trapezius strength test. Image Published under License from www.shoulderdoc.co.uk and www.shoulderpedia.org

Computed tomography (CT) and magnetic resonant imaging (MRI) are rarely needed but may be useful to rule out other diagnoses, such as neurofibromatosis-related injury [17], disk disease and radiculopathy [18], mass lesions [10] or scapular muscle detachment [12].

Discussion of the Case

The index case represents an iatrogenic injury to the spinal accessory nerve leading to trapezius palsy. EMG and NCV studies were confirmatory. In diagnosing such unusual presentations, a cluster approach remains essential as over-reliance on clinical examination or neurophysiology on its own is insufficient.

Summary

Trapezius weakness and palsy are rare. Weakness can have a debilitating effect on upper limb function. The weakness can occur from a range of mechanisms and pathology. Traumatic, iatrogenic and prolonged lifting have been described as potential events leading onto this condition. A detailed, thorough history and examination supported by EMG and NCV studies is paramount to gain an accurate diagnosis. MRI scan of the scapular region and spine is useful to rule our scapular muscle detachment or mechanical reasons for neural compromise. A summary of the main diagnostic clusters is listed in Table 18.3.

Table 18.3 Summary of diagnostic clusters for trapezius weakness

Clinical history
1. Trauma—direct blow or traction
2. Iatrogenic—neck biopsy/ surgery
3. Developmental—Sprengle's deformity
4. Insidious onset of weakness of the arm and/or shoulder girdle
5. Pain over trapezius referral pattern: occiput, lateral aspect of head, superior to ear, tip of jaw, spinous processes to medial border of scapula and along spine of scapula. Asymmetry of the shoulder girdle
Conventional examination
6. Loss of contour over the trapezius muscle bulk
7. Superior border scapula winging and drooping of the shoulder
Special tests
8. Triangle Test
9. Specific strength testing for upper, mid and lower trapezius
Investigations
10. NCS/EMG studies for the spinal accessory nerve and trapezius

References

1. Palastanga N, Field D, Soames R. Anatomy and human movement structure and function. 2nd ed. UK: Butterworth-Heinemann; 1994.
2. Kim JH, Choi KY, Lee KH, Lee DJ, Park BJ, Rho YS. Motor innervation of the trapezius muscle: intraoperative motor conduction study during neck dissection. ORL J Otorhinolaryngol Relat Spec. 2014;76:8–12.
3. Martin RM, Fish DE. Scapular winging: anatomical review, diagnosis and treatments. Curr Rev Muscoskelet Med. 2008;1(1):1–11.
4. Frame MK. Anatomy and biomechanics of the shoulder. In: Donatelli RA, editor. Clinics in physical therapy, physical therapy of the shoulder. Edinburgh: Churchill Livingstone; 1991. p. 1–18.
5. Magee DJ. Orthopaedic physical assessment. 5th ed. Philadelphia, PA: W. B. Saunders; 2008.
6. Bagg SD, Forrest WJ. Electromyographic study of the scapular rotators during arm abduction in the scapular plane. Am J Phys Med. 1986;65(3):111–24.
7. Magarey ME, Jones MA. Dynamic evaluation and early management of altered motor control around the shoulder complex. Man Ther. 2003;8(4):195–206.
8. Lee S, Savin DD, Shah NR, Bronsnick D, Goldberg B. Scapular winging: evaluation and treatment. J Bone Joint Surg Am. 2015;97(20):1708–16.
9. Nakamichi K, Tachibana S. Iatrogenic injury of the spinal accessory nerve. Results of repair. J Bone Joint Surg Am. 1998;80:1616–21.
10. Wiater JM, Bigliani LU. Spinal accessory nerve injury. Clinical Orthop Relat Res. 1999;368:5–16.
11. Symes A, Ellis H. Variations in the surface anatomy of the spinal accessory nerve in the posterior triangle. Surg Radiol Anat. 2005;27(5):404–8.
12. Kibler WB, Sciascia A, Uhl T. Medial scapular muscle detachment: clinical presentation and surgical treatment. J Shoulder Elb Surg. 2014;23(1):58–67.

13. Buschbacher RM. Practical guide to musculoskeletal disorders diagnosis and rehabilitation. 2nd ed. UK: Butterworth-Heinemann; 2002.
14. Chan PK, Hems TE. Clinical signs of accessory nerve palsy. J Trauma. 2006;60:1142–4.
15. Levy O, Relwani JG, Mullett H, Haddo O, Even T. The active elevation lag sign and the triangle sign: new clinical signs of trapezius palsy. J Shoulder Elb Surg. 2009;18(4):573–6.
16. Friedenberg SM, Zimprich T, Harper CM. The natural history of the long thoracic and spinal accessory neuropathies. Muscle Nerve. 2002;25:535–9.
17. Van Tuijl JH, Schmid A, Van Kranen-Mastenbroek VHJM, Faber CG, Vles JSH. Isolated spinal accessory neuropathy in an adolescent: a case study. Eur J Paediatr Neurol. 2006;10(2):83–5.
18. Makin GJ, Brown WF, Ebers GC. C7 radiculopathy: importance of scapular winging in clinical diagnosis. J Neurol Neurosurg Psychiatry. 1986;49(6):640–4.

Chapter 19
Pectoralis Major

U. Butt

Case Example

A 25-year male presents with sudden onset pain and deformity over the anterior chest wall. He describes himself as a "fitness enthusiast" and sustained this injury while performing a bench press at the gym. Clinical examination revealed bruising over the medial aspect of the arm and also over the chest wall. There was a loss of definition of the anterior axially fold with a positive "dropped nipple" sign.

Introduction

The pectorals major comprises clavicular and sternal components, the latter forming the bulk of the muscle [1–3]. It is a large fan-shaped muscle inserting into the lateral crista of the bicipital groove in a J-shaped fashion. The arrangement of the fibres near the insertion is such that the inferior fibres form the deep arm of the "J", hence producing a rolled inferior margin. This rounded inferior margin forms the bulk of the anterior axillary fold. The sternal component forms the majority of the tendinous attachment and lies deep to the clavicular part at the humeral insertion [1–3].

The pectoralis major (PM) is important for maximal power activity of the shoulder. It primarily acts as an adductor and internal rotator of the arm. Rupture of the pectoralis major (PM) tendon is a relatively rare but important condition. It has been gaining wider traction in the literature and reported incidence is rising possibly as a result of increased public interest in health, fitness and strenuous sporting activity [1–3]. It is easily misdiagnosed, particularly as it often presents to non-specialists in the first instance.

U. Butt
Salford Royal NHS Foundation Trust, Salford, UK
e-mail: usmanbutt02@yahoo.co.uk

© Springer International Publishing AG 2017

P. Monga, L. Funk (eds.), *Diagnostic Clusters in Shoulder Conditions*,
DOI 10.1007/978-3-319-57334-2_19

Pillar 1: Clinical History

The clinical history and presentation are paramount in the diagnosis of ruptures of the pectoralis major (PM) tendon. Attention to the salient features in the history should arouse clinical suspicion, facilitating early diagnosis and management for improved outcomes and satisfaction [1–3].

The injury classically occurs in young, active and muscular males aged between 20–40 years old. Concurrent use of anabolic steroids is frequently observed. The patient typically gives a history of engaging in a strenuous activity with the arm abducted, extended and externally rotated at the time of injury. As the tendon fails, the patient may hear or feel a "pop", with the subsequent onset of pain and bruising around the medial arm and chest wall [1–3]. The bench-press is the most commonly associated activity with PM ruptures, though the condition has been described in association with many activities including wrestling, boxing, rugby, martial arts and gymnastics [3–7].

The importance of the history and mechanism of injury in the aetiology of these injuries cannot be overstated, especially since the physical examination findings can be equivocal in certain cases, such as partial tears and muscle belly tears. The mechanism of injury also sheds light on how these injuries occur; the PM tendon tends to rupture in a predictable sequence when eccentrically loaded with the inferior segments failing first [6]. In partial tears, the upper part (clavicular head) tends to be spared and can deceive the unsuspecting clinician not attentive to the finer points in the history (Fig. 19.1). Bony avulsion of the tendon has also been described [8] though this is exceptionally rare.

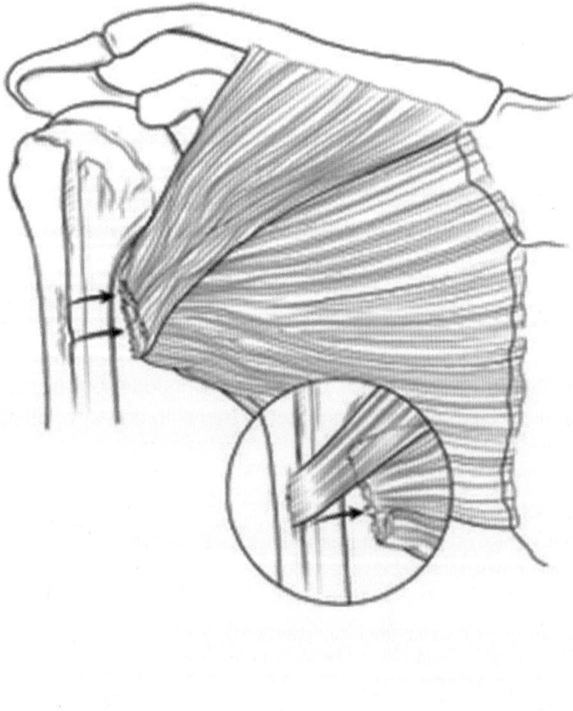

Fig. 19.1 Patho-anatomy of pectorals major tears. Reproduced from Provencher et al. [3]

Patients may describe a weakness in the shoulder when undertaking certain activities requiring adduction of the arm. This may not be apparent initially in the acute stage, but in the case of acute-on-chronic or chronic tears, patients will describe an inability to bench-press weights they previously could or may encounter difficulties in more mundane activities such as gathering a ball from the ground or even fluffing pillows.

Given the cohort of patients that this injury commonly affects, the chest wall asymmetry that results can give rise to major cosmetic concerns. Indeed this may be the primary reason for presentation.

While the vast majority of PM ruptures occur in the young male demographic described, there are less frequent reports described in females and those of varying age [9]. A second focal incidence is described in elderly patients that can occur in association with relatively stressful activities such as manual transfers [10].

Pillar 2: Physical Examination

In the acute setting, ecchymosis may be present along the medial aspect of the upper arm in the region of the PM insertion and along the chest wall in the region of the muscle belly. Swelling in these areas may be notable as a result of bleeding and haematoma formation, as well as from the bunched up and medially retracted PM muscle belly. There is likely to be pain exacerbated by attempted active or passive motion of the arm. These findings tend to develop within the first few hours following injury and may take up to 3–6 weeks to resolve [3].

It is imperative that one looks at the contour of the anterior axillary fold which will be thinned or absent in full thickness tears (Fig. 19.2); this feature can be accentuated by passively abducting the arm or asking the patient to actively adduct their shoulders against resistance (pain allowing). [1, 2]. There may be a "dropped nipple" sign when compared to the contralateral nipple [11].

Failure to appreciate the early clues in the history and the early physical signs often leads to delays in referral for definitive management. At subsequent presentation, the early signs may be absent but the hard signs of asymmetry that include a medially retracted and/or atrophic muscle belly, loss or thinning of the anterior axillary fold and a "dropped nipple" will typically still be present. Delayed management

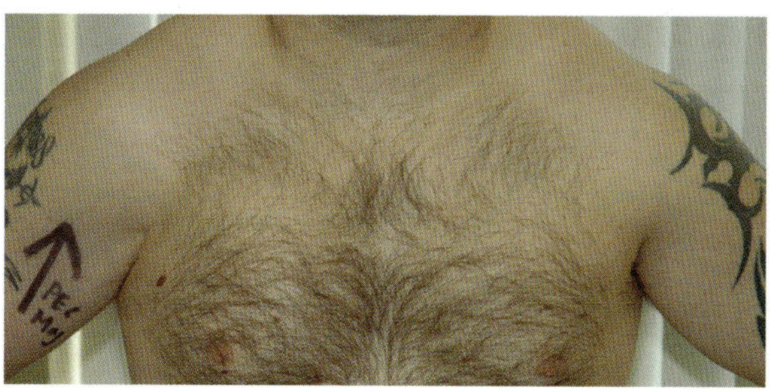

Fig. 19.2 Right sided pectoralis major rupture. Image Published under License from www.shoulderpedia.org

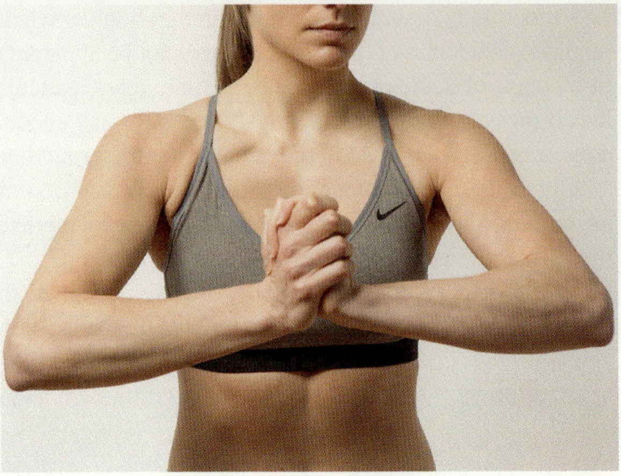

Fig. 19.3 Assessing pectoralis major using resisted adduction. Image Published under License from www.shoulderdoc.co.uk and www.shoulderpedia.org

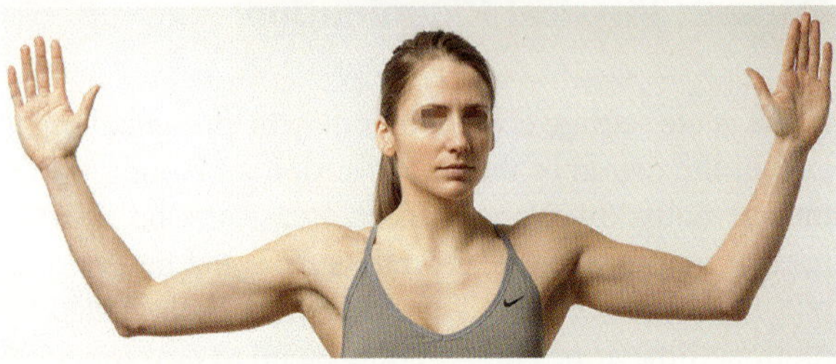

Fig. 19.4 Passive abduction to assess pectoralis major contour. Image Published under License from www.shoulderdoc.co.uk and www.shoulderpedia.org

can still yield good results and so regardless of the time of injury; it is important to make the diagnosis and refer appropriately.

Pillar 3: Special Tests

To aid in the diagnosis of PM ruptures two tests can be employed. They are designed to accentuate the altered or absent contour of the anterior axillary fold. These can be performed by asking the patient to clasp their hands and push in (resisted adduction) or by elevating the arm passively (passive abduction) (Figs. 19.3 and 19.4).

Pillar 4: Investigations

An understanding of the presenting features of PM ruptures combined with a considered and careful physical examination will frequently leave little doubt as to the diagnosis. Where uncertainty remains, adjunctive imaging can assist. However, the imaging must be focussed. If generic imaging of the shoulder is undertaken, a PM rupture will be overlooked. The true value of imaging in PM ruptures is to aid the surgeon in his/her definitive surgical planning. An MRI is useful in delineating the level of the injury in full thickness tears. Tendinous avulsions have significantly better outcomes that muscular injuries and such information can help prognosticate pre-operatively. Partial ruptures and muscular injuries can be defined preoperatively using MR scans and hence avoid unnecessary surgery in selected cases.

Plain radiographs can identify the presence of a bony avulsion and can be useful to identify other concomitant skeletal injuries or dislocations around the shoulder girdle. Specific findings have been described relating to the PM soft tissue shadow [2], however these should not be relied upon for decision-making.

Ultrasound is a readily available modality of investigation that can be useful where the diagnosis is in doubt or where there is an unacceptable delay to magnetic resonance imaging (MRI) [1–3]. However, it is operator dependent and is not of great use in surgical planning. Ultrasound is useful in assessing the post-operative integrity of a repaired pectoralis major tendon.

MRI is the imaging modality of choice [12] as it better enables complete characterisation of the tear and aids the surgeon in planning operative management. It is important for the requesting clinician to note that a standard shoulder sequence will not be sufficient to fully evaluate a PM rupture. Dedicated scanning sequences should be performed in the plane of the pectoralis muscle. This should be done in consultation with an experienced musculoskeletal radiologist to avoid inaccurate requests and unnecessary scans.

Discussion of the Case

The young man described at the start of the chapter is an example of a typical presentation of pectoralis major rupture. An early MRI scan of the anterior chest wall to include the pectoralis major confirmed the tear to be a full thickness tear of the PM sternal head. Surgery was offered and performed urgently, following a discussion regarding risks, benefits and recovery periods.

Summary

Ruptures of the pectoralis major tendon frequently present to clinicians inexperienced in their management given the relatively rarity of the condition. However, with careful attention to the mechanism of injury and presenting features, combined with an understanding of the physical signs, the diagnosis can be made confidently on clinical grounds. Even in the chronic setting, the history and physical features reliably point to the diagnosis. Imaging is helpful to confirm the diagnosis in equivocal cases, but the most important use is in surgical planning. Generic imaging of the shoulder may not detect this injury, and so imaging must be requested in consultation with a specialist musculoskeletal radiologist. A summary of diagnostic clusters for pectoralis major ruptures is described in Table 19.1.

Table 19.1 Summary of diagnostic clusters for pectorals major ruptures

Clinical history
1. Young male performing bench press exercise or other strenuous activity particularly with the arm abducted, extended and externally rotated
2. Concomitant use of steroids
3. Sudden pain and "popping" sensation upper extremity
4. Cosmetic concern
Conventional examination
5. Ecchymosis and swelling to chest wall and upper extremity
6. Loss of anterior axillary fold
7. Dropped nipple sign
Special tests
8. Passive abduction
9. Resisted adduction
Investigations
10. MRI scan (dedicated sequence)—Imaging modality of choice for diagnosis, confirmation and characterization to guide surgical management

References

1. Butt U, Mehta S, Funk L, Monga P. Pectoralis major ruptures: a review of current management. J Shoulder Elb Surg. 2015;24(4):655–62.
2. Petilon J, Ellingson CI, Sekiya JK. Pectoralis major muscle ruptures. Oper Tech Sports Med. 2005;13:162–8.
3. Provencher MT, Handfield K, Boniquit NT, Reiff SN, Sekiya JK, Romeo AA. Injuries to the pectoralis major muscle diagnosis and management. Am J Sports Med. 2010;38:1693–705.
4. Merolla G, Paladini P, Artiaco S, Tos P, et al. Surgical repair of acute and chronic pectoralis major tendon rupture: clinical and ultrasound outcomes at a mean follow-up of 5 years. Eur J Orthop Surg Traumatol. 2015;25(1):91–8.
5. Ohashi K, El-Khoury GY, Albright JP, Tearse DS. MRI of complete rupture of the pectoralis major muscle. Skelet Radiol. 1996;25:625–8.
6. Wolfe SW, Wickiewicz TL, Cavanaugh JT. Ruptures of the pectoralis major muscle an anatomic and clinical analysis. Am J Sports Med. 1992;20:587–93.
7. Zeman SC, Rosenfeld RT, Lipscomb PR. Tears of the pectoralis major muscle. Am J Sports Med. 1979;7:343–7.
8. Shepard NP, Westrick RB, Owens BD, Johnson MR. Bony avulsion injury of the pectoralis major in a 19 year-old male judo athlete. Int J Sports Phys Ther. 2013;8:862.
9. Avery DM 3rd, Carolan GF, Festa A. Pectoralis major rupture in a 49-year-old woman. Am J Orthop (Belle Mead NJ). 2014;43:E240–2.
10. Beloosesky Y, Grinblat J, Weiss A, Rosenberg PH, Weisbort M, Hendel D. Pectoralis major rupture in elderly patients: a clinical study of 13 patients. Clin Orthop Relat Res. 2003;413:164–9.
11. Shah NH, Talwalker S, Badge R, Funk L. Pectoralis major rupture in athletes: footprint technique and results. Tech Should Elbow Surg. 2010;11:4–7.
12. Lee J, Brookenthal KR, Ramsey ML, Kneeland JB, Herzog R. MR imaging assessment of the pectoralis major myotendinous unit: an MR imaging—anatomic correlative study with surgical correlation. Am J Roentgenol. 2000;174:1371–5.

Chapter 20
Latissimus Dorsi

A. Sinha

Case Example

A 28-year-old male presents after a water skiing injury. He has noticed a swelling over the posterior axillary fold along with posterior axillary and chest wall bruising. Clinical examination reveals loss of definition of the posterior axillary fold and a positive ladder test.

Introduction

The latissimus dorsi (meaning broadest muscle of the back) is a broad, thin fan-shaped muscle that spans a significant portion of the lower back and attaches on the humerus through a long flat tendon giving it a triangular shape. It has very wide origin from the Lower thoracic vertebrae (usually lower six but is known to have variations from four to eight), Lumbodorsal fascia of the lower back (which in turn originates from Lumbar Vertebrae, Sacrum & Iliac crest) and the four most inferior ribs. From this broad origin, the muscle runs obliquely, superiorly and laterally across the lower chest and its muscle fibres merge to give it a triangular shape. Before inserting onto the humerus, it forms a flat quadrilateral tendon about 7 cm long, which rotates on itself as it inserts on the proximal humerus at the intertubercular groove. Its superior fibres insert more distally, and its inferior fibres insert more proximal on the humerus (Fig. 20.1).

The insertion of latissimus dorsi can be best remembered as "The Lady Between Two Majors". As the latissimus dorsi inserts into the floor of the intertubercular groove of the humerus, the teres major inserts on the medial lip of the intertubercular groove

A. Sinha, MRCS, FRCS (Tr & Orth)
Chesterfield Royal Hospital NHS Foundation Trust, Chesterfield S44 5BL, UK
e-mail: a.sinha1@nhs.net

© Springer International Publishing AG 2017

P. Monga, L. Funk (eds.), *Diagnostic Clusters in Shoulder Conditions*,
DOI 10.1007/978-3-319-57334-2_20

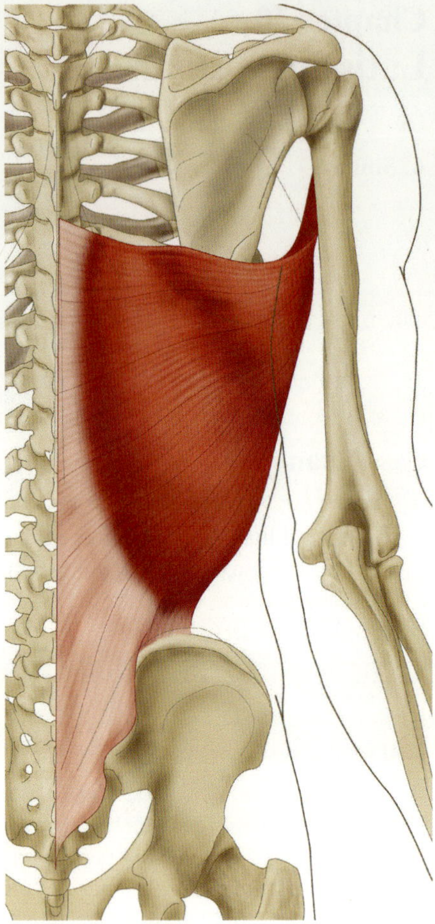

Fig. 20.1 Lattisimus dorsi anatomy. Image Published under License from www.shoulderdoc.co.uk

and the pectoralis major inserts into the lateral lip. The tendon of the teres major sometimes inserts into the tendon of the Latissimus dorsi before their humeral insertion [1].

The latissimus dorsi is supplied by the sixth, seventh, and eighth cervical nerves through the thoracodorsal (long scapular) nerve.

The latissimus dorsi is responsible for extension, adduction, horizontal abduction, flexion from an extended position and (medial) internal rotation of the shoulder. It acts to adduct the elevated arm against resistance and, in effect, pulls down on the humerus (climbing action). It also has a synergistic role in extension (posterior fibres) and lateral flexion (anterior fibres) of the lumbar spine, and assists as a muscle of both forced expiration (anterior fibres) and an accessory muscle of inspiration (posterior fibres) [2–10].

Latissmus Dorsi muscle overactivity has been associated with shoulder instability especially in multidirectional instability with abnormal muscle patterning. It can create an inferior translation of the GHJ, depending on which plane the arm is placed it will influence GHJ translation in either an anteroinferior or a posteroinferior direction leading to instability [11].

Pillar 1: Clinical History

Injury to the lattisimus dorsi is uncommon, and a majority of these reported injuries have occurred in competitive athletes, most commonly water skiers and baseball pitchers [2]. An acute latissimus dorsi tear is seen following an acute traumatic event where sudden extension force is applied on an outstretched arm. The patient usually describes a tearing sensation in the axilla and medial aspect of the upper arm close to the muscle insertion with the development of extensive bruising over the posteromedial aspect of the arm. The injury is common in pitchers and throwing athletes and usually, causes pain during release or follow-through phase [2]. The other commonly injured tendon along with lattisimus dorsi is teres major.

Pillar 2: The Conventional Examination

Physical examination demonstrates ecchymosis and bruising along the medial aspect of the upper arm and medial chest wall. In some cases, visible asymmetry of the posterior axillary fold can be seen. There is tenderness to palpation along the posterior axillary fold and reproduction of pain with resisted shoulder extension (pulling the arm down from an abducted position). On occasion, this injury can present as an axillary pseudotumour due to haematoma formation and may be confused for a sarcoma [2].

Pillar 3: Special Tests

The Ladder Test is performed in the standing position patient is asked to get his arm in 160 of abduction in the plane of the scapula and then against the resistance of examiner the patient is asked to internally rotate and extend their arm as if climbing a ladder. Weakness can be graded and compared to the contralateral side. The examiner can also place their hand along the posterior axillary fold to feel for the contraction of the muscle (Fig. 20.2).

Lattisismus Dorsi strength can be graded in the prone position. Patient's arm is placed in an adducted and internally rotated position. The patient is instructed to hold this position and while supporting the contralateral shoulder gradual and increasing force to the forearm is applied in the direction of shoulder flexion and abduction (Fig. 20.3). Power can be graded and compared to the contralateral side.

Functional test for Lattisimus dorsi involves asking the patient to place their arms on by their side and to push up and out from a seated position. In this test position, the latissimus dorsi is assisted by the triceps brachii and pectoralis muscles (Fig. 20.4). This is considered more of a functional test rather than a specific muscle test.

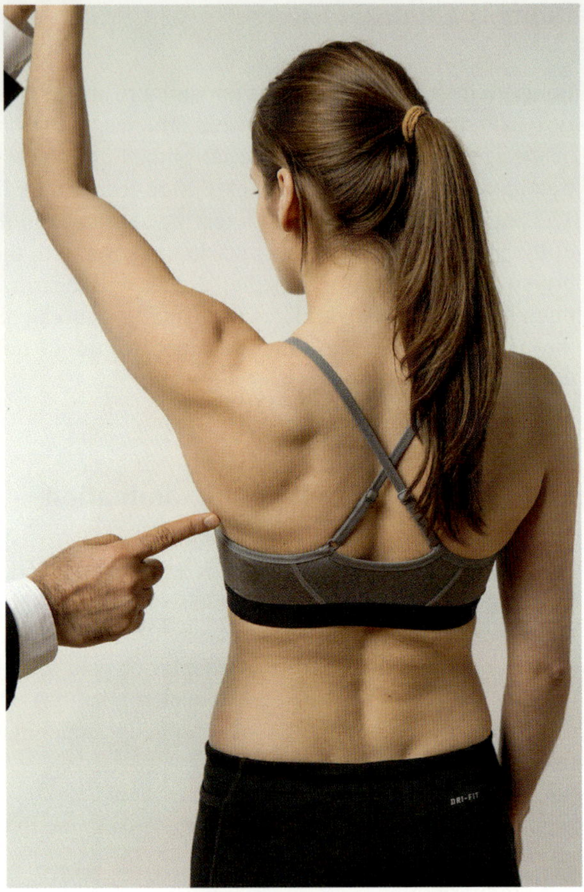

Fig. 20.2 Ladder test. Image Published under License from www.shoulderdoc.co.uk and www.shoulderpedia.org

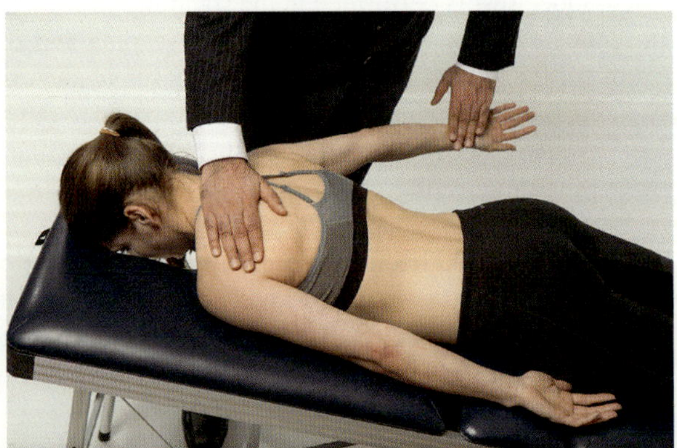

Fig. 20.3 Prone lattisimus dorsi strength test. Image Published under License from www.shoulderdoc.co.uk and www.shoulderpedia.org

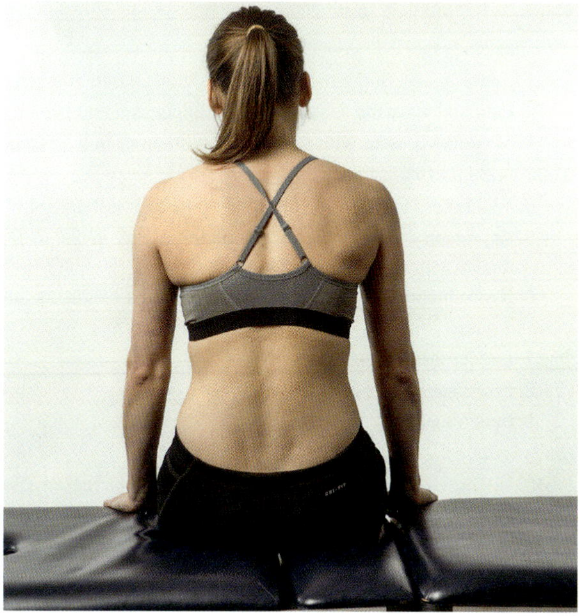

Fig. 20.4 Functional test for lattisimus dorsi. Image Published under License from www.shoulderdoc.co.uk and www.shoulderpedia.org

Pillar 4: Investigations

Initial studies used for diagnosis include plain radiographs of shoulder to rule out any bony injury. MRI is the gold standard investigation. It demonstrates low signal tendon replaced by increased T2/fluid signal intensity tendon or musculotendinous retraction, and/or intramuscular fluid [2].

In chronic cases of weakness where a definite tear is not demonstrated nerve conduction testing for thoracodorsal nerve may be useful.

Discussion of the Case

The young man described in this chapter, presenting with the waterskiing injury is suspected to have a Lattisimus Dorsi injury. Such an injury usually involves an avulsion of the tendon from the humeral attachment. As the injury is relatively rare, it is frequently missed in the initial stages. The key to early diagnosis is, in fact, the awareness of such an injury and its classic presentation. An MRI is confirmatory, and early surgical repair in an athletic individual offers best chances of recovery.

Table 20.1 Summary of diagnostic clusters for latissimus dorsi

Clinical history
1. Acute injury: Sudden extension force on an outstretched arm
2. Pain and a tearing sensation in the upper arm and posterior axillary region
3. May also present with a lump/pseudotumour in the posterior axillary fold
Conventional examination
4. Tenderness to palpation along the posterior axillary fold
5. Asymmetry, ecchymosis and sometimes a lump due to haematoma present along the medial aspect of the upper arm and posterior axillary fold
6. Reproduction of pain with resisted shoulder extension and resisted arm pull down
Special tests
7. Ladder test
8. Prone strength testing
9. Functional test
Investigations
10. MRI reveals low signal tendon replaced by increased T2/fluid signal intensity, tendon or musculotendinous retraction, and/or intramuscular fluid

Summary

Lattisimus dorsi rupture may present as an acute injury and is seen in throwing athletes due to sudden extension force on an outstretched arm. The patient presents with asymmetry, ecchymosis and tenderness to palpation along the posterior axillary fold. It can also present with a lump/pseudotumour due to haematoma formation in the posterior axillary fold or posterior chest wall. MRI is confirmatory of the diagnosis. A summary of diagnostic clusters for Lattisimus Dorsi injury is listed in Table 20.1.

References

1. Morelli M, Nagamori J, Gilbart M, Miniaci A. Latissimus dorsi tendon transfer for massive irreparable cuff tears: an anatomic study. J Shoulder Elb Surg. 2008;17(1):139–43.
2. Anderson SE, Hertel R, Johnston JO, Stauffer E, Leinweber E, Steinbach LS. Latissimus dorsi tendinosis and tear: imaging features of a pseudotumor of the upper limb in five patients. AJR Am J Roentgenol. 2005;185(5):1145–51.
3. DiGiovine N, Jobe F, Pink M, Perry J. An electromyographic analysis of the upper extremity in pitching. J Shoulder Elb Surg. 1992;1:15–25.
4. Glousman R, Jobe F, Tibone J, Moynes D, Antonelli D, Perry J. Dynamic electromyographic analysis of the throwing shoulder with glenohumeral instability. J Bone Joint Surg Am. 1988;70(2):220–6.
5. Gowan ID, Jobe FW, Tibone JE, Perry J, Moynes DR. A comparative electromyographic analysis of the shoulder during pitching: professional versus amateur pitchers. Am J Sports Med. 1987;15(6):586–90.
6. Jobe FW, Moynes DR, Tibone JE, Perry J. An EMG analysis of the shoulder in pitching: a second report. Am J Sports Med. 1984;12(3):218–20.

7. Jonsson B, Olofsson BM, Steffner LC. Function of the teres major, latissimus dorsi and pectoralis major muscles: a preliminary study. Acta Morphol Neerl Scand. 1972;9(4):275–80.
8. Pearl ML, Perry J, Torburn L, Gordon LH. An electromyographic analysis of the shoulder during cones and planes of arm motion. Clin Orthop Relat Res. 1992;284:116–27.
9. Pouliart N, Gagey O. Significance of the latissimus dorsi for shoulder instability. I: Variations in its anatomy around the humerus and scapula. Clin Anat. 2005;18(7):493–9.
10. Pouliart N, Gagey O. Significance of the latissimus dorsi for shoulder instability. II: Its influence on dislocation behavior in a sequential cut- ting protocol of the glenohumeral capsule. Clin Anat. 2005;18(7):500–9.
11. Jaggi A, Noorani A, Malone A, Cowan J, Lambert S, Bayley I. Muscle activation patterns in patients with recurrent shoulder instability. Int J Shoulder Surg. 2012;6(4):101–7.

Chapter 21
Serratus Anterior

Jill Thomas, Sarah Russell, and Jill Walton

Case Example

A 30-year-old man presents with aching around the right shoulder. He describes the onset of such an aching following a prolonged unaccustomed hike 3 months ago when he carried a heavy backpack and camping gear for 3 days in the Scottish Highlands. Although he had no direct injury as such since then the shoulder has never been "right". Examination reveals winging of the scapula. The elevation of the shoulder is limited to 120° with marked exaggeration of winging when testing in an OKC (open kinetic chain) position.

Introduction

Serratus anterior (SA) is a large muscle covering the side of the thorax, it forms the medial wall of the axilla, sitting between the ribs and the scapula. A loose fascia covers both the superior and the deep aspects of the muscle, to facilitate smooth movements of the scapula.

Serratus anterior originates from just beyond the mid-axillary line, to the outer surface of the upper eight or nine ribs, and into the intervening intercostal fascia. The muscle fibres run posteriorly inserting into the costal surface of the scapula medial border, between the superior and inferior angles. It is worth noting that the attachments are not evenly distributed along the medial border. The uppermost passes almost horizontally attaching at the superior angle, the lower four attach to the inferior angle, with the remaining spread along the medial border [1] (Fig. 21.1). Due to its location underneath the scapula, only the digitations of the

J. Thomas (✉) • S. Russell • J. Walton
Wrightington Hospital, Wigan, UK
e-mail: jill.thomas@wwl.nhs.uk

© Springer International Publishing AG 2017

P. Monga, L. Funk (eds.), *Diagnostic Clusters in Shoulder Conditions*,
DOI 10.1007/978-3-319-57334-2_21

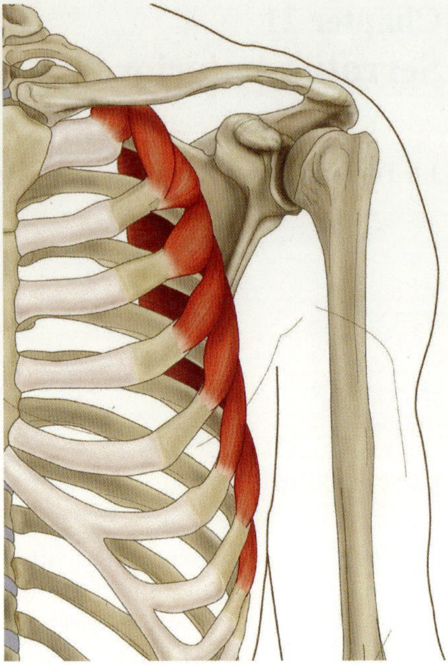

Fig. 21.1 Serratus Anterior Anatomy. Image Published under License from www.shoulderdoc.co.uk

serratus anterior may be palpable or visible in a muscular patient. These run forwards in the region of the midaxillary line and can be identified most easily when contracting.

Serratus anterior is supplied by the long thoracic nerve (C5, 6, 7). The upper two components of the muscle are innervated by C5, the next two by C6, and the remaining four by C7. This nerve has a particularly superficial course, inferior to the clavicle and the first rib, traversing onto the lateral chest wall in the mid-axillary line, therefore making it more susceptible to injury [2]. The skin over the palpable parts of the muscle (medial axilla) is supplied by the nerves originating from T3 to T7 [1].

Serratus anterior is a major protractor of the shoulder girdle and plays a vital role in activities that drive forwards the scapula, such as pushing and punching movements. This can be observed with well-developed athletes such as boxers. Serratus Anterior contracts strongly to stabilise the medial border of the scapula in upper limb function holding it to the chest wall as the arm moves into flexion, or when the upper limb is loaded in front of the body. Failure to perform this action results in the medial border standing away from the chest wall and is described as 'winging' [2]; this severely affects the function and mobility of the upper limb.

The lower components of serratus anterior work with trapezius as a force couple to rotate the scapula to position the glenoid fossa to face upwards, to enable a greater range of glenohumeral movement. As a force couple, the counteracting muscles demonstrate obvious action when a movement is loaded or performed quickly [3], one muscle (agonist) acts concentrically, whereas the other, the antagonist, acts eccentrically in a controlled, harmonised fashion, to produce a smooth movement. Also, these muscles may work by co-contraction or co-activation to provide a stabilising effect and joint control [3]. The role of serratus anterior as a force couple with trapezius continues throughout shoulder range motion and is of particular importance in the overhead position [4, 5]. Weakness is characteristic of a long thoracic nerve palsy. Long thoracic nerve palsy causes the scapula to elevate and move medially with the inferior angle rotating medially resulting in winging of the scapula [3].

Pillar 1: Clinical History

Serratus Anterior weakness can occur following trauma, due to a viral illness, or a result of a congenital deformity. A thorough, detailed history should be taken to determine the onset of symptoms. The function of serratus anterior should be fully assessed when a patient presents with a new onset of winging of the medial border of the scapula. Palsy of SA is the most common cause of scapular winging and is associated with medial border winging [2].

Scapular winging was first documented in the literature in 1723 [6]. The winging appearance can be attributed to SA or trapezius weakness [2]. While earlier studies have failed to identify a prevalence of scapular winging, more recent studies have identified a significantly higher number of cases. It is believed that this may be due to examiner error, for example not adequately undressing the patient to allow full visualisation of the scapulae [2].

Trauma can result in serratus anterior weakness following a direct blow to the scapula-thoracic area, compression of the scapula against the chest wall, or an upper limb traction injury [3]. Injury can also occur through prolonged loading and subsequent trauma [7]. This is known as a backpack injury [3]. Such patients are commonly in early-mid adulthood (age 25–45 years) [7]. Repetitive traction may cause serratus anterior palsy [8], found that as little as a 10% increase in nerve length may cause neurapraxia. Sudden scapula winging in the absence of trauma or prolonged loading may be due to a viral illness, resulting in a viral long thoracic nerve palsy [3]. A Sprengle's deformity is the most common congenital deformity of the shoulder. It results in a congenitally high or undescended scapula [3]. Identification of trauma or iatrogenic cause is particularly helpful in determining the appropriate method of management [2].

Pain originating from SA can refer proximally into the axilla, and distally along the ulnar border of the upper limb. Pain is typically centred around the levator scapulae and rhomboid minor [2]. The patient may describe a history of generalised shoulder or upper arm pain, which can worsen on elevation of the upper limb, fatigue or stiffness [2]. Pain may also be present when sitting for long periods, for example when driving, due to the prominent scapular border [2].

The principal functional limitation is difficulty in forward elevation with an extended arm, for example when lifting overhead or throwing [2].

Pillar 2: The Conventional Examination

A thorough observation of posture of the lower and upper quadrants, plus thoracic and cervical regions should be conducted. This should include analysis of the contour and tone of all relevant muscle groups [5]. It is well documented that the cervicothoracic posture influences the shoulder complex. Therefore the examiner should make considerations for this, and correct or alter the posture as required, and note the change in scapular position.

The examiner should observe and compare both scapulae for asymmetry or muscular atrophy. Any deficit in serratus anterior may lead to hypertrophy in other associated scapulothoracic contributors [9]. True scapular winging is often evident at rest, whereas pseudo-winging may only be apparent during movement of the upper limb or loading. On observation, winging is characterised by the prominence of the inferior tip, and the medial border of the scapular [7].

Serratus activity can be assessed by observing whether there is scapula winging during both elevation or loading of the upper limb and when weight-bearing through the upper limb. The scapula position and the quality of movement should be observed throughout shoulder elevation. The scapula should start in a retracted, downwardly rotated position and should move smoothly into a protracted, upwardly rotated position as the arm moves above 90 degrees of elevation [5]. This test can be progressed further with repetitions of the movement, to observe for signs of fatigue, and also by adding a load, i.e., a hand weight during the upper limb movement.

Throughout all movements the examiner should assess for asymmetry, medial border winging of the scapula, non-smooth, or uncontrolled scapular movement, any of which would be deemed as a positive test for pseudo winging or possible true winging – i.e. poor or no serratus activation.

Shoulder movements can be tested in an open kinetic chain (OKC) or closed kinetic chain (CKC) position. With OKC the hand is free (Fig. 21.2), whereas with CKC the hand remains in contact with a base, for example, a wall, table or the floor. During an OKC movement, the scapular musculature (and significantly SA) must work to control the position of the scapula about the chest wall, enabling the efficient transfer of power generated from lower limbs distally through the kinetic chain through the upper limb. If weak, the SA will be ineffective in maintaining medial border control, and protraction-upward rotation of the scapular, which limits elevation to approximately 120 degrees [7]. When observing the quality of the upper limb movement; the longer the upper limb lever or, the greater the load; the more effort will be required by the serratus and other scapula-thoracic stabilisers eliciting a more significant movement dysfunction presentation.

In the CKC position, the hand remains in contact with a surface, for example when sliding the hand up the wall into a forward elevation position (Fig. 21.3). In this position, the degree of loss of scapular control may not be as evident due to the weight distribution onto the wall. This should not be confused with assessing the scapular during weight bearing where a CKC position is adopted to load body weight through the limb. A full and accurate assessment SA will include both open and closed chain movements as well as upper limb weight-bearing.

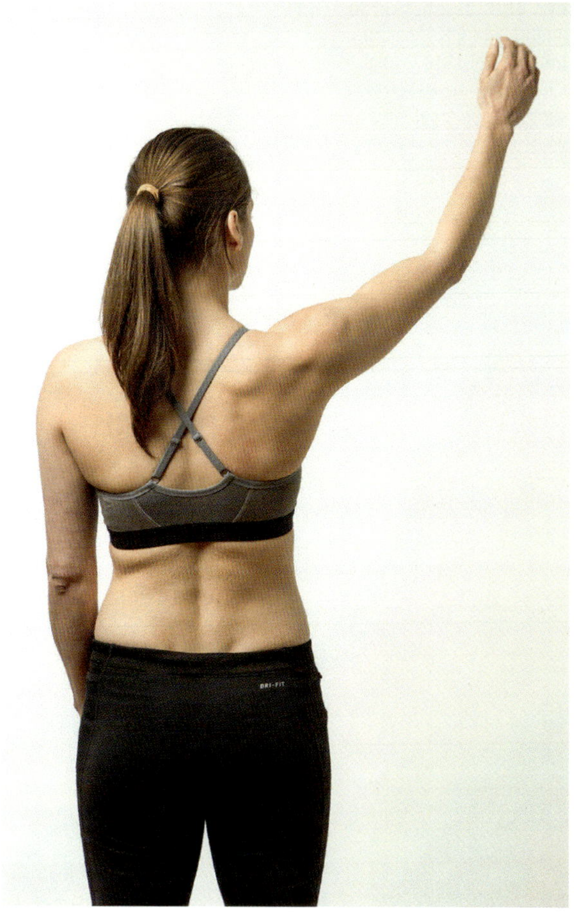

Fig. 21.2 Testing Serrates anterior in OKC position. Image Published under License from www.shoulderdoc.co.uk and www.shoulderpedia.org

SA's ability to control the scapular while weight-bearing through the upper limb can be assessed in standing with the hands weight bearing against a wall, or in four point kneeling. In standing, the patient should be approximately 1 metre away from the wall, place their hands flat against the wall, and slowly flex their elbows, to lower their chest closer to the wall (Fig. 21.4) [2]. As with non-weight bearing movement, the examiner should observe for asymmetry and in particular, winging. If one position fails to highlight weakness, an alternative weight bearing position should be tested. The movement should be repeated to assess the level of fatigue. With an incomplete palsy 5–10 repetitions may be required to elicit fatigue [2]. The test should be repeated as a movement (pushup) to fatigue. The position and movement of the scapula should be observed for signs of winging or SA fatigue. Throughout watching movement, care should be taken to note any compensatory patterns of movement that may have been adopted due to SA weakness.

Serratus anterior digitations can be felt and often seen in a muscular person. This can be felt during activation of this muscle, i.e., pushing.

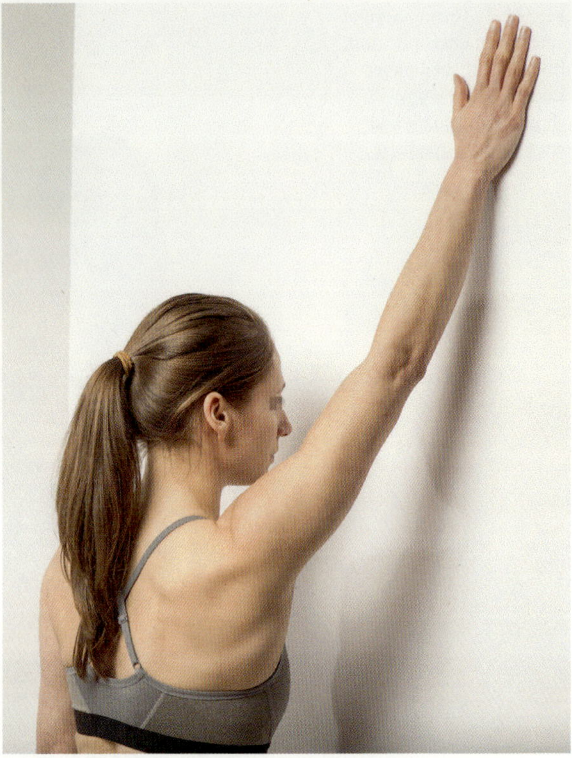

Fig. 21.3 Testing Serrats Anterior in CKC position. Image Published under License from www.shoulderdoc.co.uk and www.shoulderpedia.org

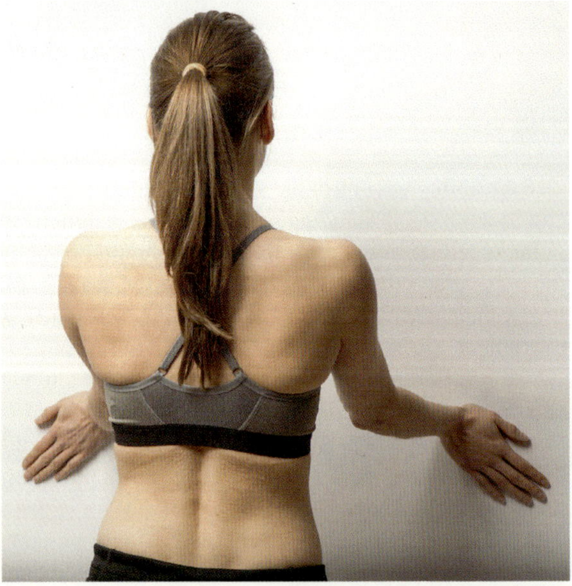

Fig. 21.4 Wall test. Image Published under License from www.shoulderdoc.co.uk and www.shoulderpedia.org

Pillar 3: Special Tests

In patients who have a winging scapula at rest, SA's ability to maintain a neutral scapula can be assessed by asking the patient to retract their scapula to neutral and maintain this position. The arm should remain by their side. A positive test is an inability to achieve a neutral scapula. In some cases, the patient may not have the proprioceptive awareness to be able to reach this position. If the test is positive, the examiner may provide manual assistance to achieve neutral, and then ask the patient to actively maintain the position.

SA weakness results in a loss of active abduction, often to 110–120° [10]. Passive assistance/stabilisation of compression of the scapula to the thorax during abduction should increase the range of active abduction [2, 7]. A scapular assistance test involves the examiner manually stabilising and facilitating the scapular to sit against the thorax, and laterally rotate as the arm moves into elevation [7]. A reduction in discomfort or an increase in arm elevation results in a positive test (Fig. 21.5).

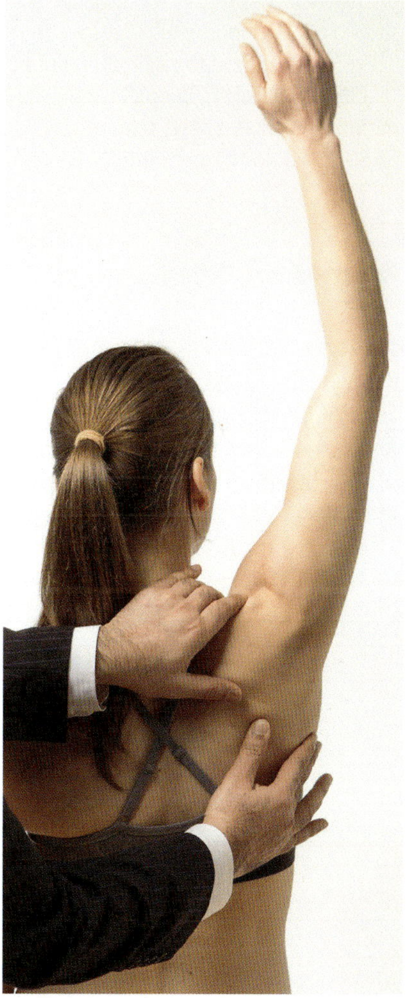

Fig. 21.5 Scapular assistance test. Image Published under License from www.shoulderdoc.co.uk and www.shoulderpedia.org

A wall test will accentuate any medial winging of the scapula, indicating SA weakness. The patient should be asked to forward flex at the shoulder to place their hands on a wall, and should then push on the wall, as in a push-up motion (Fig. 21.4) [11].

Pillar 4: Investigations

EMG is the definitive investigation for SA weakness. This should be done in conjunction with analysis of the trapezius, rhomboid, and levator scapulae [2], and should be performed at least after 4 weeks from the onset of symptoms. EMG may identify the SA weakness, but will not determine the extent nor the prognosis. Equally SA weakness may still be present in the absence of a positive EMG finding [2, 7]. It has been reported that accurate placement of the needle into SA for accurate EMG can be difficult [12]. However, this is argued that although this may be difficult in normal individuals, in those with SA weakness, the winged medial border of the scapular provides access to SA for accurate needle placement [12]. Nerve conduction studies should also be conducted. Positive findings will be demonstrated in true long thoracic nerve palsies, though again may not be positive in all cases of SA weakness.

Gleno-humeral, scapular and thoracic plain radiographs can exclude bony pathology [2]. An MRI scan of the shoulder complex can identify a structural cause of SA weakness, for example, an avulsion injury [13].

Discussion of the Case

Backpack injury to the long thoracic nerve is not uncommon. Further assessment of the patient described in the chapter involves EMG studies of the trapezius, serratus anterior, rhomboids and the elevator scapulae. A cluster approach including directed history targeted clinical examination and appropriate investigations are useful in confirming the diagnosis of serratus anterior palsy. Further management includes options of relative rest, rehabilitation and surgical decompression of the long thoracic nerve.

Summary

Serratus Anterior weakness can have a debilitating effect on upper limb function. The weakness can occur from a range of mechanisms and pathology. A detailed, thorough history and examination is paramount to gain an accurate diagnosis and to ultimately direct appropriate management. EMG and NCVs in the presence of scapular winging are confirmatory of the diagnosis. Neurophysiology assessment should specifically test for serratus anterior EMGs in cases of scapular winging. A summary of diagnostic clusters for Serratus Anterior weakness is listed in Table 21.1.

Table 21.1 Summary of diagnostic clusters for serratus anterior weakness

Clinical history
1. Trauma – direct blow/traction injury/backpack injury/compression against chest wall
2. Sudden onset following viral infection/immunisation
3. Pain over the serratus referral pattern: Axilla, ulnar border of the upper limb
4. Difficulty with heavy effort above shoulder height
Conventional examination
5. Scapula elevated and sits medially with the inferior angle rotated medially
6. Winging of the scapula on abduction and forward flexion in OKC and CKC position.
7. Difficulty abducting or forward flexing arm >90°(may be possible with lower trapezius compensation)
Special tests
8. Positive scapular assistance test
9. Wall test
Investigations
10. NCS +/– EMG confirmatory of long thoracic nerve and serratus anterior palsy

References

1. Palastanga N, Field D, Soames R. Anatomy and human movement structure and function. 2nd ed. Boston: Butterworth-Heinemann; 1994.
2. Lee S, Savin DD, Shah NR, Bronsnick D, Goldberg B. Scapular winging: evaluation and treatment. J Bone Joint Surg Am. 2015;97(20):1708–16.
3. Magee DJ. Orthopaedic physical assessment. 5th ed. St Louis, MO: Saunders; 2008.
4. Bagg SD, Forrest WJ. Electromyographic study of the scapular rotators during arm abduction in the scapular plane. Am J Phys Med. 1986;65(3):111–24.
5. Magarey ME, Jones MA. Dynamic evaluation and early management of altered motor control around the shoulder complex. Man Ther. 2003;8(4):195–206.
6. Winslow M. Sur quelques mouvements extraordinaires des omoplates et des bras, et sur une nouvelle espece de muscles. Mem Acad Royale Sci. 1723:98–112.
7. Warner JJ, Navarro RA. Serratus anterior dysfunction. Recognition and treatment. Clin Orthop Relat Res. 1998;349:139–48.
8. Bora FW, Richardson S, Black J. The biomechanical responses to tension in a peripheral nerve. J Hand Surg. 1980;5(1):21–5.
9. Safran MR. Nerve injury about the shoulder in athletes, part 2: long thoracic nerve, spinal accessory nerve, burners/stingers, thoracic outlet syndrome. Am J Sports Med. 2004;32(4):1063–79.
10. Gregg JR, Labosky D, Harty M, Lotke P, Ecker M, DiStefano V, Das M. Serratus anterior paralysis in the young athlete. J Bone Joint Surg Am. 1979;61:825–32.
11. Martin RM, Fish DE. Scapular winging: anatomical review, diagnosis and treatments. Curr Rev Muscoskelet Med. 2008;1(1):1–11.
12. Reimers CD, Kunkel M, Siever A, Kolenda H. Electromyography of the serratus anterior and subscapularis muscles: description of a technique. J Neurol Neurosurg Psychiatry. 1996;61:117–8.
13. Gaffney KM. Avulsion injury of the Serratus anterior. Clin J Sport Med. 1997;7(2):134–6.

Chapter 22
Scapular Dyskinesis

Emmet Griffiths

Case Example

A 32-year female tennis player presents with pain over the dominant right shoulder. She describes an insidious onset of symptoms for over 2 years, and her coach has noticed that the shoulder has "dropped". The pain is described anteriorly over the coracoid and also along the medial border of the scapula posteriorly. Examination reveals a prominent medial border, anteriorly tilted and protracted scapula with loss of the scapulothoracic rhythm during elevation of the arm. Elevation is also associated with pain over the scapular area.

Introduction

Scapular dyskinesis is a clinical observation of abnormal movement of the shoulder blade. It is an important sign of underlying shoulder pathology and is associated with numerous conditions. The underlying problem is one of altered muscle activation patterns in the periscapular musculature which may be due to inherent problems within the muscle, issues with the nerve supplying the muscle or altered activation as a protective mechanism to reduce pain. Many shoulder injuries can be associated with dyskinesis of the scapula [1], and it is considered an important guide to rehabilitation.

In the physiological situation, the scapula moves in the sagittal, coronal and transverse planes. This complex movement involves two planes of translation, superior/inferior and protraction/retraction and three axes of rotation (superior/inferior, internal/external and anterior/posterior). Overhead elevation involves primary

E. Griffiths
Norfolk and Norwich University Hospital, Norwich, UK
e-mail: emmetgriffiths@gmail.com

© Springer International Publishing AG 2017
P. Monga, L. Funk (eds.), *Diagnostic Clusters in Shoulder Conditions*,
DOI 10.1007/978-3-319-57334-2_22

upward rotation and secondary posterior tilting with internal and external rotation only playing a minor part until 100°of elevation [2, 3]. In abduction scapulothoracic motion plays an increasing role as the arm is abducted, in the initial 30° of abduction the movement occurs predominately at the glenohumeral joint whereas between 90 and 150° the ratio is close to 1:1 [4, 5]

There are three broad types of pathological scapular motion based on clinical observation [6], but there is often an overlap. These are inferior-medial dysfunction (Type 1), medial dysfunction (Type 2) and superior-medial dysfunction (type 3).

Inferior dysfunction is commonly associated with tight pectoralis major/minor [7] and a relative weakness of the lower trapezius and serratus anterior. Altered scapular motion via an increased posterior tilt causes increased narrowing of the subacromial space when the arm is abducted and externally rotated. This is an early common pathway in numerous shoulder disorders and as such is relatively non-specific. It is made more clinically apparent in the cocking position of throwing. The SICK scapula syndrome [6] is associated with inferior scapula prominence and is characterised by a drooping of the affected shoulder mainly in overhead athletes. It has four components, scapular malposition, inferior prominence, coracoid pain and kinetic abnormalities.

Pure medial dysfunction is made more apparent in the cocking position, and as it is associated with fatigue of the rhomboids and trapezius, this may be made more evident by repeated elevation of the arm. It may be seen in patients with underlying glenohumeral joint instability. Superior dysfunction is most often seen in patients with dysfunction of the cuff or deltoid-cuff force couple; often there is imbalance of activation

The aetiology of scapula dyskinesis is extensive and is summarised in Table 22.1. The role of intrinsic shoulder pathology may be both cause and effect further complicating management. But causative factors can be grouped into several groups. Intrinsic shoulder pathology including labral pathology, AC joint pathology, biceps tendinopathy and the sequelae of clavicle or scapular fractures are all associated with scapular dysrhythmia. Altered scapular positioning and motion have been shown to increase stress on the anterior labrum and may, therefore, increase the 'peel-back' load on the labrum [8]. Dyskinesis is frequently encountered in patients with impingement and is due to reduced upward rotation of the acromion which then increases scapular internal rotation and anterior tilt causing winging [9]. Secondly nerve dysfunction including long thoracic, spinal accessory and suprascapular nerve. Thirdly muscle pathology either primary (including kinetic chain problems) or secondary to a nerve lesion. The shoulder has an intricate pattern of static and dynamic stabilisers, and patients with multi-directional instability have been shown to have altered rotator cuff activation patterns and thus frequently display altered scapula-thoracic rhythm [10, 11]. The final group of patients who exhibit dyskinesia of the scapula are those who have specific restrictions around the shoulder related to either a tight posterior capsule (GIRD) or an overactive pectoralis muscle.

Table 22.1 Aetiology of scapular dyskinesis

Intrinsic
Labral pathology
AC Joint pathology
Biceps tendinopathy
Sequelae of clavicle or scapular fractures
Subacromial Impingement Syndrome
Snapping scapula
Glenohumeral stiffness
Adhesive capsulitis
Tight posterior capsule (GIRD)
Nerve dysfunction
Long Thoracic Nerve
Spinal Accessory Nerve
Suprascapular nerve
Spinal nerve root compression
Muscle pathology
Traumatic
Dystrophic
Disuse related weakness
Multi-directional instability

Pillar 1: Clinical History

As with any diagnosis, the first step is a focused history. The majority of shoulder disorders are associated with scapular dyskinesia, and thus the history should be quite broad. The investigation of shoulder symptoms is covered in great depth elsewhere in this book, but several intrinsic scapular pathologies should be considered. The presence of pain in the shoulder implies the existence of intrinsic shoulder pathology which may be driving the dyskinesis. The history of acute trauma points towards a structural abnormality within the shoulder girdle and the AC joint is a common culprit, nerve palsies around the shoulder are often associated with repetitive minor trauma or a preceding viral illness [12]. Previous fractures around the shoulder may be associated with malunion (e.g., clavicle) which may cause a thoracic outlet syndrome.

Pillar 2: The Conventional Examination

The diagnosis of scapular dyskinesia is however made on clinical examination. The first question is whether there is a dyskinesis or not? This is most simply assessed by viewing the scapula motion from behind. A simple yes/no answer to this observation has been shown to have good reliability and reproducibility [13]. There are several features to assess during this observation, firstly the presence of any prominence of the scapula at rest, secondly any jerking movement during elevation or abduction (including asymmetry and shrugging) and finally an accelerated dropping of the arm during the downward phase. The arm movement should be repeated several times to assess for fatiguability and should include both forward elevation and abduction. Many other tests have been described including the lateral scapula slide test (a static measurement of the distance between the inferior angle of the scapula and the nearest spinous process), but these have poor validity and reproducibility [14].

Having discerned the presence of scapula dyskinesis, the examination then continues to try to elucidate potential causes.

Inspection may show wasting of specific muscles around the shoulder girdle pointing towards a neurological lesion and the resting position of the scapula should also be assessed as an overactive pectoralis will protract it. Exaggeration of the normal thoracic kyphosis may also lead to susceptibility to scapula dysrhythmia [15]. Dynamic assessment during abduction and elevation may identify a 'hitch' (associated with subacromial pathology) or an audible crepitus.

A rare diagnosis of snapping scapula may be identified by palpitating for crepitus as the arm is abducted and elevated. Palpation may also identify areas of pain which may be driving the dysrhythmia most notably ACJ pathology.

The range of movement of the arm should be completely assessed with particular care taken to examine for an internal rotation deficit (GIRD). Multiple different methods of determining internal rotation should be utilised in all patients to allow comprehensive assessment, particularly bearing in mind that different parts of the capsule will restrict rotation in different arm positions [16]. This includes internal rotation at 90° abduction (Fig. 22.1) and the spinal level that can be reached up to the back (Fig. 2.7).

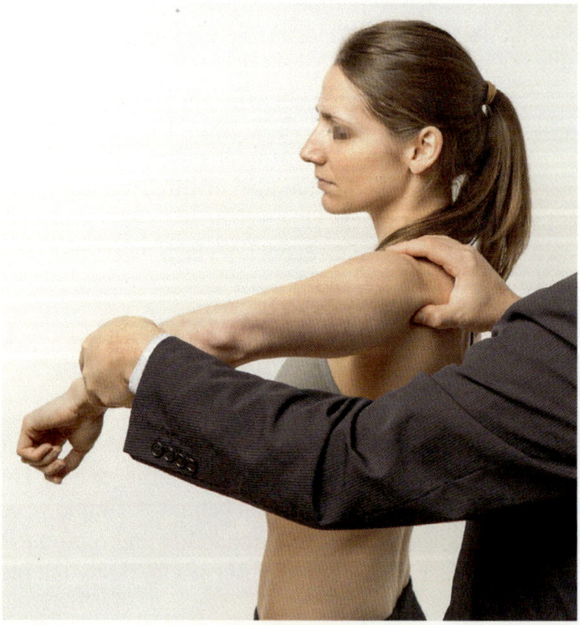

Fig. 22.1 GIRD assessment with the arm in 90° abduction. Image Published under License from www.shoulderdoc.co.uk and www.shoulderpedia.org

Examination of the periscapular muscles is vital in defining a cause for the dyskinesia. The muscle strength of serratus anterior, middle and lower trapezius are necessary to assess as these are key stabilisers of the lateral scapula [17]. Similarly, the rhomboids should be examined. An overactive pectoralis tendon may be manually impaired improving the movement of the shoulder and confirming its role. Other dynamic stabilising tests including the deliberate activation of the rotator cuff during elevation may have a stabilising effect and point towards appropriate therapy.

Pillar 3 Special Tests

Two specific tests have been described for the assessment of dyskinesia of the scapula. The scapular assistance test involves manually assisting scapula upward rotation and tilting and assessing for a reduction in pain (Fig. 21.5). It implies that any impingement is secondary to scapula dyskinesis. To achieve this, the examiner places one hand on the trapezius and the second at the inferior-medial tip of the scapula. The patient is then asked to elevate the arm, and the examiner uses manual pressure to assist the normal upward rotation of the scapula. A reduction in the pain in the shoulder caused by abnormal movement is a positive test result. This may identify the scapular dysrhythmia as a causative factor in the patient's symptoms. It has been shown to have acceptable levels of reliability and reproducibility [18].

The second test identifies those patients in whom the stability of the scapula is to blame for shoulder weakness. The scapular retraction test involves manually stabilising the scapula in a retracted position and assessing the impact on pain and strength in elevation of the affected limb. To achieve this, the examiner manually stabilises the inferior-medial scapula, and the patient actively flexes and abducts the arm. (Fig. 22.2) Unfortunately, the reliability and predictive value of this test has been questioned [19].

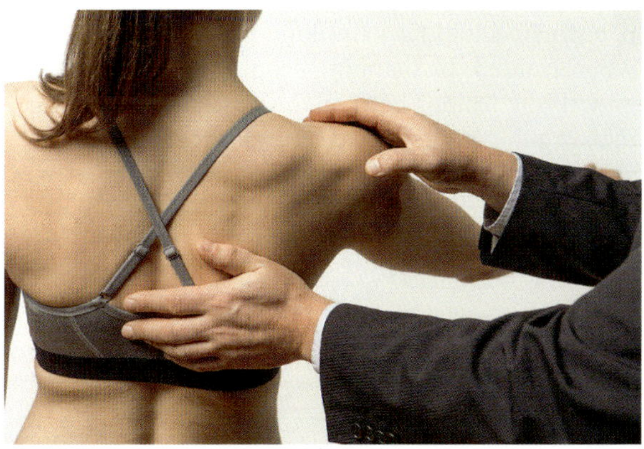

Fig. 22.2 Stabilising the inferomedial angle of the retracted scapular in the scapular retraction test. Image Published under License from www.shoulderdoc.co.uk and www.shoulderpedia.org

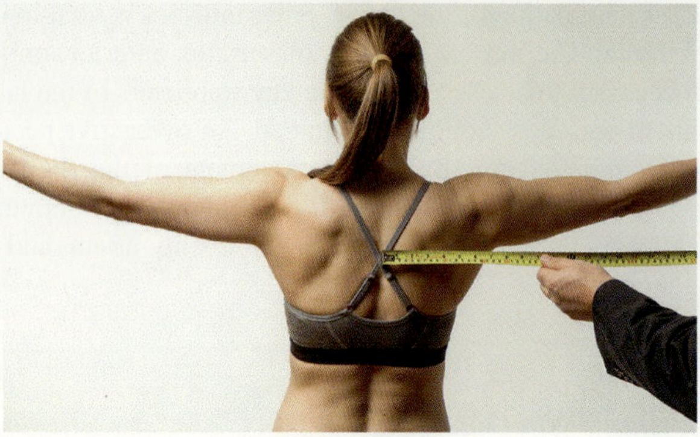

Fig. 22.3 Lateral Scapular Slide Test at 90° abduction. Image Published under License from www.shoulderdoc.co.uk and www.shoulderpedia.org

Similarly, the lateral scapula slide test has been shown to be poorly reliable. [20]. In this test, the examiner measures the distance from the medial border of the scapula to a fixed point of the spine at three positions of abduction, 0°, 45° and 90° (Fig. 22.3). The distance of the affected side is compared to the asymptomatic side, and a difference of more than 1.5 cm is a positive result.

Scapula winging may be provoked by wall press test (Fig. 21.4) and may point to weakness of serratus anterior as a causative factor. This may be related to long thoracic nerve compression (either proximally in the medial scalene or distally at the crows foot in the axilla). This may be further confirmed by the scratch collapse test. The suprascapular nerve may be assessed by Thompson's test if indicated and thoracic outlet may be confirmed clinically by standard tests (e.g., Roos).

Pillar 4: Investigations

There are no specific investigations for scapula dyskinesis, as it is a clinical observation. Thus the investigations are governed by the presumed diagnosis. A simple radiograph will identify ACJ pathology and clavicular malunion and if intrinsic shoulder pathology is suspected then MRI or MRI arthrogram may we warranted. In snapping scapula, a MRI should be requested to examine for underlying lesions both on the posterior chest wall and also the undersurface of the scapula. In suspected neurological cases EMG studies of specific muscles should be undertaken to confirm the pattern of weakness and thus the specific nerve lesion.

Discussion of the Case

The index patient described earlier in the chapter presents with scapular dyskinesia. Scapular assisted test, wall test, scapular retraction test and lateral scapular slide test were positive. She underwent further investigations in the form of MR Scan of her shoulder to rule out any structural abnormalities. Non-operative management such as specialist physiotherapy remains the mainstay for management.

Summary

Scapular dyskinesis is a clinical observation. The diagnosis of the underlying condition leading to scapular dyskinesia relies on a detailed history, careful clinical examination and appropriately directed investigations. Similarly, the management of scapula dyskinesis is targeted at the underlying diagnosis. In most cases even when there is a defined structural pathology there is a degree of secondary muscular patterning disorder. Thus the management of these complex patients requires a multidisciplinary approach. Summary of diagnostic clusters for scapular dyskinesis are listed in Table 22.2.

Table 22.2 Short list of cluster items for scapula dyskinesis

History
1. Focused history as per aetiology (Table 22.1)
Conventional Examination
2. Combined observation —Does this patient have Scapula dysrhythmia? (consensus statement)
3. Examination as directed by aetiology (Table 22.1)
Special Tests
4. Wall Test
5. Scapula assistance test
6. Scapula retraction test
7. Lateral scapula slide test
Investigations (As directed by Aetiology)
8. Radiological Investigations of scapula/shoulder/spine – Radiographs/CT scan/MRI scan
9. EMG studies
10. Diagnostic guided injections (Snapping scapula)

References

1. Kibler WB, McMullen J. Scapular dyskinesis and its relation to shoulder pain. J Am Acad Orthop Surg. 2003;11:142–51.
2. Ludewig PM, et al. Motion of the shoulder complex during multiplaner humeral elevation. J Bone Joint Surg Am. 2009;91:378–89.
3. McClure PW, et al. Direct 3-dimensional measurement of scapular kinematics during dynamic movements in vivo. J Shoulder Elb Surg. 2001;10:269–77.
4. Doody SG, et al. Shoulder movements during abduction in the scapular plane. Arch Phys Med Rehabil. 1970;51(10):595–604.
5. Bagg SD, Forrest Wj A. biomechanical analysis of scapular rotation during arm abduction in the scapular plane. Arch Phys Med Rehabil. 1988;67(6):238–45.
6. Kibler WB, Sciascia A. Current concepts: scapular dyskinesis. Br J Sports Med. 2010;44:300–5.
7. Borstad JD, Ludewig PM. The effect of long versus short pectoralis minor resting length on scapular kinematics in healthy individuals. J Orthop Sports Phys Ther. 2005;35(4):227–38.
8. Burkhart SS, Morgan CD, Kibler WB. The disabled throwing shoulder: spectrum of pathology Part I: pathoanatomy and biomechanics. Arthroscopy. 2003;19:404–20.
9. Ludewig PM, Cook TM. Alterations in shoulder kinematics and associated muscle activity in people with symptoms of shoulder impingement. Phys Ther. 2000;80:276–91.
10. Ogston JB, Ludewig PM. Differences in 3-dimensional shoulder kinematics between persons with multidirectional instability and asymptomatic controls. Am J Sports Med. 2007;35:1361–70.
11. Illyés A, Kiss RM. Kinematic and muscle activity characteristics of multidirectional shoulder joint instability during elevation. Knee Surg Sports Traumatol Arthrosc. 2006;14:673–85.
12. Martin RM. Scapular winging: anatomical review, diagnosis, and treatments. Curr Rev Musculoskelet Med. 2008;1:1–11.
13. Uhl TL, Kibler WB, Gecewich B, et al. Evaluation of clinical assessment methods for scapular dyskinesis. Arthroscopy. 2009;25:1240–8.
14. Wright AA, Wassinger CA, Frank M, et al. Diagnostic accuracy of scapular physical examination tests for shoulder disorders: a systematic review. Br J Sports Med. 2013;47(14):886–92.
15. Kebaetse M, McClure PW, Pratt N. Thoracic position effect on shoulder range of motion, strength, and three-dimensional scapular kinematics. Arch Phys Med Rehabil. 1999;80:945–50.
16. Gerber C, Werner CM, Macy JC, et al. Effect of selective capsulorrhaphy on the passive range of motion of the glenohumeral joint. J Bone Joint Surg Am. 2003;85:48–55.
17. Ludewig PM, Hoff MS, Osowski EE, et al. Relative balance of serratus anterior and upper trapezius muscle activity during push-up exercises. Am J Sports Med. 2004;32:484–93.
18. Rabin A, Irrgang JJ, Fitzgerald GK, et al. The intertester reliability of the scapular assistance test. J Orthop Sports Phys Ther. 2006;36:653–60.
19. Kibler WB, Sciascia AD, Dome DC. Evaluation of apparent and absolute supraspinatus strength in patients with shoulder injury using the scapular retraction test. Am J Sports Med. 2006;34:1643–7.
20. Odom CJ, Taylor AB, Hurd CE, Denegar CR. Measurement of scapular asymmetry and assessment of shoulder dysfunction using the lateral scapular slide test: a reliability and validity study. Phys Ther. 2001;81(2):799–809.

Chapter 23
Axillary Nerve Palsy

Chye Yew Ng

Case Example

A 55-year-old lady dislocated her right shoulder following a fall. It was noted that she had reduced sensation over the "regimental badge" area. She underwent closed reduction of the dislocation in casualty under sedation. After successful reduction, the patient presented with an inability to elevate her arm and persistent numbness over the regimental badge area. Active contraction of the deltoid was not possible. The swallow-tail sign was also positive.

Introduction

The axillary nerve contains nerve fibres from the C5, C6 roots. It branches off the posterior cord of the infraclavicular brachial plexus and courses superficial to the subscapularis muscle towards the axilla. It then passes through the quadrangular space, accompanied by the posterior circumflex humeral artery and vein, to reach the posterior region of the humeral neck. It divides into two main branches: the anterior branch supplies the deltoid muscle. The posterior branch supplies the teres minor, the posterior part of deltoid before terminating as the superior lateral cutaneous nerve of the arm. Due to the relatively fixed points (origin from the posterior cord and insertion into the deltoid muscle) as well as its proximity to the shoulder joint, the axillary nerve is particularly vulnerable to injury following:

- Traumatic shoulder dislocation/fracture-dislocation
- Proximal humeral fracture

C.Y. Ng, MBChB(Hons) FRCS(T&O) DipHandSurg
Consultant Hand and Peripheral Nerve Surgeon, Upper Limb Unit,
Wrightington Hospital, Hall Lane, Appley Bridge, Wigan WN6 9EP, UK
e-mail: info@nerveclinic.co.uk

© Springer International Publishing AG 2017

P. Monga, L. Funk (eds.), *Diagnostic Clusters in Shoulder Conditions*,
DOI 10.1007/978-3-319-57334-2_23

- Shoulder surgery

Pillar 1: Clinical History

The initial trauma or surgery may distract the healthcare professional from a possible associated nerve injury. A high index of suspicion is thus warranted.

Estimating the level of energy dissipated during the accident is important. A high-energy injury is more likely to lead to nerve injury. The nerve injury, which occurs, will be correspondingly more severe with a greater level of energy transferred. In cases of dislocation, determine the duration before the shoulder is relocated as the longer the delay, the greater the potential insult to the nerve.

Pain is an important symptom. Fracture or recent surgery will result in nociceptive pain that can be sharp or aching in nature. This needs to be distinguished from a neuropathic pain that signifies nerve injury. The latter feels like burning, shooting, stabbing or electric shocks. Beware that both types of pain may coexist. The patient may also complain of pins and needles, tingling sensation or numbness over the upper arm, which signifies potential nerve injury.

One needs to pay attention to the duration between the injury and the assessment. In the acute stage, expect the patient to complain of some degree of restriction due to the initial injury/surgery. In the later stage, patients with axillary nerve palsy may complain of persistent limitation or weakness in shoulder elevation. Those who are well compensated may maintain a full range of shoulder movement despite axillary nerve palsy. Instead, they may complain of shoulder fatigue due to denervated deltoid muscle.

Pillar 2: Conventional Examination

Adopting a systematic approach is essential. Start from proximal to distal when examining the individual muscles of the whole upper limb. This is followed by an assessment of the sensation, both in consideration to root values (C5 to T1) as well as dermatomes of the terminal branches. The aim is to ascertain whether the axillary nerve palsy occurs in isolation or associated with injuries to other nerves.

Axillary nerve palsy will result in paralysis of deltoid and teres minor muscles as well as a sensory loss over the superior lateral arm area. The deficit or impact due to paralysis of teres minor is more difficult to elicit. External rotation in adduction is predominantly a function of infraspinatus, which is spared in axillary nerve palsy. External rotation in abduction is predominantly a function of teres minor, but abduction is already affected by paralysis of the deltoid. In such situation, one may passively abduct the shoulder to 90° (if tolerated by the patient) and assess the power of external rotation.

The examination should focus on the deltoid muscle, but findings will vary depending on the chronicity of the nerve lesion.

Compare the muscle bulk to the opposite uninjured site. Deltoid muscle atrophy may be appreciable within a matter of weeks due to a combination of denervation and disuse. When viewed from the front, the injured shoulder appears *squared off* due to the relative prominence of the acromion. The hollowing of deltoid muscle belly may be better appreciated when seen from the side and the back of the patient. In addition, a sulcus sign due to inferior subluxation of the shoulder may be present.

Muscle contractions should be assessed by both inspection and palpation. In the acute setting, if the axillary nerve is intact, it is still possible to elicit deltoid contraction when the shoulder is adducted or when the arm is in a sling. This is achieved by asking the patient to *'push the elbow back'* while the examiner places his/her hand on the posterior deltoid to feel for any contraction.

Once the pain and swelling from the initial trauma have subsided, look for weakness in shoulder elevation. All three heads (anterior, middle and posterior) of the deltoid should be assessed in turn by asking the patient to forward flex, abduct and extend the shoulder while muscle contractions are confirmed by inspection and palpation. Palpation is of particular importance, as there are other shoulder girdle muscles that could initiate the same movements. The passive range of movement should also be examined carefully, looking for evidence of adhesive capsulitis.

Sensibility to light touch over the upper arm (regimental badge area) is compared to the contralateral normal side. Always examine the normal side first to establish a baseline. A 0–10 score (0 being no feeling and 10 being full normal sensation) is a straightforward and practical way of documenting loss/recovery of sensation.

Remember to palpate the radial and brachial pulses to ensure adequacy of perfusion.

One needs to bear in mind that rotator cuff tears following shoulder dislocations occur more frequently in patients with increasing age. With co-existing nerve injury, examination becomes more challenging, and the employment of MRI is particularly valuable in these circumstances.

Pillar 3: Special Tests

Beware that in spite of deltoid paralysis, shoulder abduction may still be preserved in patients with intact rotator cuffs and suprascapular nerve function and who are well rehabilitated. Compared to active abduction, the following clinical tests are more sensitive and specific to demonstrating deltoid paralysis:

Swallowtail Sign [1]:

The test specifically assesses the function of the posterior deltoid fibres, which are key to achieving humeral extension dorsal to the scapular plane. This test is performed by asking the patient to actively extend the shoulders such that both arms project to the back akin to the swallowtail, while the examiner observes from the side (Fig. 23.1). The test is positive if there is a significant lag of extension of the injured shoulder compared to the normal side. It may also be used to monitor recovery of the deltoid muscle.

Abduction in Internal Rotation Sign [2]:

This test is performed by asking the patient to abduct both shoulders in internal rotation (Fig. 23.2). If there is less than full abduction in the injured side, the examiner passively abducts the injured shoulder to the maximum and asks the patient to maintain the position when the examiner releases the limb. Any lag in abduction is attributable to deltoid palsy.

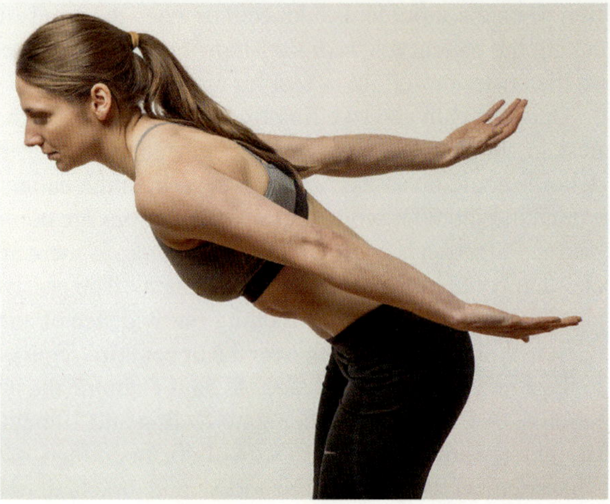

Fig. 23.1 Swallowtail sign. Image Published under License from_www. shoulderdoc.co.uk and www.shoulderpedia.org

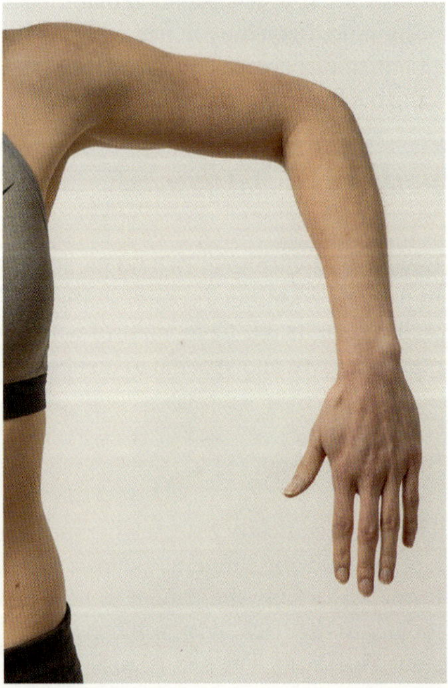

Fig. 23.2 Abduction in internal rotation sign. Image Published under License from www. shoulderdoc.co.uk and www.shoulderpedia.org

Pillar 4: Investigations

When assessing for potential axillary nerve injury, a review of radiographs of the shoulder at the time of trauma is useful to establish the position of the humeral head and the displacement of fracture fragments, if present. Post-manipulation or –surgery radiographs are essential to confirm congruency of the joint and to assess the position of the implant.

In the case of nerve injury and restricted motion, MRI of the shoulder is useful particularly to evaluate the conditions of the rotator cuffs and the infraclavicular brachial plexus. Denervated muscles will show high signal intensity in STIR and T2-weighted sequences.

Neurophysiology is the definitive investigation for the diagnosis of axillary nerve injury. Testing is recommended to be performed at least 3 weeks after injury. If the test is performed too early, a false negative result may be obtained.

Motor nerve conduction studies (NCS) of the axillary nerve may show increased latency and decreased amplitude on the injured side compared to the contralateral normal side. During electromyography (EMG), a needle electrode is used to measure the intrinsic electrical activity of muscle fibres. Insertional, spontaneous and volitional activities of the muscle are noted. Spontaneous activity, prominent fibrillations and positive sharp waves are indicative of active denervation; while high amplitude long duration motor unit potentials are indicative of chronic denervation.

Case Discussion

The index patient described in the chapter not only has features of axillary nerve injury but also has a high risk of developing rotator cuff tears with dislocations in this age group (Chaps.14–16). An MRI scan of the shoulder confirmed a rotator cuff tear. Neurophysiological studies (EMG and NCS) were deferred to 3 weeks and confirmed an axillary nerve injury. The presence of a rotator cuff tear in the absence of a functional deltoid converts this situation into a "flail" shoulder with no residual mechanism of achieving active movements. Early surgical repair of the rotator cuff is warranted in such circumstances, while the definitive plan (observation or exploration) for the nerve injury is decided. Early consultation with a peripheral nerve injury unit is recommended.

Summary

Axillary nerve injury should be suspected in all cases of shoulder trauma and should be actively excluded. Clinical examination is usually confirmatory of such an injury, although partial injuries may require neurophysiological studies to confirm the

Table 23.1 Summary of diagnostic clusters for axillary nerve injury

History
1. Trauma: Dislocation / proximal humeral fracture with significant medial displacement
2. Shoulder weakness/fatigue
3. Numbness in upper arm
Conventional examination
4. Deltoid paralysis
5. Muscle atrophy (may be appreciable within weeks due to a combination of denervation and disuse)
6. Reduced sensibility over upper arm (regimental badge)
Special tests
7. Swallowtail sign
8. Abduction in internal rotation sign
Investigations
9. MRI
10. Neurophysiology

diagnosis. A summary of diagnostic clusters for axillary nerve injury is presented in Table 23.1. Neurophysiological studies are also useful in prognostication and monitoring nerve recovery.

References

1. Nishijima N, Yamamuro K, Fujio K, Ohba M. The swallow-tail sign: a test of deltoid function. J Bone Joint Surg Br. 1995;77(1):152–3.
2. Bertelli JA, Ghizoni MF. Abduction in internal rotation: a test for the diagnosis of axillary nerve palsy. J Hand Surg Am. 2011;36(12):2017–23.

Chapter 24
Suprascapular Neuropathy

Daniel Henderson and Simon Boyle

Case Example

A 27-year-old man presents with aching and weakness of the dominant right shoulder. He plays cricket semi-professionally and is a medium pace bowler. He doesn't recollect a discreet injury. Examination reveals a wasting of the infrascapular fossa and palpation shows posterior joint line discomfort. The infraspinatus is very weak on clinical testing.

Introduction

Suprascapular neuropathy is an uncommon, yet important cause of shoulder symptoms presenting to clinicians. Meta-analyses have found that an isolated suprascapular nerve entrapment is responsible for shoulder pain in only 1–2% of cases, most frequently in males under 40. It is perhaps for this reason that this diagnosis is often forgotten in the differential diagnosis of the painful shoulder [1]. Paralysis of the supraspinatus and infraspinatus as a result of suprascapular nerve pathology was first described by Thomas in 1936 however it is only in recent years that significant improvements in the awareness, understanding and investigation of this pathology have been made. Modern arthroscopic techniques have made treatment of compression of the nerve increasingly viable with minimal morbidity particularly when identified early [2, 3].

D. Henderson
Alps Surgery Institute, Annecy, France

S. Boyle (✉)
York Teaching Hospital, York YO31 8HE, UK
e-mail: simon.boyle@york.nhs.uk

© Springer International Publishing AG 2017

P. Monga, L. Funk (eds.), *Diagnostic Clusters in Shoulder Conditions*,
DOI 10.1007/978-3-319-57334-2_24

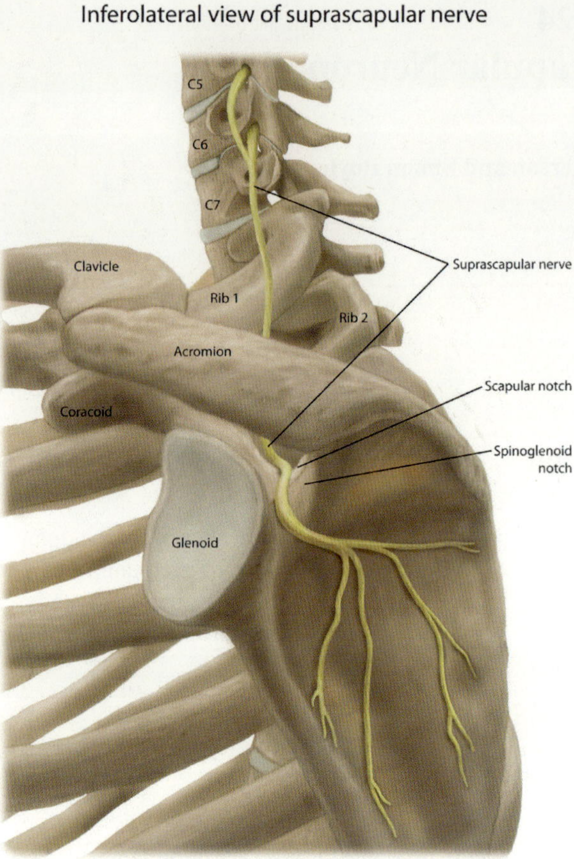

Fig. 24.1 Course of Suprascapular Nerve. Image Published under License from www.shoulder-doc.co.uk

An appreciation of the anatomy of the nerve is vital in the understanding of the different ways in which symptoms may present. The proximal course of the suprascapular nerve runs from its origin at the upper trunk of the brachial plexus and enters the posterior triangle of the neck deep to trapezius where it emerges in the supraspinous fossa. To gain entry to this region of the scapula, it passes through the suprascapular notch; a bony depression bordered superiorly by the transverse scapular ligament. Distal to this point, the nerve supplies motor branches to supraspinatus, as well as receiving afferents from the acromioclavicular and glenohumeral joints [4, 5]. The nerve then continues around the lateral border of the scapular spine, passing under the spinoglenoid ligament in the spinoglenoid notch after which it divides into its terminal motor branches to infraspinatus (Fig. 24.1). An anatomical variant exists in around 15% patients, where a cutaneous branch of the nerve supplies the skin overlying the proximal lateral third of the upper arm [6, 7].

The suprascapular nerve also carries nociceptive pain fibres from multiple structures in the shoulder joint. These include the subacromial bursa, AC joint, the coracohumeral ligament and adjacent capsule, the posterior capsule and the posterior cuff insertion.

Due to its unyielding passage through the fixed anatomical structures of the suprascapular and spinoglenoid notches, the suprascapular nerve is particularly prone to compression, traction injury and entrapment. Penetrating trauma to the neck and posterior shoulder, as well as spinal approaches through the posterior triangle of the neck, place the nerve at risk of injury in its proximal course. The suprascapular notch itself is subject to significant anatomical variation, with six morphological types described [8]. These vary in shape from the rather more nerve-friendly shallow C-shaped notches right up to those notches which are completely enclosed by an ossified transverse scapular ligament. The more constrained notch variants permit very little nerve displacement, making the nerve more vulnerable to compression by ganglion cysts, lipomas, osteochondromas and other mass lesions [8, 9]. The spinoglenoid notch serves as a further site for possible nerve compression. Its proximity to the glenoid rim places the nerve at risk of compression from expanding spinoglenoid notch cysts that may arise from labral tears [10, 11].

The suprascapular nerve is also at risk of traction injuries throughout its course across the scapula, with the two points that again pose the greatest risk to the nerve being the sharp edges of the suprascapular notch and the sharp turn taken by the nerve as it passes out of the supraspinous fossa. Movements of the arm involving scapular retraction with cross arm adduction or hyperabduction increase the tension on the nerve. Athletes involved in sports that require repetitive overhead activities e.g. volleyball are particularly prone to this kind of nerve injury. In such sports, the internal rotation and adduction seen during the follow-through phase of throwing leads to increased tension in the posterior capsular attachment of the spinoglenoid ligament leading to friction on the nerve at that site [12, 13].

Similarly, in massive rotator cuff tears, tethering or a change of direction of the branches of the nerve may occur when a torn rotator cuff has retracted. This can lead to altered suprascapular nerve function [13–15].

This appreciation of the unique anatomy and course of the SSN is a key factor in understanding the diagnostic clusters that present due to a suprascapular neuropathy. The typical sites of nerve compromise each relate to a specific cluster of clinical signs and symptoms. For example, nerve lesions in the spinoglenoid notch cause infraspinatus dysfunction while sparing supraspinatus, whereas pathology at the suprascapular notch affects both.

Pillar 1 Clinical History

Suprascapular nerve pathology is a rare isolated abnormality and was historically found to be a diagnosis of exclusion. The clinical history and examination signs are often non-specific and as such an index of suspicion is needed to aid in making this diagnosis. Most patients may present with a dull aching shoulder pain. This pain is often difficult for patients to localise and can be exacerbated by overhead movements. This can be constant and similar in nature to impingement type discomfort.

A further symptom may be vague posterior shoulder pain. When the discomfort associated with suprascapular nerve pathology does localise itself, it is usually over the posterior aspect of the shoulder [16]. This most likely reflects the pattern of nociceptive afferents and cutaneous sensation that contribute to the suprascapular nerve. Pain is less of a feature when the compression exists at or below the level of the spinoglenoid notch as the nerve is predominantly motor at this level.

Weakness is one of the most common features in the history of patients presenting with a suprascapular nerve dysfunction. This may be a late symptom and leads to patients describing difficulty in elevating the arm in movements such as forward flexion and abduction and maintaining power with any activities requiring external rotation. This is particularly disabling for manual and overhead occupations as well as overhead sports.

Fatigue with overhead activities reflects the early, often subclinical weakness resulting from nerve dysfunction. Patients who are involved in professions requiring repeated overhead tasks such as painting and decorating, cleaning, joinery and electricians, report increasing fatigue with their day-to-day work. This is usually progressive and leads to activity modification.

There is commonly a history of repetitive strain or prolonged overhead activities in patients who present with an isolated suprascapular nerve lesion. This is believed to be secondary to a traction or repetitive microtrauma mechanism leading to neuropathy. This most frequently affects the nerve at the level of the suprascapular notch or spinoglenoid notch. Sports such as tennis or volleyball are the most commonly implicated due to the repetitive and extreme nature of the arm positions required for these activities. The spinoglenoid ligament is known to tighten when the shoulder is in the overhead position for throwing which adds a further mechanism for nerve insult [17]. Vigorous activities such as horse riding or even household tasks such as cleaning can result in nerve dysfunction.

Direct trauma is an infrequent cause of direct suprascapular nerve injury but should always be considered in cases of shoulder weakness particularly after high-energy injuries. Fractures affecting the scapula can lead to nerve injury, particularly given the relatively unyielding course of the nerve. This is especially true where displaced fracture lines extend to the suprascapular notch.

Even less common are nerve injuries that occur as a result of surgery. This could include procedures on the posterior triangle of the neck or as a consequence of a posterior surgical approach the scapula. Certain stabilisation procedures and shoulder arthroscopy procedures can put the nerve at risk.

A history of a rotator cuff tear or its surgical repair is relevant in the diagnosis of suprascapular nerve disorders. The suprascapular nerve course is affected by both retracted rotator cuff tears and from the surgical reduction of chronically retracted cuff tears. In retracted supraspinatus tears, the nerve comes under increasing tension as the retraction approaches 2–3 cm [18]. The surgical advancement of chronically retracted rotator cuff tears may likewise place the nerve under tension. Just 1–3 cm of lateral advancement could lead to nerve dysfunction following repair [5, 19].

Pillar 2: Clinical Examination

Patients with suspected suprascapular nerve pathology should always undergo a thorough examination of the cervical spine and shoulder. This should follow the routine of Look, Feel, Move and Special tests. This will help exclude or identify associated pathologies such as cervical nerve root compression, labral tears and cysts and rotator cuff tears. A neurological assessment of the upper limb may reveal signs of a brachial plexopathy such as Parsonage-Turner syndrome. The following clusters should raise the examiner's suspicions of a suprascapular nerve disorder.

When both supraspinatus and infraspinatus muscles are seen to have undergone atrophy, the examiner should be suspicious of a proximal lesion of the nerve. The site of injury is most commonly at the level of the suprascapular notch. In some cases, tenderness on deep palpation behind the midpoint of the clavicle may be found.

In cases where there is isolated infraspinatus wasting, the nerve is likely to be injured distal to the suprascapular notch. This most frequently occurs at the level of the spinoglenoid notch. The examiner should be vigilant in examining for labral lesions, which may give rise to cysts as these can extend backwards to compress the nerve as it passes around the spine of the scapula. Tenderness and a reproduction of symptoms may be elicited with deep palpation of the posterior joint line or at the level of the spine of the scapula.

Cross-body adduction with internal rotation may reproduce pain in the posterior shoulder as a result of tensioning of the spinoglenoid ligament although this test has low sensitivity and specificity [17].

Patients may describe weakness in abduction, and this can be tested by contracting the muscle against gravity or an externally applied resistance force. It is useful to record this with an MRC grading and compare this to the opposite side.

Muscle testing of infraspinatus is difficult to assess in isolation. Muscle power testing in external rotation can be evaluated with the elbow at the side with the forearm perpendicular to the body Fig. (15.1). Further testing of resisted external rotation with the shoulder in 90 abduction and externally rotated may reveal differences between both shoulders and is useful in isolating Teres minor function Fig. (17.3).

Pillar 3: Special Tests

The suprascapular nerve stretch test was described by Laurent Lafosse, and is performed with the clinician stood behind the patient. The head is gently rotated away from the affected shoulder and held by the clinician. The clinician's other hand is then used to retract the shoulder (Fig. 24.2). A positive test results in an increase in pain in the posterior shoulder [20].

Injection of the suprascapular notch under image guidance assists in localising this region as a potential site of compression for the nerve. An injection here which relieves any shoulder symptoms guides further investigation for nerve pathology in this area and is a relative indication for release of the nerve, even where electrodiagnostic studies are normal [21].

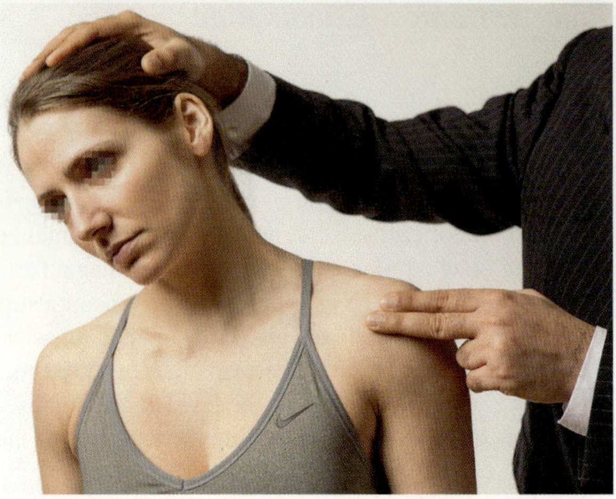

Fig. 24.2 Suprascapular nerve stretch test. Image Published under License from www.shoulderdoc.co.uk and www.shoulderpedia.org

As with suprascapular notch injections, a spinoglenoid notch injection which completely resolves all shoulder symptoms should lead to further investigation and consideration of surgical release.

Pillar 4: Investigations

Standard x-rays of the shoulder should be obtained to include AP and axillary views. These can be used to assess for osseous shoulder pathologies such as osteoarthritis, cuff tear arthropathy, tumours, fractures and mal-unions. A Stryker notch view (beam angled 15–30° cephalad) better visualises the suprascapular notch allowing the assessment of its morphology and to determine the presence of a bony bar superiorly [22].

Computerised tomography has a role in the visualisation of the suprascapular notch where bone abnormalities are suspected but where these are not clear on plain x-ray images. It is the investigation of choice where a fracture has been the cause of the nerve dysfunction.

MRI as an imaging modality provides excellent evaluation of the soft tissues around the shoulder and can be used to visualise the course of the nerve. The rotator cuff can be assessed for tears, and muscle atrophy, cysts, soft tissue tumours or any other compressive causes for nerve injury may be identified [23, 24]. The sensitivity of magnetic resonance imaging for detecting labral lesions is increased with the addition of arthrography [25].

Electrodiagnostic studies are indicated in cases where the diagnosis of shoulder pain remains unclear or where there is clinical or MRI confirmation of muscle wasting and weakness in the absence of a rotator cuff tear [26]. EMG studies can assess for denervation of the supraspinatus and infraspinatus muscles as well as any sharp waves or fibrillations. Motor velocities and latencies can be determined. However, the use of sensory velocities are less reliable due to variations in nerve anatomy. The clinical suspicion of a suprascapular nerve lesion should always be communicated to the neurophysiologist when requesting the investigations. Ideally, the investigator should be experienced in assessing the suprascapular nerve, and a comparison should always be made with the opposite shoulder.

Discussion of the Case

The case discussed earlier in the chapter underwent an MR Arthrogram scan of the shoulder which revealed a spinoglenoid cyst associated with a posterior labral tear. The Neurophysiology studies confirmed infraspinatus palsy and a suprascapular nerve lesion. Such spinoglenoid cysts are commonly associated with posterior labral tears and may compress the terminal branches of the suprascapular nerve to the infraspinatus. Arthroscopic decompression of the cyst and posterior labral repair should be considered to relieve external compression on the nerve.

Summary

Disorders of the suprascapular nerve are uncommon, but identification of these diagnostic clusters in the evaluation of the painful shoulder should significantly raise the index of suspicion. This is particularly true in the classical scenario of an overhead worker complaining of dull posterior shoulder aching pain with fatigue and a feeling of weakness. This combined with Supraspinatus and Infraspinatus muscle atrophy and weakness in abduction/external rotation should lead to further investigations, with an MRI scan and electrodiagnostic studies guiding appropriate treatment of any underlying pathology identified. A summary of diagnostic clusters for suprascapular neuropathy are presented in Table 24.1.

Table 24.1 Summary of diagnostic clusters for Suprascapular neuropathy

Clinical history
1. Dull aching or vague posterior shoulder pain
2. Weakness
3. Fatigue with overhead activities
4. Repetitive strain–overhead sports
5. Massive cuff tears
Conventional examination
6. Muscle wasting & weakness of supraspinatus and infraspinatus–suprascapular notch lesion
7. Muscle wasting & weakness of infraspinatus only–spinoglenoid notch lesion
Special test
8. SSN stretch test
Investigations
9. MRI scan—Nerve, labrum, cysts, cuff tendons, cuff muscle,
10. Neurophysiology (electromyography—EMG)

References

1. Zehetgruber H, Noske H, Lang T, Wurnig C. Suprascapular nerve entrapment. A meta-analysis. Int Orthop. 2002;26(6):339–43.
2. Thomas A. La paralysie du muscle sous-epineux. Presse Med. 1936;64:1283–4.
3. Lafosse L, Tomasi A, Corbett S, Baier G, Willems K, Gobezie R. Arthroscopic release of suprascapular nerve entrapment at the suprascapular notch: technique and preliminary results. Arthroscopy. 2007;23(1):34–42.
4. Tubbs RS, Smyth MD, Salter G, Oakes WJ. Anomalous traversement of the suprascapular artery through the suprascapular notch: a possible mechanism for undiagnosed shoulder pain? Med Sci Monit. 2003;9(3):BR116–9.
5. Warner JP, Krushell RJ, Masquelet A, Gerber C. Anatomy and relationships of the suprascapular nerve: anatomical constraints to mobilization of the supraspinatus and infraspinatus muscles in the management of massive rotator-cuff tears. J Bone Joint Surg Am. 1992;74(1):36–45.
6. Horiguchi M. The cutaneous branch of some human suprascapular nerves. J Anat. 1980;130(Pt 1):191–5.
7. Ajmani ML. The cutaneous branch of the human suprascapular nerve. J Anat. 1994;185(Pt 2):439–42.
8. Rengachary SS, Burr D, Lucas S, Hassanein KM, Mohn MP, Matzke H. Suprascapular entrapment neuropathy: a clinical, anatomical, and comparative study. Part 2: Anatomical study. Neurosurgery. 1979;5(4):447–51.
9. Ticker JB, Djurasovic M, Strauch RJ, April EW, Pollock RG, Flatow EL, et al. The incidence of ganglion cysts and other variations in anatomy along the course of the suprascapular nerve. J Shoulder Elb Surg. 1998;7(5):472–8.
10. Semmler A, von Falkenhausen M, Schöder R. Suprascapular nerve entrapment by a spinoglenoid cyst. Neurology. 2008;70:890.
11. Lee BC, Yegappan M, Thiagarajan P. Suprascapular nerve neuropathy secondary to spinoglenoid notch ganglion cyst: case reports and review of literature. Ann Acad Med Singap. 2007;36:1032–5.
12. Plancher KD, Peterson RK, Johnston JC, Luke TA. The spinoglenoid ligament. Anatomy, morphology, and histological findings. J Bone Joint Surg Am. 2005;87(2):361–5.
13. Safran MR. Nerve injury about the shoulder in athletes. Part 1: Suprascapular nerve and axillary nerve. Am J Sports Med. 2004;32(3):803–19.
14. Boykin RE, Friedman DJ, Higgins LD, Warner JJ. Suprascapular neuropathy. J Bone Joint Surg Am. 2010;92-A(13):2348–64.
15. Collin P, Treseder T, Ladermann A, Benkalfate T, Mourtada R, Courage O, et al. Neuropathy of the suprascapular nerve and massive rotator cuff tears: a prospective electromyographic study. J Shoulder Elb Surg. 2014;23(1):28–34.
16. Martin SD, Warren RF, Martin TL, Kennedy K, O'Brien SJ, Wickiewicz TL. Suprascapular neuropathy. Results of non-operative treatment. J Bone Joint Surg Am. 1997;79(8):1159–65.
17. Plancher KD, Luke TA, Peterson RK, Yacoubian SV. Posterior shoulder pain: a dynamic study of the spinoglenoid ligament and treatment with arthroscopic release of the scapular tunnel. Arthroscopy. 2007;23:991–8.
18. Albritton MJ, Graham RD, Richards RS II, Basamania CJ. An anatomic study of the effects on the suprascapular nerve due to retraction of the supraspinatus muscle after a rotator cuff tear. J Shoulder Elb Surg. 2003;12(5):497–500.
19. Greiner A, Golser K, Wambacher M, Kralinger F, Sperner G. The course of the suprascapular nerve in the supraspinatus fossa and its vulnerability in muscle advancement. J Shoulder Elb Surg. 2003;12:256–9.
20. Lafosse L, Piper K, Lanz U. Arthroscopic suprascapular nerve release: indications and technique. J Shoulder Elb Surg. 2011;20:S9–S13.
21. Shah AA, Butler RB, Sung SY, Wells JH, Higgins LD, Warner JJ. Clinical outcomes of suprascapular nerve decompression. J Shoulder Elb Surg. 2011;20(6):975–82.

22. Polguj M, Sibinski M, Grzegorzewski A, Waszczykowski M, Majos A, Topol M. Morphological and radiological study of ossified superior transverse scapular ligament as potential risk factor of suprascapular nerve entrapment. Biomed Res Int. 2014;2014:613601.
23. Inokuchi W, Ogawa K, Horiuchi Y. Magnetic resonance imaging of suprascapular nerve palsy. J Shoulder Elb Surg. 1998;7:223–7.
24. Ahlawat S, Wadhwa V, Belzberg AJ, Batra K, Chhabra A. Spectrum of suprascapular nerve lesions: normal and abnormal neuromuscular imaging appearances on 3-T MR neurography. Am J Roentgenol. 2015;204(3):589–601.
25. Magee T. 3-T MRI of the shoulder: is MR arthrography necessary? Am J Roentgenol. 2009;192:86–92.
26. Bredella MA, Tirman PF, Fritz RC, Wischer TK, Stork A, Genant HK. Denervation syndromes of the shoulder girdle: MR imaging with electrophysiologic correlation. Skelet Radiol. 1999;28:567–72.

Chapter 25
Brachial Plexus Palsy

Dariush Nikkhah and Sohail Akhtar

Case Example

A 22-year-old motorcyclist presents with multiple rib injuries, a clavicle fracture and weakness of the upper limb. He has numbness of the right upper limb involving the upper plexus distribution, a positive Horner's sign and weakness on testing for deltoid, supraspinatus and infraspinatus.

Introduction

Brachial plexus palsy is a devastating condition, resulting in profound motor and sensory loss to the upper extremity. Direct injury to the plexus is the most common cause of palsy whether this is an open or closed injury. In our modern world with ever evolving high energy environments, injuries are often as a result of road traffic accidents and the group most commonly affected is the young male patient [1]. Other than high-energy injuries the aetiology for brachial plexus palsy is varied and includes obstetric injury, penetrating trauma, iatrogenic injury from direct surgical injury or post radiotherapy injury and tumours. The nature of injury in brachial plexus palsy can vary from traction, crush, compression or sharp injuries [1]. The clinician must also be aware that brachial plexus palsy may not occur in isolation and can include damage to other vital structures; this is especially true in high-velocity trauma.

D. Nikkhah, M.R.C.S. (✉)
Barts and The Royal London Hospital, London, UK
e-mail: dariushnikkhah@hotmail.com

S. Akhtar, F.R.C.S.
Wrightington Upper Limb Unit, Wigan, UK

© Springer International Publishing AG 2017

P. Monga, L. Funk (eds.), *Diagnostic Clusters in Shoulder Conditions*,
DOI 10.1007/978-3-319-57334-2_25

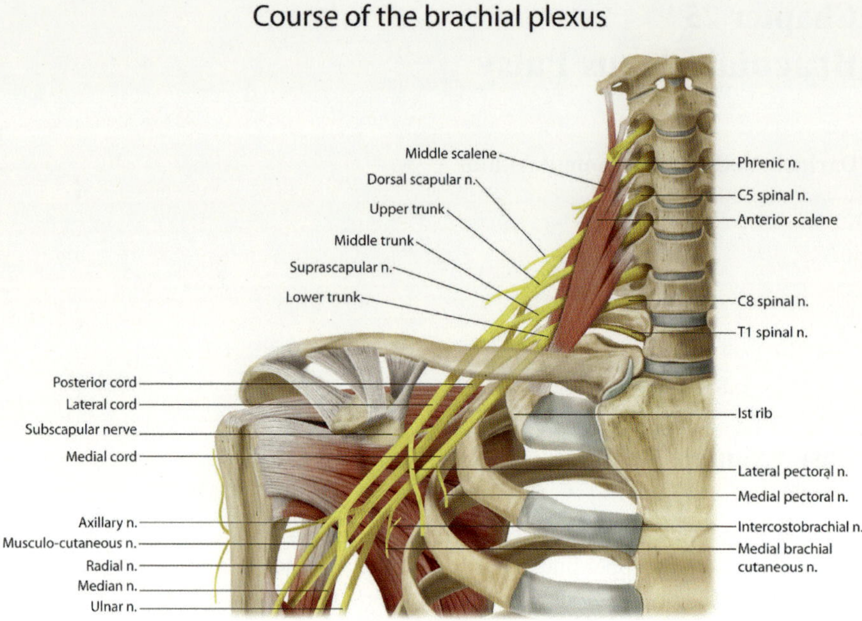

Fig. 25.1 Brachial plexus anatomy. Image Published under License from www.shoulderdoc.co.uk

Knowledge of the anatomy of the brachial plexus is key in understanding its normal action and clinical presentations of injury. The anatomy of the brachial plexus corresponds to a branching pattern of roots, trunks, divisions, cords, terminal branches and ultimately leading to the peripheral nerves (Fig. 25.1). Each section of the brachial plexus is located in its own anatomical domain. The roots travel in the upper neck between the anterior and middle scalene muscles. The three trunks are located in the posterior cervical triangle. The upper trunk is formed by the union of C5 and C6 (so called Erb's point) and the lower trunk C8 and T1; the middle trunk is the continuation of C7. All three trunks divide into anterior and posterior divisions beneath the clavicle. The divisions then travel underneath the pectoralis minor where they form three cords [1]. The cords are named in relation to their position relative to the axillary artery. The lateral and medial cords join to form the median nerve, the musculocutaneous and ulnar nerves are terminal branches of the lateral and medial cords respectively. The radial and axillary nerves are terminal cord branches of the posterior cord.

Certain patterns are more predominant in brachial plexus injuries with supraclavicular lesions being more common (75% cases) than infraclavicular lesions [2]. The roots and trunks are more commonly injured than the divisions, cords and branches [2]. Traction injuries can cause either upper plexus lesions C5, C6 or lower plexus injuries C8-T1, or in some instances total plexus injuries C5-T1.

Pillar 1: Clinical History

The clinical history should start by gaining an understanding of the *mechanism* [3] including gauging the magnitude of force involved in the injury. The mechanism and force correlate closely with the modality of treatment as an example sharp injuries may be repaired primarily however in cases where there is a significant zone of trauma, primary repair may not be possible and nerves may have to be tagged for later repair with autologous nerve grafts.

The clinician should also determine the evolution of sensory and motor deficits and whether there has been any improvement or deterioration in motor function with time [4]. Serial examination is, therefore, key in providing prognosis and guiding management.

Associated injuries should also be documented, particularly in high-velocity injuries that may have resulted in multiple ribs, cervical spine and extremity fractures. Other symptoms to explore with the patient is pain. Severe, unremitting burning pain is characteristic of nerve root avulsion [4]. The *duration since* injury is necessary to determine; presently there is evolving debate regarding when best to surgically intervene in a closed brachial plexus injury. Historically, delayed surgical exploration until at least 6 months after injury was routine [4] however over the last 10 years there has been a move to surgically explore within 4 weeks of injury in the belief that earlier nerve repair yields better functional outcomes [5, 6].

The *age* of the patient is also an important factor in children and young adults <20 years tend to do better in terms of nerve recovery [5].

Pillar 2: Conventional Examination

In a patient involved in a high-energy injury, it is important to follow ATLS principles and exclude or stabilise life-threatening injuries. Brachial plexus palsy can occur in conjunction with significant trauma [2]. Once these have been excluded or treated one can move on to looking into brachial plexus function in a more detailed fashion. Examination of the Brachial Plexus should stick to the well-trodden paradigm of *look, feel, move*.

One should *look* for asymmetry, scars and muscle atrophy in the upper body [3].

In neonates who have obstetric brachial plexus palsy physical examination is more challenging. Any asymmetry or unusual posture of the upper limb may be suggestive of brachial plexus palsy. Reflex tests such as the *Moro test* or the *Fencer test* are useful investigations to determine the presence of brachial plexus palsy.

The clinician should *feel* the supraclavicular and infraclavicular areas for evidence of any expanding masses that could be compressing the plexus. Furthermore, the clavicle can be assessed for possible fractures and the chest wall for surgical emphysema that may be suggestive of pneumothorax.

Following this *movement* of the individual muscle groups supplied by the brachial plexus are assessed through their active and passive range of motion. The MRC (Medical Research Council) scale (M0-M5) is used to gauge muscle power from proximal to distal.

Pillar 3 Special Tests (Neurological Assessment)

The key to making a diagnosis in such complex situations is pattern recognition. Initially, it is useful to proceed systematically trying to work out the level of neurological deficit and whether this injury falls into common patterns of nerve injury as described in Table 25.1. *Upper plexus injuries* (C5-7) tend to result in glenohumeral joint subluxation, loss of shoulder abduction, external rotation and elbow flexion [7]. *Lower Plexus injuries* (C8-TI) present with weakened wrist and finger flexion and loss of the intrinsic muscles of the hand [7]. *Complete plexus injury* (C5-T1) presents with an insensate flail upper limb and glenohumeral joint subluxation. Also, increased tone and deep tendon reflexes should be assessed as these would help exclude any associated head or spinal cord injury.

On a cooperative patient, the clinician can make a detailed assessment of the terminal branches off the brachial plexus. The radial, ulnar and median nerves can be assessed with wrist and finger motion [2]. When assessing motor function one must also assess neighbouring cranial nerves such as the spinal accessory nerve (XI) which has been described as an extra-plexus nerve transfer. This nerve innervates the trapezius muscle and can be damaged in addition to the brachial plexus in severe

Table 25.1 Common patterns of neurological injury

Finding	Inference
Weak trapezius	Cranial nerve - spinal accessory N XI Injury at posterior triangle of neck
Bilateral neurological deficit	Cervical spine injury
Asymmetric neurological deficit	Nerve root/brachial plexus or peripheral nerve injury
Horner's syndrome	Pre-ganglionic injury
Weak rhomboids	Dorsal scapular nerve injury (pre-ganglionic)
Weak Serratus anterior	Long thoracic nerve injury (preganglionic)
Sensory loss C5-7, loss of shoulder abduction, external rotation and elbow flexion	Upper plexus
Sensory loss C8-T1, weakened wrist and finger flexion and loss of the intrinsic muscles of the hand	Lower plexus
Insensate flail upper limb and glenohumeral joint subluxation.	Complete plexus
Weak supraspinatus and infraspinatus	Suprascapular nerve injury (upper trunk)
Loss of extension of wrist, elbow and shoulder	Posterior cord injury
Loss of flexion of elbow	Lateral cord injury
Isolated peripheral nerve involvement	Lesion distal to brachial plexus

head and neck trauma. Trapezial paralysis will result in an inability to shrug and abduct the shoulder with the rotation of the scapula.

A preganglionic injury which occurs due to root avulsion proximal to the dorsal root ganglion (DRG) will most likely be treated by nerve transfers instead of primary neurorrhaphy (primary repair of the nerve ends) or nerve grafting as these are not possible. In contrast, post-ganglionic injuries can be managed with nerve grafting or primary repair. There are better outcomes associated with post-ganglionic injuries compared to root avulsion injuries. Clinically it is possible to determine whether the injury to the brachial plexus is pre or post-ganglionic. An injury to the long thoracic nerve (LTN) or dorsal scapular nerve is suggestive of a pre-ganglionic lesion [2]. Clinically a lesion to the LTN (C5-C7) results in scapular winging. The dorsal scapular nerve (C4-C5) innervates the rhomboid muscles and if injured then on inspection of the patient's back there will be visible atrophy of this muscle group [2]. Horner's syndrome which manifests as miosis, ptosis, enophthalmos and dry eyes is also another clinical sign of preganglionic disruption to the plexus. The sympathetic outflow of the head and neck is in close proximity with the T1 nerve root. Therefore avulsion of the T1 nerve root results in injury to the sympathetic ganglion and results in Horner's syndrome [2].

From the trunk level, the only nerve that can be examined is the suprascapular nerve (C5-C6) which results in atrophy of the infraspinatus and supraspinatus muscles, with increased visibility of the scapular spine [1]. The infraspinatus can be assessed by bending the elbow in flexion and resisting external rotation. The lateral and medial pectoral nerves, innervate the clavicular and sternal heads of the pectoralis major muscle and come off the lateral and medial cords of the plexus [2]. The pectoralis major muscle can be palpated for bulk and contraction by forced adduction by the patient.

If the patient has an inability to flex the elbow, this is suggestive of a C5-C6 lesion affecting the musculocutaneous nerve coming off the lateral cord. Failure to extend the elbow is indicative of a high radial nerve injury coming off the posterior cord (C5-T1). The posterior cord has several branches that come off in addition to the radial nerve. The axillary nerve comes off the posterior cord and innervates the deltoid, which enables shoulder abduction. Therefore an inability to extend the wrist, elbow and shoulder is suggestive of a posterior cord lesion [2].Another important branch coming off the posterior cord is the thoracodorsal nerve which innervates the latissimus dorsi (LD) muscle; this nerve can also be used as an Intra plexus nerve transfer. The anterior border of the LD can be palpated in the posterior axillary fold and can be accentuated by forced adduction by asking the patient to hold their hands to their hip or provide a forced cough [2].

A weakness of the intrinsic muscles of the hand, weakened wrist and finger flexion is suggestive of a lower brachial plexus injury (C8-T1). The patient will not be able to adduct and abduct the fingers with evidence of wasting of the interosseous muscles.

Physical examination should also include a thorough assessment of the sensory dermatomes of the upper limb (Fig. 25.2). Moving and static two-point discrimination can also be helpful in objectively determining lesions of the terminal branches of the brachial plexus. Vascular rupture of the subclavian artery can occur in high-velocity trauma [4] and therefore the vascular state of the upper limb should be assessed using simple palpation of peripheral pulses or a hand held doppler. One should also feel for any thrills and auscultate for any bruits that may be evidence of axillary or subclavian artery dissection or rupture.

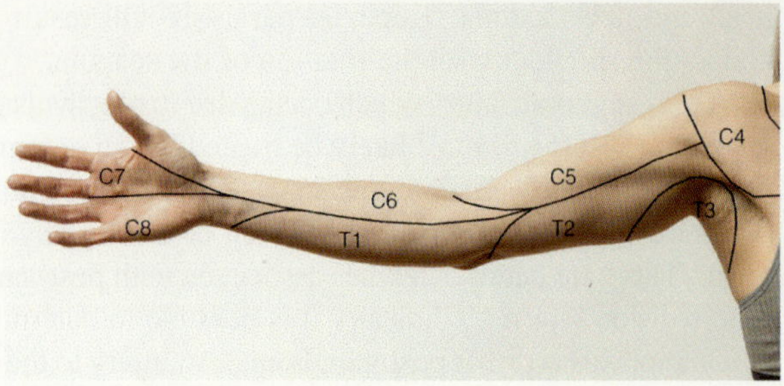

Fig. 25.2 Upper limb dermatomes. Image Published under License from www.shoulderdoc.co.uk and www.shoulderpedia.org

Nerve recovery can be assessed by percussion; the *Tinel sign* involves percussing over the nerve, paraesthesia occurs over the site of the recovering nerve lesion. With time if the lesion recovers then the Tinel sign advances [1]. It is suggested that nerve regeneration occurs at 1 mm a day and is a slow process after primary nerve repair. In cases of preganglionic rupture where there has been avulsion from the cord, the percussion test would reveal no pain and predicts a much poorer prognosis.

The multiply injured patient may have their brachial plexus palsy overlooked. Associated shoulder girdle injury, first rib injuries, axillary artery injuries may be the only clues of brachial plexus palsy in the sedated patient on ITU [2].

Pillar 4: Investigations

Radiological imaging can be used to determine gross anatomical disruption of the brachial plexus such as root avulsion as well as picking out associated injuries and giving an impression of the energy of the injury. With intrinsic nerve injury as apposed to gross anatomical nerve disruption sophisticated electrical studies can shed light on the physiological function of the nerve.

Radiographic evaluation should include standard radiographs of the cervical spine, clavicle, shoulder, scapula and chest. Cervical radiographs that reveal fractures of spinous processes, transverse processes and vertebral bodies are suggestive of preganglionic injuries. A plain radiograph of the chest (CXR) should be performed to exclude pneumothorax, and can at the same time delineate any clavicular or glenohumeral joint fractures or dislocations. Phrenic nerve injury (C3 - C5) will result in an elevated hemidiaphragm which would be visible on an inspiratory CXR. Phrenic nerve injury is also suggestive of a preganglionic injury to the brachial plexus. CXR should also be used to assess for rib fractures as intercostal nerves may be utilised as extraplexus nerve transfers in the patient's future treatment, and rib fractures is a contraindication for this surgical reconstructive option [2].

Myelography was initially described to determine the nature of avulsion injuries in the brachial plexus, and since then CT myelography has been developed to help evaluation the level of nerve root injury. CT myelography has a sensitivity of 95% and specificity of 98% [1]. Root avulsion results in dural tears, which scar and develop into pseudo meningoceles that can be visualised with CT myelography. However, this process usually takes up to a month to develop and therefore CT myelography is best performed at this stage [1, 8]. In contrast, MRI is a non-invasive approach to assessing root avulsion and does not need to be delayed like CT myelography. Furthermore, MRI provides a global picture of the brachial plexus and MR Neurography has currently become the most useful tool for assessing brachial plexus injuries.

Nerve conduction studies (NCS) and needle electromyography (EMG) provide additional preoperative and intraoperative assessment of brachial plexus palsy [9]. These studies serve as an adjunct to clinical examination, history and imaging modalities described earlier. For closed plexus injuries, EMG and NCS can be performed after 3 weeks. EMG tests muscles during activity and at rest and helps identify denervation changes in the muscle and can be seen as fibrillation potentials [2]. EMG also has a potential to show increased motor unit potentials which are suggestive of nerve recovery with a reduction in fibrillation potentials in reinnervated muscle [2]. Serial EMGs should be performed to assess for recovery. This is useful in low-velocity injuries where on clinical examination there are signs of recovery *e.g. advancing Tinel's sign* that is suggestive of gradual recovery.

NCS can accurately localise nerve lesions to a few centimetres [9] and can be used in the intraoperative setting to demonstrate sensory nerve action potentials (SNAPs). This can clarify whether the lesion is preganglionic or postganglionic [1]. The recording of SNAPs from the peripheral nerves indicates the presence of root avulsion, and therefore recovery is not possible, and surgical exploration is warranted [1]. The DRG lies outside of the spinal cord and is therefore not injured in root avulsion injuries. In contrast, if the avulsion occurs distal to the DRG, the sensory axons undergo Wallerian degeneration, and no SNAPs are recorded [1].

Discussion of the Case

High-energy injuries are commonly associated with brachial plexus injuries. The patient described in this chapter has an upper plexus preganglionic injury, perhaps nerve root avulsion. An MR scan of the spine and MR of the brachial plexus followed by deferred neurophysiological tests (EMG/NCV) at 3 weeks confirmed the diagnosis.

Summary

The diagnosis and subsequent management of brachial plexus palsy require a systematic history and serial examination as discussed in this chapter. With methodical clinical examination in the cooperative patient, one can localise the nerve lesion. This initial assessment along with serial examination will accurately provide a prognosis for the condition and guide a clinician as to how and when to proceed with treatment. Additional imaging and electrophysiological tests serve as useful preoperative and intraoperative adjuncts in the management of these injuries. A summary of diagnostic clusters for a brachial plexus injury is provided in Table 25.2. A debate regarding the merits of early surgical intervention has been developing over the last decade; this decision requires an understanding of the mechanism along with clinical progression and results of imaging.

Table 25.2 Summary of diagnostic clusters for brachial plexus

Clinical history
1. Mechanism of injury to plexus [1] crush [2] traction [3] compression [4] open
2. Obstetric—Shoulder dystocia
3. Nature of any pain, severe, unremitting burning pain characteristic of nerve root avulsion
4. Any additional injuries sustained (vascular, chest, fractures)
Conventional examination
5. Inspection look for asymmetry, scars, muscle atrophy
Special tests
6. Schematic neurological assessment: Dermatomes, individual muscles and as per Table 25.1
7. Tinel sign—Percussion at the site of nerve repair or injury— Paraesthesia occurs at the site of nerve regeneration
8. Horner's sign—Indicates avulsion of the T1 root
Investigations
9. MR of brachial plexus and spine
10. Nerve conduction tests after 3 weeks can differentiate pre- from post-ganglionic injuries

Conflict of Interest None.

References

1. Tung TH, Mackinnon SE. Brachial plexus injuries. Clin Plast Surg. 2003;30(2):269–87.
2. Moran SL, Steinmann SP, Shin AY. Adult brachial plexus injuries: mechanism, patterns of injury, and physical diagnosis. Hand Clin. 2005;21(1):13–24.
3. Terzis JK, Papakonstantinou KC. The surgical treatment of brachial plexus injuries in adults. Plast Reconstr Surg. 2000;106(5):1097–122. quiz 123-4
4. Thornton DK, S. A clinical approach to the management of brachial plexus and peripheral nerve injury. Surgery. 2009;28(2):79–84.
5. Jivan S, Kumar N, Wiberg M, Kay S. The influence of pre-surgical delay on functional outcome after reconstruction of brachial plexus injuries. J Plast Reconstr Aesthet Surg. 2009;62(4):472–9.
6. Birch R. Timing of surgical reconstruction for closed traumatic injury to the supraclavicular brachial plexus. J Hand Surg Eur. 2014;40(6):562–7.
7. Chuang D. Brachial plexus injuries: adult and Paediatric. In: Neligan P, editor. Plastic surgery. 3rd ed. China: Elsevier; 2015.
8. Birch R. Brachial plexus injuries. J Bone Joint Surg Br. 1996;78(6):986–92.
9. Harper CM. Preoperative and intraoperative electrophysiologic assessment of brachial plexus injuries. Hand Clin. 2005;21(1):39–46. vi

Part IV
Shoulder Instability Clusters

Chapter 26
Atraumatic Instability

Julia Walton, Sarah Russell, and Jill Thomas

Case Example

A 17-year-old girl attends with her anxious parents with a history of recurrent subluxations of her shoulder for the past 2 years. There is no history of any significant traumatic event and no true dislocations, requiring relocation. Both the parents are busy TV "celebrities" and are busy professionals. The girl describes recurrent dislocations in different directions. On active forward flexion, she has a reproducible posterior subluxation of her shoulder in the midrange. Her Beighton score is 7/9, sulcus sign is positive, and one can see abnormal muscle patterning behaviour and scapular dyskinesia on arm elevation.

Introduction

Atraumatic shoulder instability is a subgroup of shoulder instability that presents without a traumatic primary cause. There is a delicate balance between the structural stability provided at the glenohumeral joint, and dynamic stability. Dynamic stability is provided by muscular activation and locally by the rotator cuff, which centralises the humeral head on the glenoid, and from the scapula-thoracic region. Additionally, stability and strength is gained from the rest of the musculoskeletal system also known as the kinetic chain [1].

Management and diagnosis should assess the degree of trauma, the extent of structural damage, any abnormal muscle recruitment, and the full kinetic chain.

J. Walton (✉) • S. Russell • J. Thomas
Wrightington Hospital, Wigan, UK
e-mail: julia.walton@wwl.nhs.uk

© Springer International Publishing AG 2017

P. Monga, L. Funk (eds.), *Diagnostic Clusters in Shoulder Conditions*,
DOI 10.1007/978-3-319-57334-2_26

The Stanmore classification system recognises a continuum and coexistence of these pathologies, which can occur and can be graphically displayed as a triangle [2] (Fig. 26.1).

The polar instability pathologies are called Type I (traumatic instability) Type II (atraumatic instability) and Type III (atraumatic neurological dysfunctional or muscle patterning). Patients are classified according to the history and clinical examination findings. An unstable shoulder can sit anywhere along this continuum, and its position can change along an axis. Ongoing assessment is essential to ensure appropriate management. Atraumatic Instability (Polar Type II) is a clinical manifestation involving a vast spectrum of underlying causes or associated presentations. The atraumatic unstable shoulder can present clinically as uni- or multi-directional, often involving shoulder joint hyperlaxity and possible repetitive end of range stresses. The patient may also present with abnormal muscle patterning Polar type II/III) with an ability to voluntarily dislocate their shoulder which can manifest in an involuntary shoulder instability. Atraumatic unstable shoulders may also have additional damage to the capsulo-labral structures (Polar Type II/I) as seen in the traumatic instability cohort (Table 26.1).

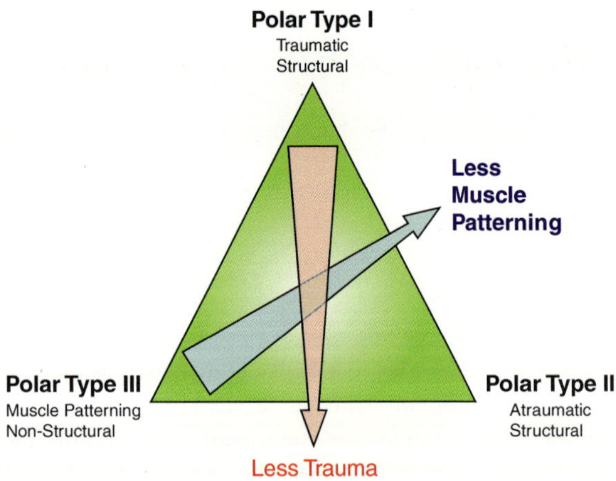

Fig. 26.1 The Stanmore Instability Triangle

Table 26.1 Common Clinical manifestations of atraumatic instability

Uni/multidirectional
Hyperlaxity at shoulder or generally
Voluntary instability with associated abnormal muscle patterning
Underlying anatomical or neural deflect/pathology
Dysfunctional motor development
Possible Psychological factors e.g. secondary gain
Repetitive end of range shoulder movements e.g. thrower
Capsulo-labral structural damage
Pain
Weakness

The challenge clinically is to identify the contributing factors and devise a patient-specific rehabilitation programme to target the most relevant issues.

Pillar 1: History

Atraumatic shoulder instability often presents between the ages of 10–35 years old, with pain and instability on activity, without any substantial history of trauma. It can present uni- or bilaterally. Patients may report a variety of instability symptoms from subclinical instability, less obvious glenohumeral instability to recurring shoulder dislocations.

Atraumatic Instability can present with unidirectional dislocations/subluxation or as instability in more than one direction. Even though the term multidirectional instability (MDI) is often used, the definition of MDI does not have a consensus and as a result, may lead to confusion. Excessive laxity of the glenohumeral joint should only be classed as an instability if the patient reports actual symptoms of instability. It is far more useful and accurate to state the directions of instability when making a diagnosis [3].

Patients with atraumatic shoulder instability commonly describe a feeling of the shoulder "coming out" or "slipping out" during certain activities or even at rest. They may also report apprehension, weakness and possible catching, occasionally with numbness, which has been described as the dead arm syndrome [4].

The clinician needs to explore the onset of symptoms and possible causes or changes in activity or lifestyle that may have predisposed to the instability symptoms. The nature of the instability and/or pain behaviour needs to be established. The aggravating and easing factors must be identified. This includes asking about the activities which cause instability and/or pain; any positions that relieve symptoms; what is the patient unable to do functionally and how they manage their instability, e.g., A&E admittance/self-relocation and any rest period or analgesia management.

It is essential to check for a history of trauma or associated condition that may contribute to their shoulder symptoms (Table 26.2). Awareness of other associated conditions is not only essential for the safe management of the atraumatic shoulder instability patient but may also contribute to their symptoms, for example, a connective tissue disorder such as Ehlers Danlos syndrome.

Table 26.2 Underlying conditions associated with atraumatic instability

Condition
Hypermobility
Ehlers Danlos syndrome
Muscular Dystrophies
Viral triggers for denervation
Nerve injury
Marfans
Gleno-humeral dysplasia

Knowledge of the patient's frequency and the dose of analgesia requirements can aid the clinician to establish the patient's pain levels and severity. An awareness of other medications such as steroids and anticoagulants is essential.

Social history is relevant to the onset of the patient's problem. This includes the patient's perspectives, experience and expectation, age, employment, home situation and details of their leisure and sporting activities [5]. Psychosocial risk factors for poor outcomes are normally associated with low back pain and may be relevant in atraumatic instability as well.

Pillar 2 The Conventional Examination

It is important to observe throughout the appointment how the shoulder functions during tasks such as getting on and off a plinth or dressing and undressing. One needs to assess if there are any indication of disuse, limb neglect, abnormal muscle activity, muscle spasm, deformity, bruising, wasting or signs for possible trophic changes present with CRPS. During assessment does the patient report any changes to their symptoms?

When palpating an atraumatic shoulder, it is essential to be guided by the history and consider the irritability and nature of any pain reported by the patient. The shoulder joint congruence, muscle contours and tone, and any asymmetry can be palpated and any tenderness of specific structures can be identified. Any neurological changes should be established. Dermatomal and myotomal assessment investigate sensory or motor changes that may occur due to compression or lesion of the associated peripheral nerve root [6]. It is also important to identify any potentially altered pain perception such as hyperalgesia, allodynia or CRPS. If the shoulder is subluxed or painful, the shoulder girdle posture can often present as downwardly rotated and depressed. Such a position can, therefore, put traction on the lower part of the brachial plexus leading to paraesthesia in the C8 dermatomal distribution.

When assessing the shoulder movement, full or excessive active and passive movement should be evaluated. The quality of the shoulder movement should also be noted. To truly determine dynamic shoulder stability through active movement it is important to assess the endurance element of upper limb movement and, if irritability allows, to repeat movements several times to see the effects of muscle fatigue around the shoulder girdle and trunk.

Abnormal muscle patterning such as inappropriately activating latissimus dorsi or pectoralis major may be observed during the assessment and can be a result of multiple factors (Table 26.3). Throughout the assessment of movement, the position of the humeral head should be observed or palpated to identify significant translation in any direction away from the central axis of rotation. Any compensatory strategies used by the patient to regain a central position to achieve a further range of motion should be noted.

Table 26.3 Factors influencing abnormal muscle patterning

A motor recruitment movement dysfunction that has resulted from recurrent 'party trick' voluntary dislocation manoeuvres;
Dysfunctional motor development;
Underlying anatomical or neural deflect/pathology;
Weakness and fatigue of other more appropriate scapular stabilisers or issues with rotator cuff recruitment;
Possible fear avoidance.

Reproducing movements that provoke the pain can be invaluable in assessing the main physical drivers of atraumatic shoulder instability. Altering the movement strategy and/or muscle recruitment to specific muscular regions, such as scapular assisting or rotator cuff recruiting with gentle external rotation may provide an effective treatment option to address the cause. These sorts of improvement strategies are vital in assessing atraumatic instability and establishing the first stage of a rehabilitation approach [7].

Pilar 3: Special tests

Signs of laxity are frequently seen in adolescents with asymptomatic shoulders. Unlike apprehension signs, which are suggestive of pathology, these signs merely assess movement of the humeral head about the glenoid [8]. Assessing the level and direction of laxity is useful in determining the appropriate diagnosis and management.

Sulcus sign is performed with the patient seated. The examiner exerts a downward pull by grasping the elbow with one hand and stabilising the shoulder girdle with the other. A significant step-off between the acromion and the humeral head indicates a positive test (Fig. 26.2).

Brighton Score [9] assesses global joint hypermobility. A score out of 9 is derived by adding, (i) passive apposition of the thumbs to the flexors aspects of the forearm, (ii) passive dorsiflexion of little fingers beyond 90° (iii) hyper-extension of the elbows beyond 10°, (iv) hyper-extension of the knees beyond 10° and (v) forward flexion of the trunk with knees straight so that palms rest easily on the floor (Fig. 26.3).

Gagey sign is an assessment of passive glenohumeral abduction with the scapula stabilised (Fig. 26.4). In a normal shoulder, such abduction is usually 90° and is an indicator of the laxity of the inferior glenohumeral ligament. An angle of over 105° is associated with lengthening and laxity of the Inferior glenohumeral ligament, usually seen in patients with joint laxity. One needs to assess the core stability of the patient using tests such as the Kibler's corkscrew test (Fig. 26.5). The patient is asked to perform a single leg squat, and the trunk control is assessed. Other tests for assessing anterior instability and posterior instability are described in the respective chapters which follow.

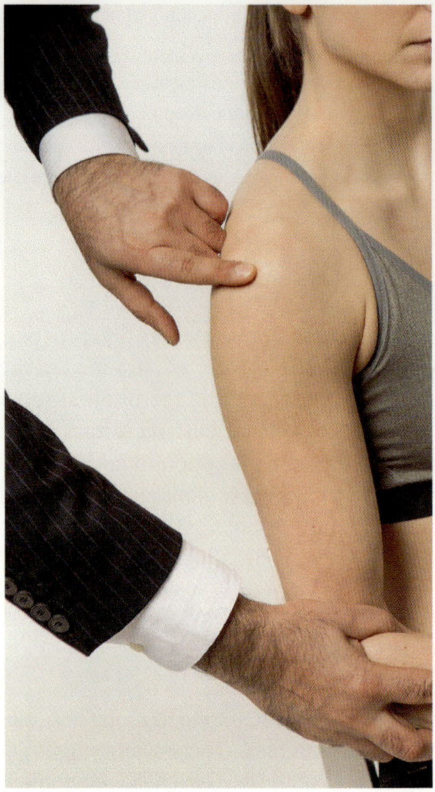

Fig. 26.2 Sulcus Sign. Image Published under License from www.shoulderdoc.co.uk and www.shoulderpedia.org

Pillar 4 Investigations

An MR arthrogram may indicate structural soft tissue and bony lesions as a result of repetitive dislocation. It may also allude to an excessively capacious capsule. A plain MRI without contrast may be inconclusive, and may not identify a labral or capsular tear. In cases of atraumatic instability, such a scan may serve as a reassurance to the patient and the therapist that there is no underlying mechanical lesion.

Arthroscopic assessment will help to determine the direction of instability and forms an essential part of assessing structural laxity and instability. A positive drive through may be present in a lax glenohumeral joint but is not necessarily specific for shoulder instability [10].

Discussion of the case

The 17 year old girl described at the start of the chapter is a "stereotypical" patient with atraumatic instability. Such patients commonly have psychosocial factors influencing the presentation, along with a natural predisposition to instability in the form of hyper laxity. It is very common to hear about relatively minor trauma setting off such episodes of instability. Appropriate management relies on effective pain

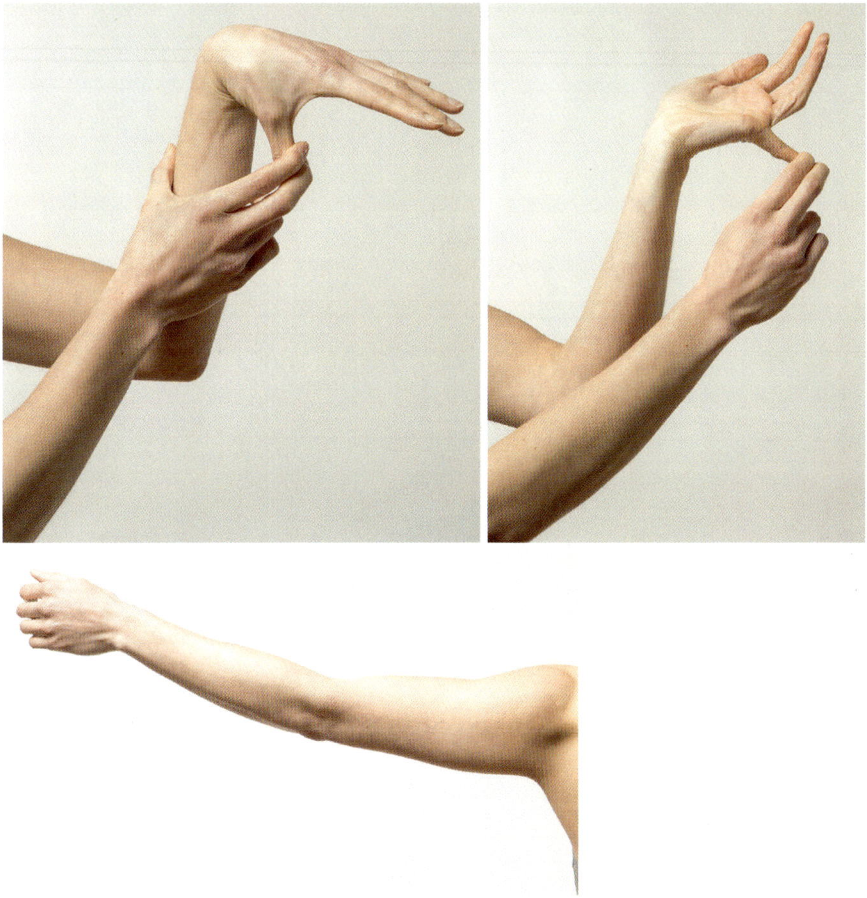

Fig. 26.3 Beighton Score; Thunb to forearm (**a**), little finger hyperextension (**b**), elbow hyperextension (**c**), Palm to floor (**d**) and knee hyperextension (**e**). Image Published under License from www.shoulderdoc.co.uk and www.shoulderpedia.org

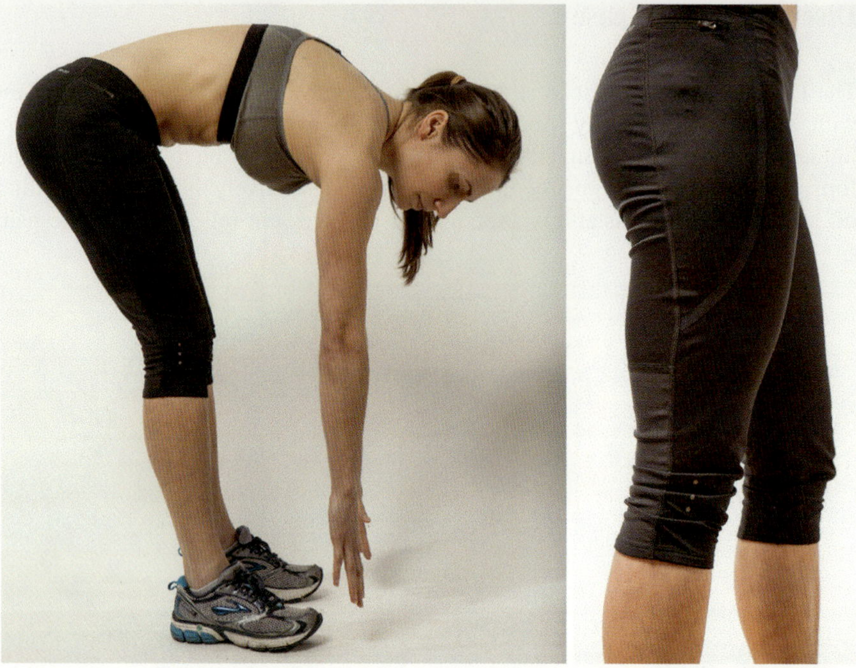

Fig.2.3 (continued)

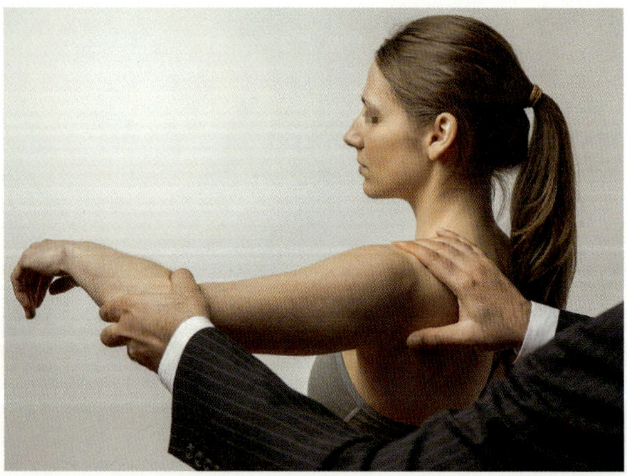

Fig. 26.4 Gagey Sign. Image Published under License from www.shoulderdoc.co.uk and www.shoulderpedia.org

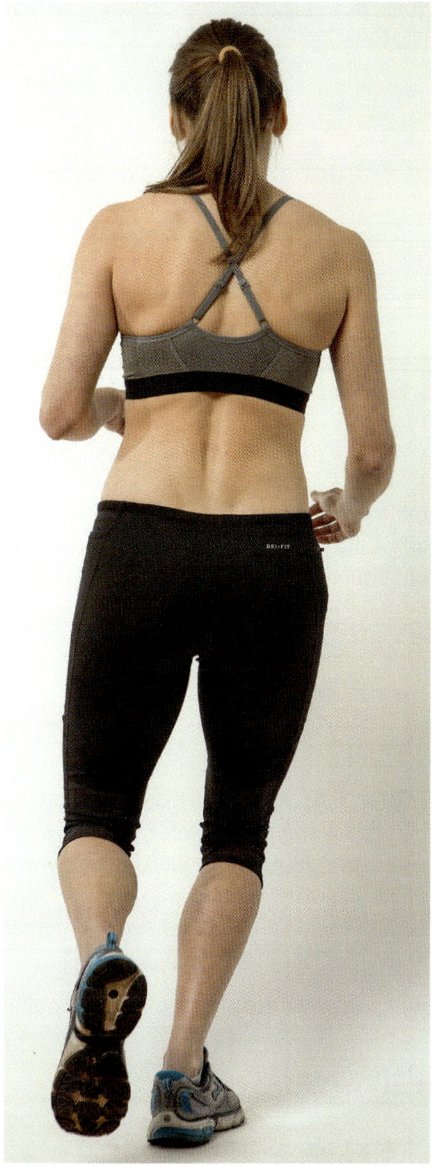

Fig. 26.5 Kibler's corkscrew test. Image Published under License from www.shoulderdoc.co.uk and www.shoulderpedia.org

Table 26.4 Summary of diagnostic clusters for atraumatic instability

Clinical History
1. Age 10–35y
2. Insidious onset- No significant trauma.
3. Recurrent dislocations or subluxations of the shoulder
4. Psychosocial associations common
Conventional Examination
5. Scapula dyskinesia
Special Tests
6. Kibler's corkscrew sign
7. Sulcus sign
8. Gagey Sign
9. Beighton's 5/9
Investigations
10. Capacious capsule on MRA

management, psychosocial support, retraining of affected overactive muscles (usually Lattisimus Dorsi and Pectorals Major) by specialist physiotherapy and ruling out structural causes of instability (MR arthrogram).

Summary

The diagnosis of atraumatic instability is primarily based on a cluster approach (Table 26.4). A detailed history should include not only aspects of pain and instability but also associated psychosocial factors, social history, previous medical treatment and expectations from physiotherapy and rehabilitation. Identification and management of associated social issues (psychologist) are key to management along with a management of structural lesions (surgery), pain management (pain specialist) and management of abnormal muscle patterning behaviour (specialist physiotherapy).

References

1. McMullen J, Uhl T. A kinetic chain approach for shoulder rehabilitation. J Athl Train. 2000;35(3):329–37.
2. Lewis A, Kitamura T, Bayley JIL. The classification of shoulder instability: new light through old windows. Curr Orthop. 2004;18:97–108.
3. McFarland EG, Kim TK, Park HB, Neira CA, Gutierrez MI. The effect of variation in definition on the diagnosis of multidirectional instability of the shoulder. J Bone Joint Surg Am. 2003;85-A(11):2138–44.
4. Magee DJ. Orthopaedic physical assessment. 5th ed. St. Louis, MO: Saunders; 2008.
5. Hengeveld E, Banks K, Maitland GD. Maitland's peripheral manipulation. 4th ed. Edinburgh: Elsevier Butterworth Heinemann; 2005.
6. Petty NJ, editor. Neuromusculoskeletal examination and assessment: a handbook for therapists. UK: Churchill Livingstone Elsevier Health Sciences; 2011. p. 466.

7. Timmons MK, Thigpen CA, Seitz AL, Karduna AR, Arnold BL, Mitchener LA. Scapular kinematics and subacromial impingement syndrome: meta-analysis. J Sport Rehabil. 2012;21(4):354–70.
8. Emery RJ, Mullaji AB. Glenohumeral joint instability in normal adolescents. Incidence and significance. J Bone Joint Surg. 1991;73-B:406–8.
9. Beighton PH, Solomon I, Soskolne CL. Articular mobility in an African population. Ann Rhem Dis. 1073;32(5):413–8.
10. McFarland EG, Neira CA, Gutierrez MI, Cosgarea AJ, Magee M. Clinical significance of the arthroscopic drive-through sign in shoulder surgery. Arthroscopy. 2001;17(1):38–43.

Chapter 27
Anterior Instability

Avanthi Mandaleson

Case Example

A 20-year-old man presents 3-months after a rugby injury. He made a tackle with his arm out to the side and felt a clunk in his shoulder. Since the acute injury has settled, he had felt that his shoulder is clunking when he played tennis and other activities with his arm overhead and extended to the side. His shoulder feels weak with a "dead arm" sensation with overhead activities or when reaching forward to lift a weight. He is otherwise fit and healthy with no evidence of generalised ligamentous laxity. On clinical assessment, the range of motion is well preserved although he feels apprehensive during terminal abduction and external rotation. Apprehension test, relocation test and anterior load and shift tests are all positive.

Introduction

The shoulder joint is an inherently unstable articulation. It is made stable through the complex capsulolabral and dynamic muscular structures that surround the shoulder.

Anterior instability is often associated with an initial traumatic event that can subsequently result in ongoing instability with lesser degrees of trauma or even normal everyday activities. The initial traumatic event can be related to a fall or contact to the arm when it is in its most vulnerable position; with the arm extended to the side and overhead. In this position, there is a long lever arm against which the

A. Mandaleson
Department of Orthopaedic Surgery, Austin Hospital, Heidelberg, Victoria, Australia
e-mail: avanthi.mandaleson2@austin.org.au

© Springer International Publishing AG 2017

P. Monga, L. Funk (eds.), *Diagnostic Clusters in Shoulder Conditions*,
DOI 10.1007/978-3-319-57334-2_27

Table 27.1 Factors affecting shoulder instability [1]

1.	Capsulolabral complex and proprioceptive mechanism
2.	Rotator cuff tears
3.	Glenohumeral joint surface contact area
4.	Central or peripheral nerve dysfunction

force directs the humeral head anteriorly and inferiorly out of the glenoid, with the least soft tissue restraint. Factors related to shoulder instability are listed in Table 27.1.

The trauma can lead to a predictable pattern of injury that may affect the static and dynamic stabilisers. Static constraints include the bony articular surfaces and ligaments. Bony injuries are caused by impaction to the anterior glenoid (bony Bankart) and/or posterior humeral head (Hill-Sachs lesion). This leads to a reduction in the articular contact surface through a range of motion, known as the 'glenoid track'. A soft tissue injury almost always occurs, even in the absence of the bony injury and can be the primary factor leading to recurrent instability. The anterior and inferior capsule with it's associated anterior and inferior glenohumeral ligaments, and labrum can be stretched and torn from the anterior rim of the glenoid which results in a loss of the deepening, suction effect and anteroinferior support to the humeral head. Recurrent dislocations can lead to further erosion of the articular surfaces and result in a cycle of increasing instability and arthrosis. Risk factors for recurrent instability include male gender, young age [2], ligamentous laxity, a large Hill-Sachs [3] or Bony Bankart [4] lesions. The natural history of anterior shoulder instability is that of arthropathy with increased rates in patients with recurrent dislocations, older age at time of primary dislocation and high energy sports [5].

Pillar 1: History

The history should broadly cover the direction of instability, duration and chronicity of symptoms and any underlying cause. These aspects of the history aim to identify the risk of recurrence and therefore help in determining the appropriate management. 96% of shoulder dislocations are associated with a traumatic event, and 4% are atraumatic [1]. Following the injury, there may be both structural and non-structural components of instability that need to be identified to allow appropriate management [1].

If a particular traumatic event marked the start of the symptoms, the nature and degree of energy involved in the trauma should be noted. The direction of force or position of the arm should be recorded. One needs to enquire whether the episode was associated with a frank dislocation that required manipulation or an X-Ray confirming dislocation or whether there was a subjective feeling of a clunk. If the details of the inciting event cannot be recalled, the position of the arm that reproduces symptoms can also aid in determining the direction of instability. High energy trauma is often associated with structural changes whereas an insidious atraumatic onset often points to non-structural causes [1]. The age of the patient at the time of initial onset is an important prognostic indicator. There is over an 80% risk of recurrence in patients younger than 20 years of age [6], which increases to over 90% if they return to sport [7], as compared with only 16% risk in patients older than 40 years [8]. Age also determines the structural damage occurring at the time of dislocation. Rotator cuff tears, greater tuberosity fractures and associated neurological injury tend to be more common over the age of 40 years [9] in contrast to capsulo-labral injuries in the younger age group.

The frequency of symptoms during periods of daily activities, work or leisure activities can inform the severity of instability. A distinction should be made between the number of episodes of frank dislocation compared with subluxations of the joint. Almost half of patients with anterior subluxation do not experience subjective instability and may complain only of pain or a "dead arm" sensation. The association of any neurological symptoms or ongoing deficit in the arm can determine the nature and timing of any treatment. Associated pain with instability episodes may imply other intra-articular pathology such as a tear of the rotator cuff or greater tuberosity fracture, which is more common in older patients. The presence of these injuries may alter the nature and timing of investigations and in fact of any surgical treatment required. Progressive pain and stiffness can also herald the development of arthritic changes, a late presentation of recurrent instability, at which point joint salvage surgery may be the only option. Other important systemic signs are the presence of other joint dislocations, voluntary dislocations or joint laxity. This may represent a collagen disorder or non-structural changes that may be best managed with targeted specialist physiotherapy. Other medical co-morbidities such as epilepsy, neurological disorders or congenital problems may also aid in identifying a cause of recurrent instability and may need to be managed for successful control of the instability.

Pillar 2: Conventional Examination

The physical examination should focus on identifying any structural pathology associated with the dislocation and features that maybe contributing to recurrent instability. A pre-reduction and post-reduction assessment should be performed specifically documenting the neurovascular status of the arm.

Both shoulders should be examined using the normal shoulder as a reference. In the immediate period, before reduction, there may be an abnormal contour of the shoulder with a sulcus over the lateral deltoid and a prominent anterior humeral head with an extremely limited range of motion. Following reduction, acute features of pain and discomfort that limit shoulder range of motion may be due to haematoma formation within the shoulder joint from intra-articular structural pathology. If there is an associated fracture, there may be obvious bruising around the shoulder girdle. Once the acute pathology has settled, especially in younger patients, there may be very few signs. Observation of the shoulder girdle from all positions may identify subtle asymmetrical shoulder posture or periscapular muscle wasting. However, there is often a normal active range of motion, no bruising or deformity and full power of the rotator cuff muscles. In the older population, where there is a greater incidence of acute rotator cuff tears, fractures or neurological injury, serial assessment should be performed to document any weakness of the rotator cuff, the range of motion deficit and neurological status of the limb. Ongoing significant pain or weakness after 3 weeks should prompt further investigation of concomitant pathology that may require surgical intervention [10]. The infraclavicular plexus is most at risk and specifically the axillary nerve, but can also involve the suprascapular, radial, ulnar nerves or the whole brachial plexus.

Signs of non-structural changes that maybe contributing to instability include an assessment of scapula position and rhythm through a range of shoulder abduction and forward elevation [11], core muscle strength and a kinetic chain assessment, any voluntary dislocation manoeuvres and signs of ligamentous laxity, with a Beighton score >6. Positive findings here are equally important to identify, to allow appropriate therapy for successful management.

Pillar 3: Special Tests

Various special tests (Table 27.2) have been described for assessment of the young patient presenting after a primary traumatic anterior dislocation or with anterior subluxation. Provocative signs are highly specific and can guide the examiner to structural pathology. Glenohumeral translation tests can vary depending on the degree of generalised ligamentous laxity and should always be compared to the normal shoulder and be taken in context with provocative signs.

Table 27.2 Special tests for shoulder instability [12]

Test	Structure tested	Assessment
Anterior drawer test [13]	Anterior capsule and ligaments	Grade 1: 0–5 mm Grade 2: 5–10 mm Grade 3: >10 mm displacement (when compared with the normal side)
Load and shift test [14]	0–60°—Superior GHL/CHL/rotator interval 60–90°—MGHL 90°—IGHL	Grade 0: Little or no movement Grade 1: Humeral head translation to the glenoid rim Grade 2: Translation over the glenoid rim with spontaneous relocation Grade 3: humeral head translation over the glenoid rim that remains dislocated
Anterior apprehension test [15]	Anteroinferior labrum or glenoid rim lesion	Positive if apprehension +/− pain
Relocation test [16]	As above	Relieves pain and tolerates external rotation

The anterior drawer test, described by Gerber [13], is aimed at grading the degree of laxity or insufficiency of the anterior capsular mechanism. The test is performed with the patient supine and relaxed. The hand of the affected shoulder is fixed in the examiner's axilla. The shoulder is held in 80–120° of abduction, 0–20° of forward elevation and 0–30° of external rotation to allow the shoulder to relax in a comfortable position. The examiner fixes the scapula by holding the scapula spine with the index and middle finger and the coracoid process with the thumb. The examiner's opposite hand grasps the upper arm to draw it anteriorly (Fig. 27.1). The presence of any click which maybe associated with labral pathology and the degree of humeral head translation should be recorded [5].

The load and shift test described by Hawkins [14] as a modification of the anterior drawer test is considered the gold standard for assessment of instability. The goal of the test is to load the humeral head into the glenoid and then translate the humeral head anteriorly. Variations of this test have been described with the patient either in the seated or supine position and with the shoulder in different degrees of abduction. With the arm in 0–60° of abduction the superior glenohumeral ligament (GHL), coracohumeral ligament (CHL) and rotator interval integrity is tested. With the shoulder in 60–90° of abduction the middle glenohumeral ligament (MGHL) is stressed, and in 90° of abduction, the inferior glenohumeral ligament (IGHL) is tested (Fig. 27.2). The translation of the humeral head can be graded as follows; Grade 0—little or no movement. Grade 1—humeral head translation to the glenoid rim. Grade 2—translation over the glenoid rim with spontaneous relocation when pressure released and Grade 3—humeral head translation over the glenoid rim that remains dislocated after the release of pressure [17]. Both are tests of translation and the results of which can be exaggerated under anaesthesia [12].

The anterior apprehension test, initially described by Rowe and Zarins [15], is performed with the patient in the sitting or supine position. The shoulder is abducted

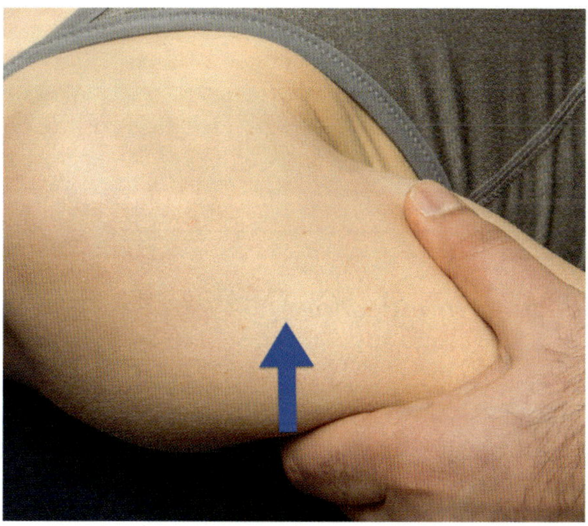

Fig. 27.1 Anterior drawer test—Anterior translational force. Image Published under License from www.shoulderdoc.co.uk and www.shoulderpedia.org

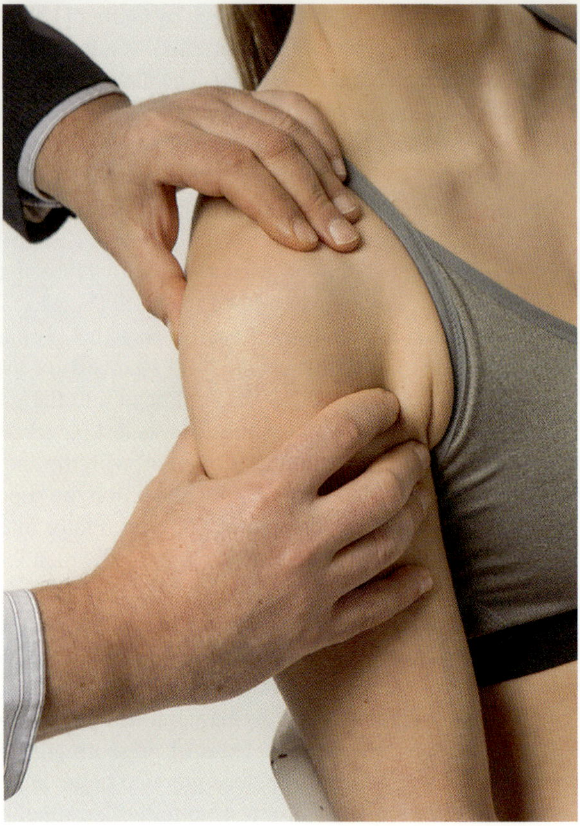

Fig. 27.2 Load and shift test. Image Published under License from www.shoulderdoc.co.uk and www.shoulderpedia.org

to 90 degrees and passively moved into the maximal external rotation, an anteriorly directed force is applied to the posterior humeral head which produces apprehension (Fig. 27.3). This is test can be coupled with a relocation test (Fig. 27.4), described by Jobe [16]. Addition of a posteriorly directed force on the anterior aspect of humeral head relieves any pain and allows further external rotation This has a 68% sensitivity, 100% specificity and positive predictive value, 78% negative predictive value and accuracy of 85% when apprehension alone was considered a positive result [11].

Pillar 4: Investigations

The role of imaging in the acute shoulder dislocation, in the first instance, is to confirm the diagnosis and direction of the dislocation and exclude any fractures. A summary of imaging techniques used for traumatic instability is listed in Table 27.3. The usual trauma series includes an AP, scapular "Y" and axillary views, assuming that

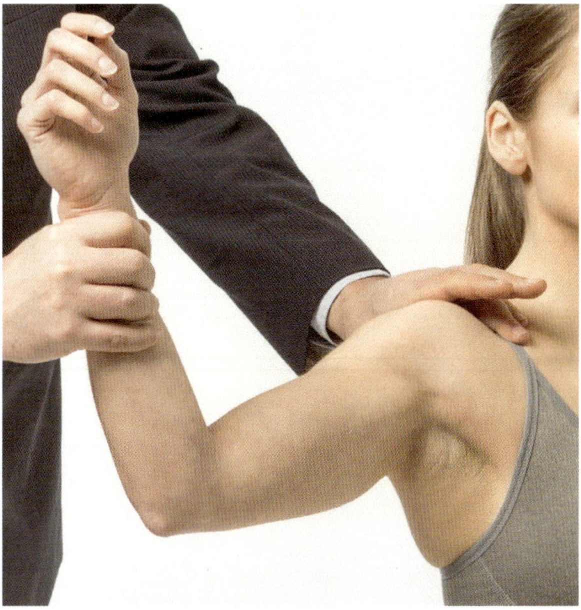

Fig. 27.3 Apprehension test. Image Published under License from www.shoulderdoc.co.uk and www.shoulderpedia.org

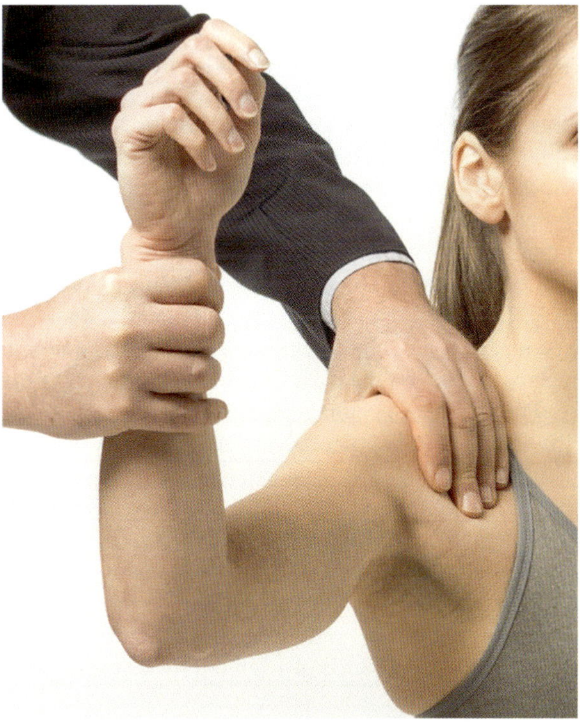

Fig. 27.4 Relocation test. Image Published under License from www.shoulderdoc.co.uk and www.shoulderpedia.org

Table 27.3 Summary of investigations

Imaging modality	Views	Pathology
X-ray	AP shoulder Axillary Scapula "Y" West point [21] Stryker notch [22]	Proximal humerus fracture Congruent articulation Bony bankart Hill-Sachs lesion
CT	Axial cuts Reconstructed images	Glenoid bone loss Glenoid version Humeral head defects
MRI	Plain/arthrography	Glenoid side:
		Bankart lesion
		Perthes lesion
		GLAD lesion
		ALPSA lesion
		Humeral side:
		HAGL lesion
	ABER views	Rotator cuff tears
		Biceps pathology
		Undisplaced anteroinferior labral tears

the patients can tolerate positioning [18]. In the acute setting, these plain radiographs are paramount to confirm that a concentric reduction has been achieved following any reduction manoeuvres. Additional views provide better visualisation of either a Hill-Sachs defect in the posterior humeral head or anterior glenoid rim defect or "bony bankart" lesion. The West Point view is a variation of the axillary view and improves visualisation of the anteroinferior glenoid rim to detect Bankart fractures. The Stryker notch view demonstrates the posterolateral margin of the humeral head, which can be useful in detecting a Hill-Sachs lesion. Both these views can be difficult to obtain in the acute setting due to pain during patient positioning [19]. If there is any doubt or if the patient is unable to tolerate positioning, cross-sectional imaging in the form of a CT should be used to guide additional manipulation or surgery on the basis of any osseous defects or interposed soft tissue [18].

Pre-operative planning should be aimed at assessing the degree of bone loss in the humeral head or glenoid, and this can be evaluated using a CT or MRI. Although Hill-Sachs lesions are the more common bony defect, however glenoid rim fractures have greater prognostic significance. The risk of recurrent instability increases with the size of the glenoid bone defect [4, 20].

MRI is now the gold standard to evaluate the degree of soft tissue injury. In the acute setting, the haemarthroses acts as a form of contrast medium to allow distension of the joint and outlining intra-articular structures. However, in the chronic setting and the absence of haemarthrosis, gadolinium-enhanced scans (arthrography) can better delineate subtle intra-capsulolabral pathology [18]. The inferior capsulolabral complex is the most commonly involved structures and can demonstrate characteristic changes on MRI. These include the Bankart lesion, Perthes lesion,

Glenoid Labral Articular Defect (GLAD) lesion, anterior labroligamentous periosteal sleeve avulsion (ALPSA) lesion and humeral avulsion of the glenohumeral ligament (HAGL) lesion. Bankart lesions are the most common and are due to detachment of the labrum from the glenoid rim. Perthes lesions are a variation of the Bankart lesion, where the scapular periosteum is lifted and stripped medially with the detached anterior labrum. GLAD lesions are also an extension of a Bankart lesion with associated articular cartilage damage, and ALPSA lesions are inferomedially displaced labral tears. HAGL lesions are the results of avulsion injury of the glenohumeral ligaments from the humeral side. Osseous injury can be identified on MRI by looking for patterns of bony contusion. This can give an indication of the direction of dislocation [18]. MRI can also assess the biceps and rotator cuff tendons, which can be a source of ongoing pain and dysfunction following traumatic dislocation in patients older than 40 years of age [10]. Provocative positioning manoeuvres such as placing the shoulder in the abducted and externally rotated (ABER) position. This has been found to improve the diagnostic accuracy of MR arthrography from 48–89% sensitivity, by improving the detection of undisplaced anteroinferior labral tears [18] although was initially described to increase the sensitivity of detecting articular-sided rotator cuff tears.

Discussion of the Case

The clinical scenario in this chapter describes a classic high energy sporting injury with the shoulder positioned and forced into a likely anteroinferior dislocation. His young age and energy of injury make him at over 80% risk of further dislocation without further treatment and over 90% risk if he returns to sport. Further clunking sensations when his arm is positioned in an overhead and externally rotated position are highly suggestive of recurrent anterior dislocation episodes. A "dead arm" sensation is also suggestive of episodes of subluxation in addition to dislocations and is most likely attributed to intra-articular pathology. Management of recurrent instability is aimed at preventing further episodes of dislocation. An MR Arthrogram is performed to identify the degree of glenoid bone loss and soft tissue injury to allow a discussion about the type of treatment required.

Summary

The diagnosis of anterior shoulder instability can be made on a directed history regarding the mechanism of injury and underlying predisposing conditions. A meticulous examination can identify subtle signs of instability and non-structural changes that can be targeted by both physiotherapy and surgical treatment options. Imaging is predominantly used for pre-operative planning to guide either a soft-tissue or a bony reconstruction. A summary of diagnostic clusters for anterior instability are listed in Table 27.4.

Table 27.4 Summary of diagnostic clusters for anterior instability

Clinical history
1. Young age
2. High energy injury (commonly seen in contact, combat and riding sports)
3. Shoulder "feels" unstable/loss of confidence
4. Dead arm sensation
5. Position of arm and direction of force levering shoulder in anterior direction
Conventional examination
6. Apprehensive at terminal abduction
Special tests
7. Positive apprehension and relocation test
8. Positive load and shift test
9. Positive anterior drawer test
Investigations
10. CT/MRI arthrogram scan for assessment of bone loss and degree of soft tissue injury to direct management

References

1. Jaggi A, Lambert S. Rehabilitation for shoulder instability. Br J Sports Med. 2010;44(5):333–40.
2. te Slaa RL, Wijffels MPJM, Brand R, Marti RK. The prognosis following acute primary glenohumeral dislocation. J Bone Joint Surg Br. 2004;86(1):58–64.
3. Hovelius L, Augustini BG, Fredin H, Johansson O, Norlin R, Thorling J. Primary anterior dislocation of the shoulder in young patients. A ten-year prospective study. J Bone Joint Surg Am. 1996;78(11):1677–84.
4. Itoi E, Lee SB, Berglund LJ, Berge LL, An KN. The effect of a glenoid defect on anteroinferior stability of the shoulder after Bankart repair: a cadaveric study. J Bone Joint Surg Am. 2000;82(1):35–46.
5. Hovelius L, Saeboe M. Neer award 2008: Arthropathy after primary anterior shoulder dislocation--223 shoulders prospectively followed up for twenty-five years. J Shoulder Elb Surg Am Shoulder Elb Surg Al. 2009;18(3):339–47.
6. Robinson CM, Howes J, Murdoch H, Will E, Graham C. Functional outcome and risk of recurrent instability after primary traumatic anterior shoulder dislocation in young patients. J Bone Joint Surg Am. 2006;88(11):2326–36.
7. Wheeler JH, Ryan JB, Arciero RA, Molinari RN. Arthroscopic versus nonoperative treatment of acute shoulder dislocations in young athletes. Arthroscopy. 1989;5(3):213–7.
8. Rowe CR. Prognosis in dislocations of the shoulder. J Bone Joint Surg Am. 1956;38-A(5):957–77.
9. Robinson CM, Shur N, Sharpe T, Ray A, Murray IR. Injuries associated with traumatic anterior glenohumeral dislocations. J Bone Joint Surg Am. 2012;94(1):18–26.
10. Sonnabend DH. Treatment of primary anterior shoulder dislocation in patients older than 40 years of age Conservative versus operative. Clin Orthop. 1994;(304):74–7.
11. Kibler BW, Sciascia A, Wilkes T. Scapular Dyskinesis and its relation to shoulder injury. J Am Acad Orthop Surg. 2012;20(6):364–72.
12. Tennent TD, Beach WR, Meyers JF. A review of the special tests associated with shoulder examination. Part II: Laxity, instability, and superior labral anterior and posterior (SLAP) lesions. Am J Sports Med. 2003;31(2):301–7.
13. Gerber C, Ganz R. Clinical assessment of instability of the shoulder. With special reference to anterior and posterior drawer tests. J Bone Joint Surg Br. 1984;66(4):551–6.
14. Hawkins RJ, Bokor DJ. Clinical evaluation of shoulder problems. In: The shoulder. Philadelphia: W. B. Saunders; 1990.

15. Rowe CR, Zarins B. Recurrent transient subluxation of the shoulder. J Bone Joint Surg Am. 1981;63(6):863–72.
16. Jobe FW, Kvitne RS, Giangarra CE. Shoulder pain in the overhand or throwing athlete. The relationship of anterior instability and rotator cuff impingement. Orthop Rev. 1989;18(9):963–75.
17. McFarland EG, Torpey BM, Curl LA. Evaluation of shoulder laxity. Sports Med Auckl NZ. 1996;22(4):264–72.
18. Bencardino JT, Gyftopoulos S, Palmer WE. Imaging in anterior Glenohumeral instability. Radiology. 2013;269(2):323–37.
19. Sanders TG, Morrison WB, Miller MD. Imaging techniques for the evaluation of glenohumeral instability. Am J Sports Med. 2000;28(3):414–34.
20. Lo IKY, Parten PM, Burkhart SS. The inverted pear glenoid: an indicator of significant glenoid bone loss. Arthrosc J Arthrosc Relat Surg Off Publ Arthrosc Assoc N Am Int Arthrosc Assoc. 2004;20(2):169–74.
21. Rokous JR, Feagin JA, Abbott HG. Modified axillary roentgenogram. A useful adjunct in the diagnosis of recurrent instability of the shoulder. Clin Orthop. 1972;82:84–6.
22. Hall RH, Isaac F, Booth CR. Dislocations of the shoulder with special reference to accompanying small fractures. J Bone Joint Surg Am. 1959;41-A(3):489–94.

Chapter 28
Posterior Instability

Abbas Rashid

Case Example

A 26-year-old rugby player describes pain and a loss of confidence in his shoulder. This follows an injury 1 month earlier when he was tackled from behind and fell forward onto a flexed elbow while holding the ball. He felt immediate pain and a tearing sensation followed by a feeling of a 'dead arm'. He was unable to continue playing and had not returned to contact since then, despite rehabilitation. He has pain at the back of his shoulder with any pressing or pushing exercises, with painful clunking from the joint. Examination reveals a full range of movement and no external signs of injury. The Jerk test and Wrightington Posterior instability test are positive.

Introduction

Posterior instability represents 2–10% of all shoulder instability [1]. Affected patients are usually men between the ages of 20–30 years who engage in overhead activity or contact sports, and there is also an association with seizures [2]. Posterior instability can be acute or chronic, recurrent or fixed, and part of a uni-, bi- or multidirectional instability problem [3]. Only a minority of patients recall an actual dislocation. The majority experience repetitive microtrauma on a background of pre-existing capsular laxity exacerbated by the development of abnormal muscle patterning [4].

A. Rashid, F.R.C.S.
University College London Hospitals NHS Trust, 250 Euston Rd, London, UK
e-mail: abbas.rashid@uclh.nhs.uk

© Springer International Publishing AG 2017

P. Monga, L. Funk (eds.), *Diagnostic Clusters in Shoulder Conditions*,
DOI 10.1007/978-3-319-57334-2_28

There are a number of static and dynamic restraints that contribute to shoulder stability. The static restraints are bones, capsulo-labral complex and rotator interval. The dynamic restraints are all the musculotendinous units crossing the glenohumeral joint. Congenital or acquired irregularities of these may increase the risk of posterior instability.

Congenital glenoid deficiency, as seen in obstetric brachial palsy, ranges from mild retroversion to severe hypoplasia of the scapular neck and posterior glenoid. Larger deficits increase the retroversion and may contribute to posterior translation of the humeral head [5, 6]. Acquired glenoid deficiency is usually due to posterior glenoid fractures from a reverse bony Bankart defect (fracture of the posteroinferior rim of the glenoid) to a larger glenoid rim fracture. Furthermore, a reverse Hill-Sachs defect (an impaction fracture of the anteromedial humeral head) greater than 30% of the articular surface may engage the posterior glenoid rim within the physiological range of motion resulting in posterior dislocation [7]. Although the posterior capsulo-labral complex is the thinnest and weakest portion of the joint capsule, it is the most important static restraint to posterior translation of the humeral head when the arm is flexed, adducted and internally rotated [8]. Traumatic structural lesions which can result in posterior instability include detachment from its glenoid attachment (reverse Bankart lesion), avulsion a sleeve of glenoid periosteum (posterior labrocapsular periosteal sleeve avulsion), avulsion from its humeral attachment (reverse HAGL) or a mid-substance tear (Kim's lesion). The rotator interval is a triangular space between the Subscapularis tendon, the Supraspinatus tendons and the base of the coracoid. Its deficiency has been shown to contribute to posterior instability making it a secondary static restraint to posterior translation of the humeral head [9]. Dynamic stability is provided by scapulohumeral balance and concavity compression mainly due to contraction of paired groups of muscles across the joint, which centre the humeral head on the glenoid during movement [10]. These force couples are between anterior vs. posterior cuff and superior cuff vs. deltoid.

Pillar 1 Clinical History

Traumatic posterior instability is commonly seen in contact sports, such as rugby, where the athlete lands on a flexed arm and suffers a longitudinal and posteriorly directed injury.

Posterior instability can also be the result of repetitive micro-trauma through overhead throwing, volleyball, tennis, swimming and weightlifting [11]. These patients commonly report aching pain along the posterior joint line in the latter stages of the sport as muscle fatigue results in loss of dynamic stability particularly during the cocking and follow-through phases of throwing when the arm is in the forward flexion, adduction and internally rotation [11].

Atraumatic instability is usually due to soft tissue abnormalities (e.g. Marfan's or Ehlers-Danlos) or bone abnormalities (e.g. idiopathic glenohumeral dysplasia or obstetric brachial palsy). A subset of patients habitually dislocate their shoulders. This volitional ability may develop into an involuntary problem and is discussed in detail in Chap. 26 [12]. The dislocations themselves are often painless, but the patients can experience aching, paraesthesia and numbness in the arm.

Pillar 2 Conventional Examination

Clinical examination should look specifically at core, muscle patterning, capsular laxity and stability.

Assessment of core includes looking at posture and the kinetic chain. The Kibler Corkscrew Test assesses core by asking the patient to perform a single leg squat (on the leg opposite the affected shoulder) [13]. If the patient is seen to corkscrew (twisting at the hip and the knee) the test is positive. Poor core stability can influence the superficial torque action of larger muscles creating instability at the shoulder girdle and can affect proprioception (Fig. 26.5) [14].

The scapula is observed in ascent and descent with dyskinesis becoming more pronounced with repetition due to fatigue of key muscles. It is important to note the resting position of the humeral head; to ensure it is not already displaced under resting muscle tone. Aberrant activation of large muscles (usually Latissimus Dorsi, Pectoralis Major and Anterior Deltoid) and simultaneous suppression of the rotator cuff at the onset of movement can undo force couples resulting in instability. The Dynamic Rotatory Stability Test assesses the cuffs ability to maintain the humeral head on the centre of the glenoid through the arc of rotation [15]. The examiner observes for humeral head translation and scapular movements during active rotating the arm in 90° of flexion.

Generalised hypermobility is assessed using the Beighton Score (Fig. 26.3) [16]. Localised capsular laxity, however, will manifest as excessive external rotation and a sulcus sign [17]. Patients with capsular laxity typically hang the arm at the extreme of their hypermobile range resulting in poor core stability and may develop a compensatory thoracic kyphosis.

Pillar 3: Special Tests

Posterior Load & Shift Test: The examiner stabilises the shoulder with one hand (between the clavicle and coracoid anteriorly and the spine of the scapula posteriorly) and holds the humeral head with the other hand (Fig. 27.2) [18]. The examiner presses the humeral head medially into the glenoid to evaluate the neutral position of the joint and translates the humeral head posteriorly assessing the excursion as +1 (humeral head translates to posterior glenoid rim), +2 (translates beyond posterior glenoid rim and reduces spontaneously) and +3 (translates beyond posterior glenoid rim and remains dislocated).

Posterior Apprehension Test: (Fig. 28.1) the examiner stabilises the shoulder with one hand and pushes the 90° flexed, adducted and internally rotated shoulder posteriorly by the elbow [19]. If the patient experiences pain and apprehension, then the result is positive.

Kim Test: the arm is abducted to 90°. The examiner then passively elevates the arm an additional 45° while applying a downward and posterior force to the upper arm with an axial load to the elbow (Fig. 28.2) [20]. Posterior subluxation with pain indicates a positive test result.

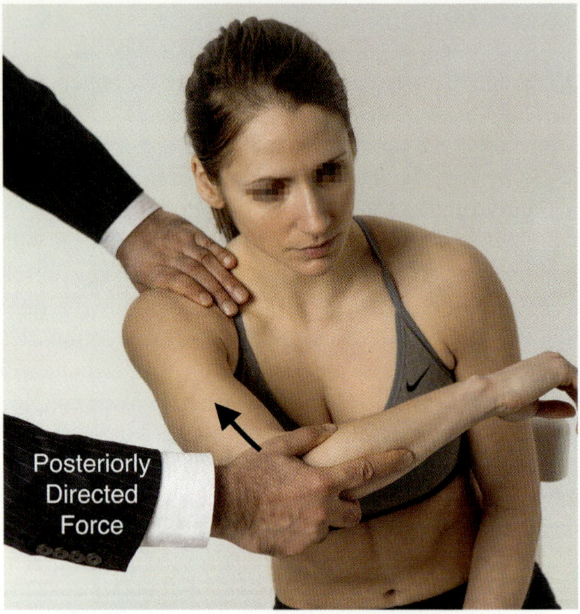

Fig. 28.1 Posterior apprehension test. Image Published under License from www.shoulderdoc.co.uk and www.shoulderpedia.org

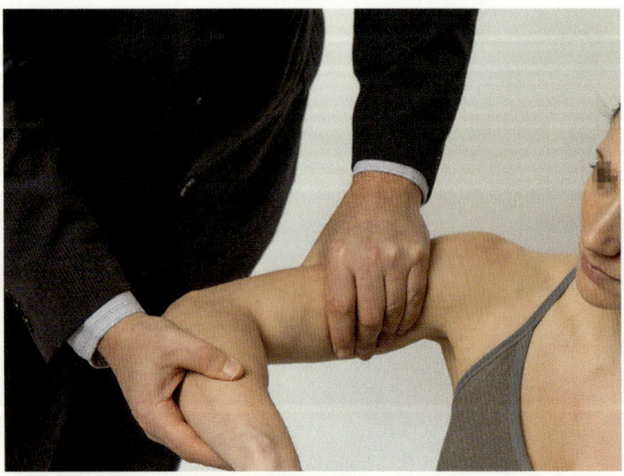

Fig. 28.2 Kim test starting position as load is applied postero-inferiorly. Image Published under License from www.shoulderdoc.co.uk and www.shoulderpedia.org

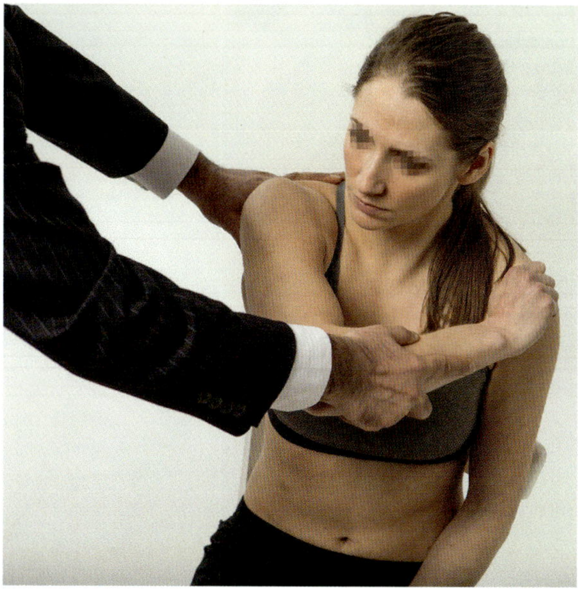

Fig. 28.3 Jerk test starting position—Further abduction leads to a relocation jerk. Image Published under License from www.shoulderdoc.co.uk and www.shoulderpedia.org

Jerk test: the examiner stabilises the scapula with one hand while holding the elbow with the other (Fig. 28.3) [21]. With the shoulder elevated 90° and internally rotated and the elbow flexed 90°, the shoulder girdle is pressed anteriorly with one hand, and the elbow pushed posteriorly with the other, causing posterior subluxation of the humeral head. The arm is then abducted as it is pushed posteriorly. If the patient experiences a sudden painful jerk as the humeral head relocates, the test is positive.

Wrightington posterior instability test [22]: In many cases of posterior instability, patients present with posterior pain and clicking instead of true dislocations. This is predominantly seen in muscular contact athletes. These patients have excess posterior laxity and translation, posterior glenohumeral joint pain in hyperabduction and external rotation. This is a form of subclinical instability. These patients will exhibit marked weakness and pain in resisted flexion in full adduction and internal rotation at 90°—a similar position to the O'Brein's test. This is probably due to posterior translation of the humeral head in the position of flexion and internal rotation, with resultant posterior cuff weakness. This test has a sensitivity of 93.8% and positive predictive value of 96.8% for traumatic posterior capsulo-labral injury of the shoulder [23] (Fig. 28.4).

Pillar 4: Investigations

Standard radiographs are usually normal. However large bony abnormalities can be found on specialised views. The Stryker Notch or axillary lateral views show a reverse Hill-Sachs defect and a West Point Axillary view show Reverse bony

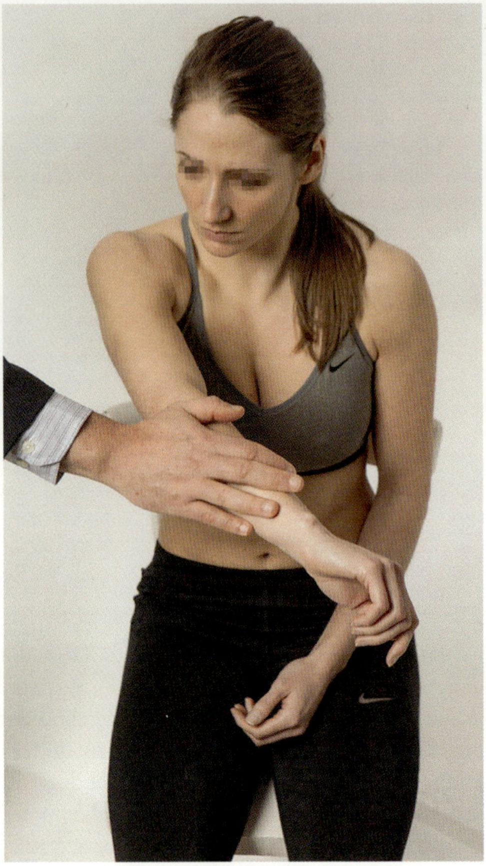

Fig. 28.4 Wrightington posterior instability test. Image Published under License from www.shoulderdoc.co.uk and www.shoulderpedia.org

Bankart defects [21, 24]. CT is useful to characterise bony defects whereas MRI is more useful for soft tissue pathology. The addition of arthrography increases sensitivity to 90–94% for labral pathology when the imaging corresponds to clinical examination [25].

In refractory cases where there is a significant disparity between the history, clinical findings and images one may need to proceed to examination under anaesthesia and/or diagnostic arthroscopy.

Discussion of the Case

Traumatic posterior instability is commonly seen in contact sports such as rugby. The athlete described at the start of the chapter had an MR arthrogram, which confirmed a posterior labral tear. Upon failure of non-operative management, he would be a candidate for arthroscopic assessment and posterior labral repair.

Table 28.1 Summary of diagnostic cluster for posterior instability

Clinical history
1. Single macro trauma: Indirect (e.g. electrocution, seizure) or direct (posterior directed impact to flexed adducted internally rotated arm).
2. Repetitive microtrauma: High impact contact sports (rugby, weight lifting).
3. Painful clicking and weakness with loading the flexed, adducted and internally rotated arm
Conventional examination
4. Posterior joint line tenderness
Special tests
5. Positive posterior drawer test.
6. Positive posterior apprehension test.
7. Positive Kim test.
8. Positive jerk test.
9. Wrightington posterior instability test
Investigations
10. MR arthrogram: Posterior labral tear or Kim's lesion

Summary

Diagnosis of posterior instability is best made using a cluster approach. Traumatic instability is commonly seen in the setting of contact sports such as rugby. Diagnosis is confirmed by clinical examination and MR arthrogram. Atraumatic posterior instability, on the other hand, is commonly associated with poor core stability, abnormal muscle patterning and hyperlaxity. A summary of diagnostic clusters related to posterior instability are presented in Table 28.1.

References

1. McLaughlin HI. Follow-up notes on articles previously published in the journal: posterior dislocation of the shoulder. J Bone Joint Surg Am. 1972;44:1477.
2. Boyd HB, Sisk TD. Recurrent posterior dislocation of the shoulder. J Bone Joint Surg Am. 1972;54(4):779–86.
3. Antoniou J, Duckworth DT, Harryman DT 2nd. 2nd Capsulolabral augmentation for the management of posteroinferior instability of the shoulder. J Bone Joint Surg Am. 2000;82(9):1220–30.
4. Sekiya JK, Cole BJ, Cohen SB. Arthroscopic treatment of multidirectional shoulder instability. In: Surgical techniques of the shoulder, elbow, and knee in sports medicine. Portland, OR: WB Saunders Co; 2008. p. 816.
5. Abrams JS, Savoie FH, Tauro JC, Bradley JP. Recent advances in the evaluation and treatment of shoulder instability: anterior, posterior, and multidirectional. Arthroscopy. 2002;18(9 Suppl 2):1–13.
6. Edelson JG. Localized glenoid hypoplasia: an anatomic variation of possible clinical significance. Clin Orthop Relat Res. 1995;321:189–95.

7. Lynch JR, Clinton JM, Dewing CB, Warme WJ, Matsen FA III. J treatment of osseous defects associated with anterior shoulder instability. Shoulder Elbow Surg. 2009;18(2):317–28.
8. Pagnani MJ, Warren RF. Stabilizers of the glenohumeral joint. J Shoulder Elb Surg. 1994;3(3):173–90.
9. Harryman DT 2nd, Sidles JA, Harris SL, Matsen FA 3rd. The role of the rotator interval capsule in passive motion and stability of the shoulder. J Bone Joint Surg Am. 1992;74(1):53–66.
10. Wang VM, Flatow EL. Pathomechanics of acquired shoulder instability: a basic science perspective. J Shoulder Elbow Surg. 2005;14(1 Suppl S):2S–11S.
11. Tibone JE, Bradley JP. The treatment of posterior subluxation in athletes. Clin Orthop Relat Res. 1993;291:124–37.
12. Rowe CR, Pierce DS, Clark JG. Voluntary dislocation of the shoulder: a preliminary report on a clinical, electromyographic, and psychiatric study of twenty-six patients. J Bone Joint Surg Am. 1973;55(3):445–60.
13. Kibler WB, Press J, Sciascia A. The role of core stability in athletic function. Sports Med. 2006;36:189–98.
14. Kibler WB. The role of the scapula in athletic shoulder function. Am J Sports Med. 1998;26:325–37.
15. Magarey ME, Jones MA. Specific evaluation of the function of force couples relevant for stabilization of the glenohumeral joint. Man Ther. 2003;8:247–53.
16. Beighton PH, Solomon L, Soskolne CL. Articular mobility in an African population. Ann Rheum Dis. 1973;32:413–7.
17. Neer CS 2nd, Foster CR. Inferior capsular shift for involuntary inferior and multidirectional instability of the shoulder. A preliminary report. J Bone Joint Surg Am. 1980;62(6):897–908.
18. Tzannes A, Murrell GA. Clinical examination of the unstable shoulder. Sports Med. 2002;32(7):447–57.
19. Gerber C, Ganz R. Clinical assessment of instability of the shoulder. With special reference to anterior and posterior drawer tests. J Bone Joint Surg Br. 1984;66(4):551–6.
20. Kim SH, Park JS, Jeong WK, Shin SK. The Kim test: a novel test for posteroinferior labral lesion of the shoulder--a comparison to the jerk test. Am J Sports Med. 2005;33(8):1188–92.
21. Tannenbaum E, Sekiya JK. Evaluation and management of posterior shoulder instability. Sports. Health. 2011;3(3):253–63.
22. Funk L, Owen JM, Bonner C. Clinical assessment of posterior shoulder joint instability. J Arthrosc Joint Surg. 2014;1(2):53–8.
23. Owen JM, Boulter T, Walton M, Funk L, Mackenzie TA. Reinterpretation of O'Brien test in posterior labral tears of the shoulder. Int J Shoulder Surg. 2015;9(1):6.
24. Itoi E, Lee SB, Amrami KK, Wenger DE, An KN. Quantitative assessment of classic anteroinferior bony Bankart lesions by radiography and computed tomography. Am J Sports Med. 2003;31(1):112–8.
25. Gusmer PB, Potter HG. Imaging of shoulder instability. Clin Sports Med. 1995;14(4):777–95.

Chapter 29
Sternoclavicular Joint Instability

Chris Peach

Case Example

A 25-year-old male lawyer presents to the clinic with painful clicking in the front of the neck. The onset of symptoms was six months ago after he fell off his bicycle in a road traffic accident. At the time he was treated in hospital for a fractured ankle and other soft tissue bruising. Gradually he has noticed a painful clicking and clunking around the medial end of the clavicle. This is now causing him pain when lying on his back at night along with having a dull aching throb constantly during the day. He is unable to do press-ups or lift weights in the gym.

Introduction

Dislocation and subsequent instability of the sternoclavicular joint is uncommon. However, for those who have an acute injury to this joint, due to the force required to disrupt the soft tissue stabilisers, there is often significant associated injury which can distract from sternoclavicular joint pathology. Thus presentation is frequently delayed, and a high index of suspicion should be had in patients presenting with painful symptoms around the medial clavicle after trauma. Despite its rarity, chronic instability is a painful and functionally disabling condition for the young patients who often present. Prompt diagnosis and treatment can quickly restore function.

C. Peach
Department of Shoulder and Elbow Surgery, University Hospital of South Manchester, Southmoor Road, Manchester M23 9LT, UK
e-mail: c.peach@doctors.org.uk

© Springer International Publishing AG 2017

P. Monga, L. Funk (eds.), *Diagnostic Clusters in Shoulder Conditions*,
DOI 10.1007/978-3-319-57334-2_29

Instability of the sternoclavicular joint can manifest itself either acutely or chronically in an anterior or posterior direction. Acute and chronic instability usually follows a traumatic injury, however atraumatic instability of the sternoclavicular joint can occur.

The sternoclavicular joint is normally very stable. Although the bony articulation is highly incongruent and imparts little bony stability, there is a dense, soft tissue envelope surrounding the joint. In fact, only half of the medial end of the clavicle is in contact with the sternum. The joint capsule has discrete thickenings posteriorly and anteriorly which form the intrinsic capsular ligaments. There are two main extrinsic ligaments, the costoclavicular and the interclavicular ligaments which contribute to the soft tissue stabilisers of the joint. As with all moving joints, stability is imparted not only by osseous and ligamentous stabilisers but also dynamically by the periarticular muscles. The sternoclavicular joint does receive some dynamic stability from the sternocleidomastoid, the sternal head of pectoralis major, sternohyoid, sternothyroid and the subclavius. Chronic instability results from injury and/or dysfunction to any one of these factors. Treatment depends on accurate diagnosis of the instability and its causes.

Pillar 1: Clinical History

There is most commonly a history of a traumatic injury [1], although atraumatic instability can occur secondary to generalised ligamentous laxity or periarticular muscular dysfunction. In all patients with a traumatic injury to the sternoclavicular joint, in particular, if this resulted in a dislocation, associated injuries should be suspected due to the forces required to dislocate the joint. Dislocation occurs due to either a direct injury to the joint or an indirect injury elsewhere on the shoulder girdle. A direct, blunt force to the anteromedial aspect of clavicle causes a posterior dislocation. If the injury is sustained on the lateral aspect of the shoulder, an anterolateral force (blow to the front of the shoulder) will cause an anterior dislocation, and a posterolateral force will cause a posterior dislocation. Falls onto an outstretched hand can drive the shoulder and clavicle medially, thus indirectly dislocating the sternoclavicular joint anteriorly [2].

In cases of posterior dislocation, patients may describe dysphagia, hoarseness or a choking feeling. Any of these features represent significant mediastinal compromise and should be treated as an emergency.

In chronic cases, patients will describe prominence of the medial clavicle (with anterior instability) and an asymmetrical hollow (in posterior instability). Other common symptoms reported are increased pain when lying supine and painful clicking particularly on overhead movement.

Pillar 2: Physical Examination

After an acute traumatic injury, patients will report pain and either an anterior prominence at the sternoclavicular joint (anterior dislocation) or a palpable defect (posterior dislocation) which can be easily compared to the contralateral side. In severe cases of posterior dislocation, due to compression of adjacent retrosternal structures, patients may display signs of venous congestion in the neck or ipsilateral arm. Patients with chronic instability may be able to demonstrate subluxation or dislocation easily.

Pillar 3: Special Tests

A sternoclavicular joint stress test is carried out by placing one hand over the spine of the scapula. The other hand is placed over the medial clavicle, and an anteriorly, posteriorly or superiorly directed force is applied which can detect either pain or abnormal movement (Fig. 29.1). This should be compared to the contralateral side. If positive, it indicates instability due to damage to the sternoclavicular joint stabilisers.

To detect symptomatic anterior or posterior instability that occurs during active movement, stand on the contralateral side of the patient's affected joint, placing the flat of your hand directly over the sternoclavicular joint. Ask the patient to forward flex their arm, and you will palpate the joint dislocating at approximately 90°of forward flexion, reducing spontaneously as the patient lowers their arm.

Pillar 4. Imaging

Plain radiography is sometimes useful in detecting a persistently dislocated sternoclavicular joint either posteriorly or anteriorly. However, it is usually difficult to obtain a clear enough view to ensure clinical certainty either to confirm or refute the diagnosis. A Heinig view is obtained with the patient lying supine and the x-ray beam angled so that it is directed perpendicularly to the joint [3]. This helps to detect anterior and posterior dislocations by the relationship of the medial clavicle to the laterally projected manubrium.

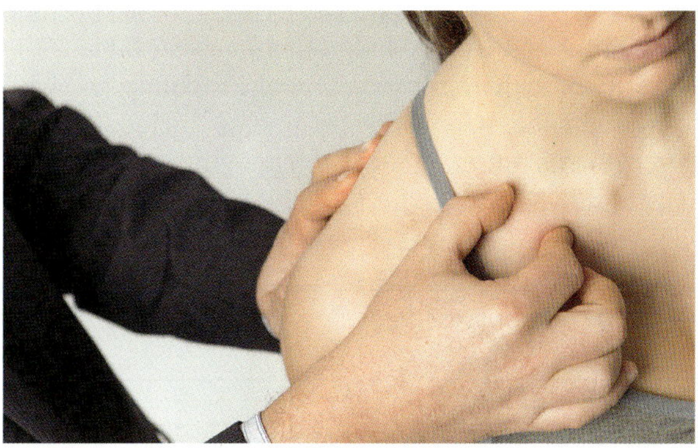

Fig. 29.1 Sternoclavicular joint stress test. Image Published under License from www.shoulderdoc.co.uk and www.shoulderpedia.org

CT scanning has superseded the use the plain radiography due to its availability in the acute setting and due to the superior resolution and the ability for 2D and 3D reconstruction of the images.

MRI scanning including MR arthrography can be useful at delineating structural abnormalities to the soft tissue restraints as well as injury to the intra-articular disc [4].

In the acute setting, CT scanning is normally used to diagnose acute dislocations. MRI scanning is used in chronic cases to define structural anomalies and aid planning of reconstructive treatment.

Discussion of the Case

Our patient demonstrates common features of a patient with chronic anterior sternoclavicular joint instability. Note that this was a high impact injury with the patient sustaining distracting injuries. In this case, it was in the lower limb, but commonly there are associated injuries around the shoulder girdle or the thoracic cage. The patient on direct questioning remembers severe bruising and grazing to the anterior aspect of his shoulder after falling off his bicycle suggesting a blunt indirect force to the front of the shoulder, producing an abnormal anterior force on the sternoclavicular joint. He also described painful clunking around the sternoclavicular joint with resulting functional impairment. Examination revealed pain and abnormal anterior translation on Sternoclavicular joint stress testing as well as a palpable anterior subluxation of the joint on active forward flexion beyond 90°. An MR Arthrogram demonstrated a split in the intra-articular disc, chondral damage to the medial end of the clavicle and disruption to the costoclavicular ligaments. He was treated with surgical reconstruction of the joint.

Summary

Sternoclavicular joint instability is an important differential diagnosis of medial clavicular pain and clicking. It can be acute or chronic and is most commonly caused by a traumatic insult to the shoulder girdle. Defining the direction of instability can be elicited by the history and on careful clinical examination. Imaging can be helpful and can exclude other causes (Table 29.1). Treatment depends on the severity of symptoms, direction of instability and whether the onset was traumatic or atraumatic. Common treatments include activity modification along with strengthening physiotherapy. Image-guided intra-articular injections can sometimes ameliorate pain from intra-articular inflammation. Patients failing to improve with conservative measures respond well to surgical stabilisation with capsular plication and ligament reconstruction.

Table 29.1 Summary of diagnostic clusters for Sternoclavicular joint instability

Clinical History	
1.	Direct injury
	a. Blunt force from anteromedial aspect of clavicle—posterior dislocation (unusual for direct force to produce anterior dislocation)
2.	Indirect injury
	a. Compression with blunt force anterolateral (anterior dislocation) or posterolateral aspect of shoulder (posterior dislocation) (Majority of cases of posterior dislocation are due to indirect force)
	b. Direct lateral compression force on shoulder e.g. fall on outstretched abducted arm driving shoulder medially
3.	Prominence medial end clavicle
4.	Painful clicking on overhead movement
Conventional Examination	
5.	Anterior prominence—anterior dislocation
6.	Palpable defect—posterior dislocation
Special Tests	
7.	Sternoclavicular joint stress test
8.	Palpable subluxation/ dislocation on forward flexion >90°
Investigations	
9.	CT scan with 3D reconstruction—good for alignment
10.	MRI—good for the sternoclavicular soft tissue restraints

References

1. de Jong KP, Sukul DM. Anterior sternoclavicular dislocation: a long-term follow-up study. J Orthop Trauma. 1990;4(4):420–3.
2. Wirth MARC. Disorders of the sternoclavicular joint. In: Rockwood Jr CA, Matsen 3rd F, Wirth MA, Lippitt SB, editors. The shoulder. 4th ed. Philadelphia: Saunders; 2009. p. 527–60.
3. Heinig CF. Retrosternal dislocation of the clavicle: Early recognition, x-ray diagnosis, and management. J Bone Joint Surg Am. 1968;50(4):825–44.
4. Brossmann J, Stabler A, Preidler KW, et al. Sternoclavicular joint: MR imaging--anatomic correlation. Radiology. 1996;198(1):193–8.

Chapter 30
Acromioclavicular Instability

Amar Malhas

Case Example

A 40-year-old cyclist presents 6 months after falling off his bike, landing on the point of his shoulder. He describes pain and a cosmetic change over the AC joint immediately after the injury. He did not seek medical attention initially but remains concerned that the "lump" hasn't settled. He has noticed a persistent weakness during overhead activities and an aching over the scapula at the end of the day. Examination reveals prominence of the lateral end clavicle and also pain on cross arm adduction. There is clear mobility felt on both anteroposterior and superoinferior stressing of the AC joint.

Introduction

Acromioclavicular joint (ACJ) dislocations are common and represent 4% of all shoulder injuries and are more common in males [1]. Such an injury is relatively common in athletes with an incidence of 9 per 1000 person-years [2]. In contact sports such as rugby or American football, the ACJ can be involved in as many as 35–41% of all shoulder injuries [3, 4] and can occur concomitantly with other shoulder injuries [3–5]. The most common classification in use for these injuries is the Rockwood Classification [6], (Fig. 30.1). In brief: Types 1 and 2 represent injury to the acromioclavicular ligaments (ACL) with preservation of the coracoclavicular ligaments (CCL); Type 3 represents disruption to the ACL and some of the CCL ligaments; Types 4 to 5 represent disruption of both the ACL and CCL with increasing displacement (posteriorly, superiorly or inferiorly) and soft tissue involvement.

A. Malhas
Royal Berkshire Hospital, Reading, UK
e-mail: amarmalhas@hotmail.com

© Springer International Publishing AG 2017

P. Monga, L. Funk (eds.), *Diagnostic Clusters in Shoulder Conditions*,
DOI 10.1007/978-3-319-57334-2_30

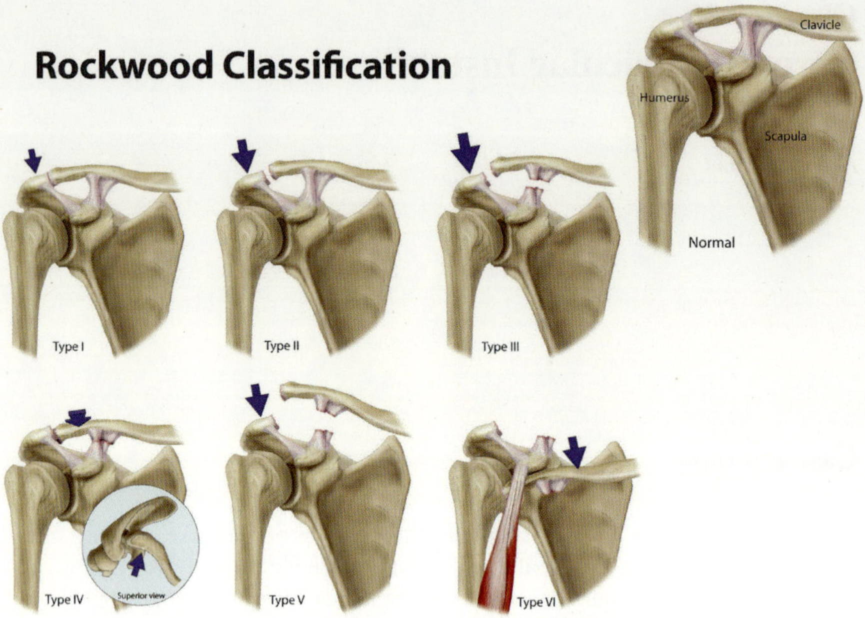

Fig. 30.1 Rockwood classification. Image Published under License from www.shoulderdoc.co.uk

The traditional consensus in the literature is that of non-operative management of most type 1–2 and operative treatment of types 4–5 with type 3 remaining controversial [7], although recent studies have shown poor reliability in classifying the injury. The diagnostic challenge is both identifying the injury and assessing the degree of instability and severity of symptoms to plan the management decisions.

Pillar 1: Clinical History

The most common mechanism for ACJ dislocation is direct trauma applied to the lateral aspect of the acromion with the arm adducted across the body [7]. Although this can occur with any fall, this is most commonly seen in rugby and football players following a tackle [3, 4]. The force applied will sequentially damage and disrupt the ACJ capsule, then the trapezoid and conoid ligaments [8, 9]. Indirect mechanisms of injury (such as a fall onto the elbow) are less common, but do occur and have an association with a separate injury (such as a cuff tear, labral lesion and glenoid fracture). In this mechanism, it is thought that the proximal humerus is driven up to the acromion, shearing the ACJ and damaging the glenohumeral joint [8, 9]. In higher energy injuries with a greater degree of soft tissue damage and disruption, there is a higher risk of other injuries within the shoulder [5].

Patients will typically complain of pain directly over the ACJ following such an injury and will often point directly to the ACJ. Also, if the lateral end of the clavicle is prominent, patients will often complain of a cosmetic change. In cases of chronic ACJ instability, there is often on-going pain and discomfort over the ACJ but also around the periscapular musculature [10, 11]. Complaints of ACJ tenderness, in the chronic setting, may be less prominent and the pain is more diffuse over the neck, back and shoulder region [8]. The chronic instability often leads to complaints by the patient of being unable to return to sport or suffering difficulty in heavy manual or repetitive work (particularly with overhead activities) [8, 12]. They often complain of fatiguability in the shoulder, particularly in overhead activities [8]. However, in patients over the age of 40, a rotator cuff tear is a more common cause of loss of overhead activity and should be ruled out [11].

Pillar 2: Conventional Examination

In an appropriately exposed patient, a general inspection will often reveal asymmetry of the shoulder contour [8, 10, 11]. There may be a "step-off" sign (Fig. 30.2) denoted by the inferior subluxation of the shoulder girdle leading to a prominent lateral clavicle and a protracted scapula, particularly in type 3–6 injuries [8]. There may not be any deformity in type 1 and 2 injuries. In the acute setting, there may even be visible bruising and swelling around the region. Asking the patient to hold a weight, or pulling the patient's arm inferiorly has been described to distract the ACJ and make it easier to spot on general inspection [8].

Palpation over the ACJ often elicits pain, particularly in the acute setting. It has been demonstrated that ACJ tenderness has a high sensitivity of about 96% and is, therefore, a useful sign but its specificity is around 10% and therefore needs to be used in the context of the overall clinical picture [13]. The differential diagnosis can include ACJ osteoarthritis (in older patients), or osteonecrosis of the lateral clavicle (in younger patients) [11, 14]. Often, in the chronic setting, ACJ tenderness can diminish, and the pain is more generalised around the shoulder and peri-scapula region so tenderness on palpation may be less useful [8]. In severe ligament disruption, palpation can demonstrate increased mobility of the lateral clavicle with a so-called "piano-key" sign [14].

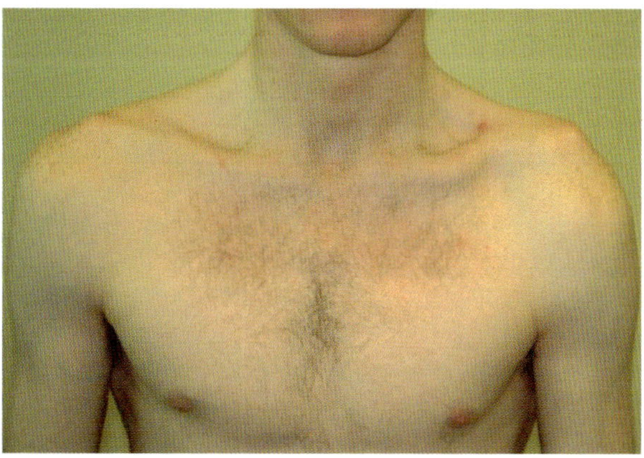

Fig. 30.2 Step off sign following an AC joint injury. Image Published under License from www.shoulderdoc.co.uk

In the acute setting, dynamic assessment on active movement can be challenging [8]. Often the soft tissue tenderness and pain can restrict the patient's range of movement due to pain and make an acute assessment challenging. Patients with chronic injuries tend to demonstrate visible scapular dyskinesia and a reduced range of movement when compared to the other side [15, 16]. These are best viewed during active elevation with the observer standing behind the patient to detect asymmetry. In type 3–5 injuries, a clinically demonstrable dyskinesia was found to affect 73% of patients and cause a reduction in the overall range of movement [17]. Since the lateralising support of the clavicle is no longer present, the scapula drifts into internal rotation, and protraction in addition to the well-described inferior drift. This abnormal position can predispose the patient to impingement and reduced the perceived cuff strength on clinical testing [16]. Rockwood Type 2 injuries may also cause a dynamic alteration in movement, although far more subtle and less pronounced. There may also be a "clicking" sensation or a palpable crepitus. There may be a subtle difference in arm elevation and a reduced arm function [16].

Pillar 3: Special Tests

There are many special tests described in the literature [8, 13, 14]. In essence, there are two types of presentation, based on Rockwood type, and each has a different clinical priority.

Presentation 1

The first presentation occurs in type 1 and 2 ACJ injuries in the acute or sub-acute setting. The clinical priority is that of correctly localising the problem to the ACJ and achieving a correct diagnosis, as often the radiographs can be normal. No individual test will provide an accurate diagnosis, and a cluster of tests is required [10].

Cross-body adduction test—the arm is forward flexed to 90°, and the shoulder is then passively adducted to its natural limit, and the test is positive if it elicits pain, crepitus or instability (Fig. 8.1). In a comparative study, this test has been shown to have a sensitivity of 77% and specificity of 79% [10]. Unlike many ACJ test for arthritis, it will also elucidate any underlying instability with abnormal movement.

The active compression test of O'Brien (Fig. 7.1). This test involves resisted forward flexion with the arm at 90° and 10° adduction from the sagittal plane (with the arm in full internal and external rotation). Although widely used as a test for superior labral anterior to posterior lesions (SLAP), it also compresses the ACJ and will highlight pain from this joint. This test is one of the most specific with a specificity of 94%. However, the sensitivity is as low as 41%. A combination of both tests will therefore efficiently aid the clinical examination.

The Paxinos test [13] is described as the examiner hooking the thumb around the scapula spine and the index and middle finger around the mid-shaft of the clavicle and squeezing (Fig. 8.1). Tenderness or pain is considered positive and has a reported sensitivity of 79% [13]. A similar variation has been described using both hands to achieve the same posterior shear force on the ACJ [11].

The acromioclavicular distraction test [8] involves distraction in the vertical plane by applying downwards and upward force on the arm at rest to elucidate the vertical instability. The acromioclavicular distraction test [8] is positive when abnormal movement is suggested and would imply increasing involvement of the trapezoid than the conoid ligament [18]. (Fig. 30.3) A posteriorly unstable joint with some preservation of anterior and vertical stability may suggest a lower grade injury with some conservation of the CCL complex.

Presentation 2

With Rockwood type 3 or higher grade injuries, the clinical deformity is evident. The clavicle is prominent due to the dropped and protracted scapula.

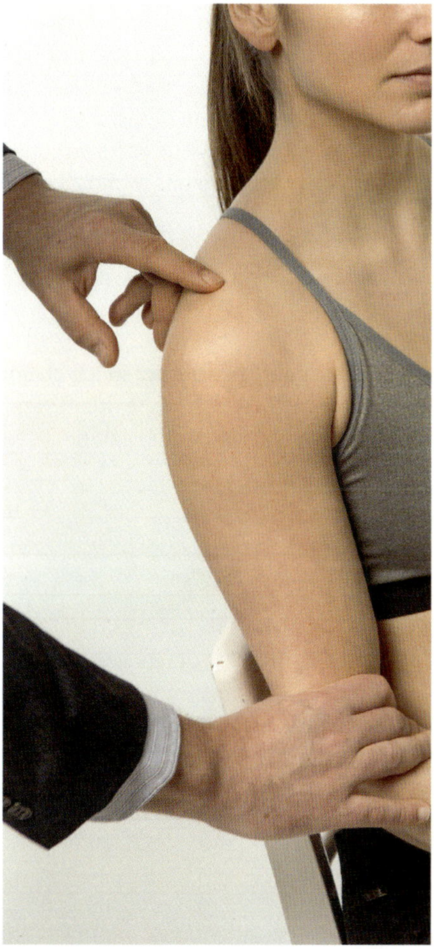

Fig. 30.3 Acromioclavicular distraction test. Image Published under License from www.shoulderdoc.co.uk and www.shoulderpedia.org

Pillar 4: Investigations

Plain film radiographs will demonstrate the injury in type 3–6 dislocations and rule out clavicle fractures and bony injury. A Zanka view [18] has been classically described with a 10–15° cephalic tilted anterosuperior view to give the best assessment of the ACJ in that plane (Fig. 8.4). An Axillary lateral can be useful in demonstrating the horizontal displacement of the ACJ. Attempts have been made to distract the joint and highlight the injury by hanging weights on the arms [8]. In practice, these do not add much value.

MRI scans can demonstrate soft tissue and associated injuries [8, 9, 14]. MRI can be performed with sagittal and coronal planes aligned to the axis of the lateral clavicle to be able to differentiate between the types of injury and the structures disrupted [19]. They can distinguish between type 1,2 and 3 in the acute situation [19]. There is some concern that MRI scans may overestimate the injury and often the clinical picture does not always correlate with the severity of the injury [18]. The consensus seems to be that an MRI scan may be an option in a low-grade injury that fails to settle [9, 18].

When compared to CT and ultrasound imaging modalities, an MRI scan (in the plane of the clavicle) was found to be the most accurate imaging modality [19]. Further imaging is therefore rarely required unless there is evidence of a fracture, mal-union or non-union of the clavicle, in which case a CT may be useful. The decision to offer the patient reconstructive surgery is, therefore, clinical and only requires plain radiographs in most cases.

Discussion of the Case

The cyclist described earlier in the chapter presents with a chronic AC joint dislocation. Clinical diagnosis is evident, and radiographs confirm the diagnosis. This patient would be a potential candidate for AC joint reconstruction, upon failure of a non-operative trial.

Summary

ACJ injuries are best diagnosed using a cluster approach as initial radiographs for low-grade injuries may not be conclusive. For chronic ACJ injuries, clinical examination is sufficient to make a diagnosis, and the cluster approach is useful in determining further management. A summary of diagnostic cluster for AC joint instability is presented in Table 30.1.

Table 30.1 Summary of diagnostic cluster for AC joint instability

Clinical history	
1.	A history of trauma involving a direct blow to the shoulder or indirect injury by falling onto an elbow
2.	Pain over the acromioclavicular region
3.	Loss of shoulder contour with a prominent lateral clavicle
Conventional examination	
4.	Prominent lateral clavicle with a "step off" and/or "piano-key" sign
5.	Dropped and abnormal scapula rhythm on shoulder elevation
Special tests	
6.	Cross-body adduction test
7.	Active compression (O'Brien's) test
8.	Acromioclavicular shear (or Paxinos) test
9.	Acromioclavicular joint distraction test
Investigations	
10.	Plain film radiographs: 10–15° cephalic tilted anteroposterior view (Zanka view) and axillary radiograph

References

1. Nordqvist A, Petersson CJ. Incidence and causes of shoulder girdle injuries in an urban population. J Shoulder Elb Surg. 1995;4(2):107–12.
2. Pallis M, Cameron KL, Svoboda SJ, Owens BD. Epidemiology of acromioclavicular joint injury in young athletes. Am J Sports Med. 2012;40(9):2072–7.
3. Kaplan LD, Flanigan DC, Norwig J, Jost P, Bradley J. Prevalence and variance of shoulder injuries in elite collegiate football players. Am J Sports Med. 2005;33(8):1142–6.
4. Headey J, Brooks JH, Kemp SP. The epidemiology of shoulder injuries in English professional rugby union. Am J Sports Med. 2007;35(9):1537–43.
5. Pauly S, Kraus N, Greiner S, Scheibel M. Prevalence and pattern of glenohumeral injuries among acute high-grade acromioclavicular joint instabilities. J Shoulder Elb Surg. 2013;22(6):760–6.
6. Williams GR, Nguyen VD, Rockwood CA. Classification and radiographic analysis of acromioclavicular dislocations. Appl Radiol. 1989;18:29–34.
7. Yewlett A, Dearden P, Ferran NA, Evans RO, Kulkani R. Acromioclavicular joint dislocation: diagnosis and management. Shoulder Elbow. 2012;4(2):81–6.
8. Rockwood CA Jr, Matsen FA III, Wirth MA, Lippitt SB. The shoulder. Philadelphia, US: Elsevier Health Sciences Saunders. 2009.
9. Tauber M. Management of acute acromioclavicular joint dislocations: current concepts. Arch Orthop Trauma Surg. 2013;133(7):985–95.
10. Chronopoulos E, Kim TK, Park HB, Ashenbrenner D, McFarland EG. Diagnostic value of physical tests for isolated chronic acromioclavicular lesions. Am J Sports Med. 2004;32(3):655–61.
11. BurBanK KM, Stevenson JH, Czarnecki GR, Dorfman J. Chronic shoulder pain: Part I. Evaluation and diagnosis. Am Fam Physician. 2008;77(4):453–60.
12. Weinstein DM, McCann PD, Mcllveen SJ, Flatow EL, Bigliani LU. Surgical treatment of complete acromioclavicular dislocations. Am J Sports Med. 1995;23(3):324–31.
13. Walton J, Mahajan S, Paxinos A, Marshall J, Bryant C, Shnier R, Quinn R, Murrell GA. Diagnostic values of tests for acromioclavicular joint pain. J Bone Joint Surg. 2004;86(4):807–12.

14. Fraser-Moodie JA, Shortt NL, Robinson CM. Injuries to the acromioclavicular joint. J Bone Joint Surg Br. 2008;90(6):697–707.
15. Limb D. Examination techniques in orthopaedics. In: Harris N, Ali F, editors. Examination of the shoulder. Cambridge: Cambridge University Press; 2014. p. 9.
16. Kibler BW, Sciascia A, Wilkes T. Scapular dyskinesis and its relation to shoulder injury. J Am Acad Orthop Surg. 2012;20(6):364–72.
17. Gumina S, Carbone S, Postacchini F. Scapular dyskinesis and SICK scapula syndrome in patients with chronic type III acromioclavicular dislocation. Arthroscopy. 2009;25(1):40–5.
18. Zanca P. Shoulder pain: involvement of the Acromioclavicular joint: (analysis of 1000 cases). Am J Roentgenol. 1971;112(3):493–506.
19. Alyas F, Curtis M, Speed C, Saifuddin A, Connell DMR. Imaging appearances of Acromioclavicular joint dislocation 1. Radiographics. 2008;28(2):463–79.

Index

© Springer International Publishing AG 2018

P. Monga, L. Funk (eds.), *Diagnostic Clusters in Shoulder Conditions*,
DOI 10.1007/978-3-319-57334-2

Printed by Printforce, the Netherlands